# SMART FOOD

Also by Dr. Arthur Winter and Ruth Winter

*Brain Workout*

# SMART FOOD

*Diet and Nutrition for Maximum Brain Power*

Arthur Winter, M.D., F.I.C.S.,
and
Ruth Winter, M.S.

ST. MARTIN'S GRIFFIN

NEW YORK

This book describes current research and theories about the effect of diet and nutrients on brain function. Before you make any radical changes in your diet, consult your own physician.

Names and other identifying characteristics in this book's case histories have been changed to protect privacy.

A previous edition of this work was published under the title *Eat Right, Be Bright* by St. Martin's Press, 1988.

Design by Nancy Resnick

Library of Congress Cataloging-in-Publication Data

Winter, Arthur.
    Smart food : diet and nutrition for maximum brain power / by Arthur Winter and Ruth Winter.
        p.    cm.
    Rev. ed. of: Eat right, be bright. New York : St. Martin's Press. c1988.
    Includes bibliographical references.
    ISBN 0-312-20013-7
    1. Intellect.   2. Nutrition.   3. Brain.   4. Appetite.
5. Nootropic agents.   6. Dietary supplements.   I. Winter, Ruth.
II. Winter, Arthur. Eat right, be bright.   III. Title.
QP398.W56       1999
613.2—dc21                                                    98-48688
                                                                  CIP

First St. Martin's Griffin Edition: April 1999

10  9  8  7  6  5  4  3  2  1

To
Robin, Craig, Grant,
Jonathan, Samantha, Hunter,
and Katelynd

# Contents

# Introduction

Imagine holding a lemon in your hand, cutting it open, and then sucking it.

Did you begin to salivate?

This is just a small example of how the sight, smell, taste, and texture of foods can cause your brain to release digestive chemicals and elicit hormonal, heart, and kidney responses. This phenomenon is believed to be nature's way of priming your body to better absorb and use the nutrients you eat.[1]

When you actually do sit down to a meal, your brain receives feedback from various organs as it is fueled up. What you choose to ingest, therefore, has a profound influence on your central nervous system and thus on your ability to think, your mood, your energy and, in fact, your survival.

The concept that diet can affect the condition of your body is not new. Ever since a Scottish naval surgeon cured scurvy by giving lemons and limes to sailors (forever after known as "limeys") modern physicians have accepted the fact that *major* nutritional deficiencies can lead to severe alterations in behavior. What is new is the recognition that *minor* vitamin and mineral deficiencies can affect the condition of the body or brain, or can alter one's mood or ability to perform!

It is also only recently that modern scientists have begun to believe that specific foods or their absence may affect our brains and hence our thoughts and behavior. What is fueling all this interest in food and the brain relates to:

- The discovery of neurotransmitters, the chemical agents that send messages between brain cells.

- The discovery that neurotransmitters can be derived from the food we eat.

The interaction of food and the brain, however, is extremely complicated. Start with the simple questions:

- Why do we eat?
- When do we eat?
- Why do we choose the foods we do?

Most of us eat three meals a day—breakfast, lunch, and dinner—but what about coffee breaks and snacks after school, in front of the TV, and at bedtime? Are we hungry or do we eat out of habit, boredom, or the need for comfort?

Where are the hunger and satiety centers in the brain and how much voluntary control do we have over our choices of food? Are the eating disorders anorexia (in which there is self-starvation) and obesity (in which there is eating beyond need) culturally or bio-chemically induced?

There are chemical additives, intentional and unintentional, present in our food and drink. These additives may affect the brain. Certainly, no one would disagree that lead in the diet is toxic to brain cells, but what about color additives? Artificial sweeteners? Preservatives? Pesticides? More than ten thousand chemicals in the marketplace have yet to be tested for their possibly toxic effects on the brain.

Just as there is great interest in the safety of the edibles we buy, there is a growing interest in the preventive and healing power of nutrients. Therapeutic uses of food date back at least several thousand years to ancient Egypt, where onions were recommended to induce sleep, almonds and cabbage to prevent hangovers, lemons to protect against the evil eye, and salt to stimulate passion. The ancient Greeks also staunchly believed that diet was an integral part of the treatment of both physical and psychological illness. Folk medicine is rich in food prescriptions. Who hasn't heard that eating oysters will enhance one's sexual desire and performance? This may be just myth, but in fact oysters are rich in zinc and scientists have discovered that a zinc deficiency interferes with sexual function.

More than eight hundred years ago, Maimonides, a famous Jewish physician who practiced in Cordova, Spain, and his contemporaries believed that humans could modulate their moods and appetites by using specific food items. Today it is being rediscovered that diet does indeed affect thought and behavior. The brain/food link is not new to us modern humans, either. We know from experience that we can use food to alter our moods. Caffeine is the most common psychoactive (mind- or mood-altering) drug in the world. Ice cream and candy are typically used as rewards or consolations. Steak and potatoes make some men feel manlier, just as losing weight may help raise a woman's self-esteem.

The correlations between food, dietary supplements, and the brain, however, are often hard to make because behavioral changes are subtle and there are confounding factors such as culture and stress. Food represents tradition, reward, and love. It is the focal point of most social gatherings. It is a cultural obsession on which Americans spend millions of dollars each year on books, devices, and special diets. Nevertheless, as anyone who has had a hangover from too much alcohol or irritability due to hunger knows, what we eat and drink can influence how our brains function and, subsequently, our intellect and our behavior.

This book, written by a neurosurgeon and a veteran science writer, describes the burgeoning research on the effects of diet on the brain and, conversely, of the brain on diet. It spotlights the brain and belly chemicals that cause us to eat or stop eating; and the nutrients that affect our mental prowess and our moods. We hope it will give you not only food for thought but also thoughts about your food, because you really are what you eat.

Arthur Winter, M.D., F.I.C.S., and Ruth Winter, M.S.

# 1

# Your Brain-Belly Connection

Do you eat when you are nervous or do you find it impossible to swallow a bite?

Are there "butterflies" in your stomach when you have to give a speech, take an exam, or go through a rite of passage?

How is your control of your bladder and bowels when you are terribly frightened?

While scientists are just now trying to identify the neurochemical connections between gut and brain, we all experience this interaction "in the pit of our stomachs" under periods of high emotion. In such instances, we are conscious of what is happening between our bellies and brains. Most of the time, however, we are unaware of this interaction. We may be in a "bad mood" and not realize it is because we skipped breakfast. Our nerves may be "on edge" because we had that third cup of coffee or we may feel sleepy after a "heavy meal" and still not make the connection between our central nervous systems and substances we ingested.

Our mental function is directly related to what we eat or don't eat because our brains are chemical factories that produce dozens of different psychoactive drugs. We eat the starter materials for these brain chemicals which we make into the chemicals that affect our intelligence, memory, mood, appetite, and weight control.

Our digestive systems also are chemical factories. In the linings of the esophagus, stomach, small intestine and colon, there are millions of nerve cells that send out stop-and-go messages to our brains. The components of this digestive control center are lumped under the title the *enteric* (from the Greek *entera* meaning bowels) *nervous system*. Current thinking among a number of scientists is that there is a "brain" in the gut, independent from the brain encased in the skull and that the enteric nervous system may be able to learn and remember independently of *the central nervous system.*

Developmental biologists point out there is a clump of tissue, the *neural crest*—that forms early in the embryo. One section turns into the central nervous system. Another piece migrates to become the enteric nervous system. Later, the two nervous systems are connected via a telephonelike wire, the *vagus nerve.*

Until relatively recently, people thought that the gut's muscles and sensory nerves were wired directly to the brain and that the brain controlled the gut through the vagus nerve. When scientists began to count nerve fibers in the gut, they found it contained more than 100 million—more than those of the spinal cord—yet the vagus nerve is "wired" to carry only a couple of thousand nerve fibers. The interaction between belly and brain via the vagus nerve is still somewhat mysterious.

**Why do an increasing number of researchers believe there is a second brain in our bellies?**

Dr. Michael Gershon, professor of anatomy and cell biology at Columbia Presbyterian Medical Center, New York City, says the gut can work independently of the brain and spinal cord: "In an experiment in 1917, Swiss researchers excised a gut from a pig and blew into it. The isolated gut blew back. We now know that we can take gut tissue and put it in a nutrient solution and it will live for weeks. It has sensors so that if you touch it, it wiggles. This is due to a type of cell that responds to pressure and stimulation. These cells are found only in the gut and nowhere else in the body. That means the gut can function when cut off completely from the brain and spinal cord. Other organs of the body—for example, the bladder, the kidneys, the heart—cannot."[1]

**Why did this talent of the gut evolve?**

Dr. Gershon says, "It is very simple. The gut does hard work. It takes in food, breaks it down, and digests it. This requires very complicated organic chemistry. For instance, the gut must produce the right amount of enzymes, send instructions to the pancreas to spurt more insulin for processing sugar or the gall bladder to secrete bile, and so forth. While all this is happening, the gut must protect its lining to keep all the nasty stuff from getting into the body because nothing we eat is sterile."

The gut is "hard wired" and sends nerves directly to the gall bladder, for example, or the pancreas. It only takes about three percent of its instructions from the brain, according to Dr. Gershon. "If it had to have nerve connections to the brain for all the jobs it does, then the brain would have to be enormous and the trunk line between the gut and brain would take up the whole body."

## Nerve Receiving Message

The brain in your head is very dependent upon the abilities of the brain in your belly. For you to survive, your belly must feed your brain by providing nutrients that will enable it to carry out its duties.

One of the major functions of your central nervous system is communication—communication within its various parts—with the rest of your body, and with the outside world. Your brain has its own private "postal system." Each of your individual nerve cells, or *neurons,* can communicate with thousands of other cells by chemical messengers called *neurotransmitters.* Your body creates these brainy postal "employees" from substances in our diets. There are two ways neurotransmitters deliver their information between nerve cells:

1. Electrodynamically by "wire" in the brain and elsewhere in the body.
2. Chemically, like a bottle tossed in the ocean.

Within nerve cells, signals are sent predominantly by wire (electrodynamically); conversely, the signals that are transmitted from one nerve cell to another "shoot the rapids" to carry a message across the gap between them—a process called *synapsis.* Since nerve cells do not touch one another, nature provided this chemical "message-carrying" system as well as the electronic "Internet" setup. The brain's communication service has an amazing capacity to deliver. It was not long ago that it was believed messages could be sent only between adjoining nerves. Now it is known that nerves can issue substances that travel throughout the body, affecting other nerves at distant sites. It has also been recently discovered that a single nerve is capable of sending out several messages, not just one, as previously believed.

You can alter the levels and functions of neurotransmitter messages with drugs such as antidepressants, which elevate your mood; tranquilizers, which calm you down; and stimulants that increase your alertness. *Your diet can also alter your mood and your ability to think—perhaps not as dramatically as drugs but usually a lot more safely.*

Since nature provided two of many important organs—ovaries, testes, lungs, kidneys, etc.—it seems to have also provided two brains—one to concentrate on obtaining food and the other as the master control system. The enteric nervous system regulates the normal activity of the digestive system and prepares it for whatever its future may hold, whether a forthcoming meal you might ingest or some dangerous creature that might try to ingest you. Just imag-

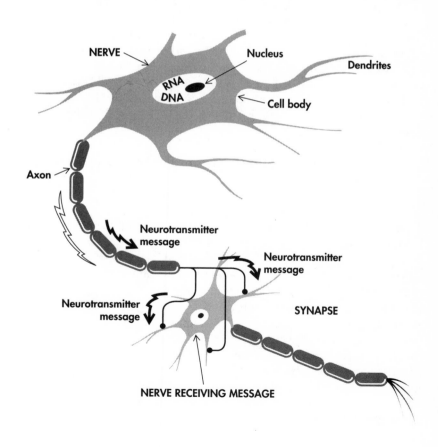

ine how your stomach feels when you are hungry and anticipating your favorite meal. Then recall how your intestines react when you become really scared.

## Brain-Belly Interaction

It has been reported within the current scientific literature that nearly every chemical order the brain sends out can be found in the gut. Major brain messengers—neurotransmitters—are there, as well as self-made opiates called *endorphins* that are similar to popular tranquilizers such as Valium and Xanax.

There is no doubt that both your stomach and your brain secrete these powerful messengers that affect your behavior. More than sixty-five neurotransmitters have been identified at this writing, and it is believed that many more have yet to be discovered. The correlation between diet, neurotransmitters, and brain function is often inconclusive and controversial. What is agreed upon, however, is that in order for a chemical messenger in your brain to be manufactured from a substance in food, four things must happen:

1. The substance must be absorbed through your gastrointestinal tract.
2. It must be carried by your blood to a specific area in your brain.
3. Enzymes, the workhorses of your body, must convert it into a specific neurotransmitter.
4. Once manufactured, the neurotransmitter must be stored in the proper place and be available for release when needed.

The central computer in the brain that receives information about the nutrients you ingest is your *hypothalamus,* a tiny bunch of nerve cells that weighs less than four grams. It has a big job. It integrates information about your weight, temperature, activity level, season, reproductive cycle (if you are female), and then it computes how much food you need.

At first, scientists did not believe that foods could alter the levels of neurotransmitters, because the manufacture of these highly potent brain chemicals must be exquisitely regulated; any interference with them can cause all sorts of problems, ranging from memory loss and depression to muscle paralysis and inability to speak. It is now known, however, that foods can modify the production of neurotransmitters and result in changes in brain function, mood, and behavior that are often predictable.

## The Meal Messengers—Hormones and Neurotransmitters

The link between your brain's hypothalamus and your gastrointestinal tract is the object of much research today, as previously mentioned. Researchers now want to know why chemical "signals" commonly found in our intestines are also in our brains. These include:

Gastrin, a hormone secreted by the lower part of your stomach when it is full of food. It then travels into your bloodstream and acts on the upper part of your stomach to stimulate the production of gastric acid. Gastrin is one of the gut proteins recently found in the brain. To determine if gastrin in the brain might influence digestion, researchers at the University of Western Ontario injected it into the hypothalamus of rats and then measured stomach acid secretion. Gastrin consistently caused stomach acid secretion to double or triple within fifteen minutes. In contrast, injection of other chemical signals common to the gut and brain did not increase stomach acid.[2] The researchers believe that brain gastrin influences the gut by acting as a neurotransmitter on that telephone cable, the vagus nerve, communicating between the belly and brain. When the investigators severed the vagus nerve in rats, brain gastrin did not increase stomach acid.

CCK (cholecystokinin), a hormone produced by the small intestine during the movement of food from the stomach into the intestine. It causes the contraction of the gallbladder, thus releasing bile into the small intestine that aids digestion. It acts as a powerful suppressant of normal eating. CCK also appears to act on the vagus nerve and is found in many places in the brain. Administration of CCK to human volunteers reduced meal duration and intake.[3] CCK is sold in health food stores as an appetite suppressant, but many researchers believe that its ability to cause nausea is its real effectiveness in dulling hunger. At this writing, Glaxo Wellcome is working on a medication that mimics CCK to inhibit eating.[4] Researchers at the Geriatric Research, Education and Clinical Center, St. Louis Department of Veterans Affairs, MO, theorize that CCK has an effect on both feeding and memory. They point out that lack of sufficient CCK and some other hormones may be at the root of the lack of appetite in aging.[5]

*Norepinephrine* is a neurotransmitter that decreases food intake in animals when injected into the brain's hypothalamus. Norepinephrine levels increase in the same area when food is injected into the duodenum (the beginning of the small intestine). These results are consistent with the belief that satiety is affected by neurotransmitters in the brain that become activated when food enters the small intestine.[6] Your brain then gets the message "you're full of food." Another bit of evidence that norepinephrine may affect satiety is related to the fact that amphetamines, very similar in structure to norepinephrine, were once highly successful "diet pills" until their side effects and abuse caused the FDA to forbid their use. Knoll Pharmaceuticals is working on a medication that boosts serotonin and norepinephrine in the brain to cut appetite. At this writing, early reports were that the average weight loss was 9 percent with some people achieving over 20 percent and some none. It reportedly increases the feeling of fullness and speeds up the rate at which bodies burn calories.[7]

*Serotonin,* which regulates mood, may also be involved in the production of satiety, several studies have shown. It has been reported that overweight people have a lower level of serotonin in their brains, which may be a reason why they have trouble in stopping eating. A lot of people eat when they are depressed and it is theorized that they are instinctively trying to raise their self-produced antidepressant, serotonin. Studies of food intake with fenfluramine, a once widely used prescription diet pill with a structure similar to serotonin, demonstrated that fenfluramine can suppress food intake.[8] Dr. Gershon says there is much more serotonin in the gut than in the brain and that serotonin sweeps down through and around the bowel.

*Vasoactive intestinal peptide (VIP)* is present in both your brain and your gut. Its duties include lowering your blood pressure by causing dilation of blood vessels, suppressing secretion of your stomach acid, and stimulating secretions in your small intestine and colon. VIP is believed to be a neurotransmitter that plays a role in arousal, a state of mind necessary when hunting food.

*Calcitonin* is a calcium-lowering hormone released from your thyroid and by your gut after a meal. It has been shown to have a potent hunger-dampening effect.

*Corticotrophin-releasing factor (CRF)* causes the release of "stress" hormones from your adrenal gland that increase your heart rate and blood pressure and cause the release of a number of hormones from your pituitary gland. Stress, as we all know from experience, can result in increased eating or loss of appetite. When CRF is injected into the brains of rats, it results in increased grooming activity, a known response to stress. It also suppresses drinking and feeding behavior under a variety of conditions. Patients with anorexia nervosa, self-starvation, have been found to have an overactive hypothalamus, pituitary gland, and adrenal gland, suggesting the basic defect may be an increase in CRF. Similarly, depressed patients, who often have a poor appetite, also have an overproduction of pituitary and adrenal gland hormones, suggesting the possibility of CRF malfunction. Thus it would appear that stress can either produce overeating through activation of the neurotransmitters in the brain or decreased eating through an increase in CRF.[9]

*Leptin.* A naturally occurring hormone that is believed to dampen appetite. There was a great deal of excitement about the discovery of this hormone and its gene in the early '90s. The weight-reducing effects of leptin are believed to be due to its signaling the size of the body's fat stores. This belly-brain interaction involves the hypothalamus.[10] "When we found leptin in 1995, we suspected it acted in the hypothalamus, a region of the brain known to regulate food intake and body weight," says Jeffrey Friedman, M.D., Ph.D., a professor at Rockefeller University. "In our current work, we have determined that there are at least six different forms of the leptin receptor, known as Ob-R." Friedman and his colleagues have found Ob-Rb is mutant in diabetic (db) mice, which are consequently massively obese and resist leptin. "Leptin may modulate the activity of neuropeptide Y, glucagon-like peptide 1 and other peptides and neurotransmitters that are known to affect feeding behavior in the hypothalamus," Friedman explains. "Leptin also may affect other tissues that have Ob-Rb receptors, including fat."

Several companies are working on products. Amgen has clinical trials at UCLA, as of this writing, and Hoffman–La Roche is looking at leptin receptors in the brain to make them work more effectively.

*Neuropeptide Y (NPY)*. A neurotransmitter believed to play a role in carbohydrate craving. Pfizer has a neuropeptide Y blocker in early human testing at this writing.

Columbia's Dr. Gershon says that the receptors on the cells that receive neurotransmitters that are native to both the brain and gut may cause the substances to stimulate or block different reactions. He points out that there are more nerve cells in the gut than in the spinal cord. "The gut handles the messy job of digestion while the brain is the grand master that reacts to Mozart and is the central control center. It wouldn't be able to do its job if it had to deal with the duties of the gut."

## More About Stress and Digestion

Stress affects many body processes and the digestive and central nervous systems are no exception. Researchers have found that if the stress is short-lived, the changes in stress hormone levels will be transient and unlikely to induce a breakdown response. If, on the other hand, the stress is intense or applied for an extended period of time, changes in the hormonal system can lead to a breakdown of body substances, such as proteins. Not everybody, however, reacts equally to the same stress so what upsets your stomach when you are stressed out may not upset someone else's.

Although precise signals that initiate the speedup of metabolism under stress are unknown, clues point to the role of the brain. A wide variety of stresses stimulate the hypothalamus, the area of the brain involved in eating behavior and in sending commands to the pituitary gland to relay a message to the adrenal glands to release stress hormones. The stress hormones are then carried in the blood and are fed back to the brain saying, "Quick, release your own stress neurotransmitters." This system makes sense. Your adrenals prepare your body to fight or flee by making your heart beat faster and your muscles tense up, and then your brain decides whether to stand and fight or to beat a hasty retreat with your well-prepared body.

These circulating stress chemicals also affect sugar and fat metabolism. They interfere with energy storage and protein metabolism. So you can see stress can affect your body's use of food and certain foods can affect your stress levels.

How much the brain in the belly and the brain in the head converse chemically and electronically is a matter of intense study and debate among scientists at this writing. Just as scientists argue about what portion of behavior is due to nurture (family environment) and what is due to nature (genetics), so too do they argue about the belly–brain connection.

Dr. Gershon points out that for years people who had ulcers or difficulty in swallowing or chronic abdominal pains were told their problems were psychosomatic—all in their heads. They were told to obtain psychiatric treatment or were given tranquilizers by their family physicians.

He says physicians were right in ascribing these problems to the brain, but they blamed the wrong one. Many gastrointestinal disorders such as colitis and irritable bowel syndrome originate from problems within the gut's brain, he says. And the current wisdom is that germs cause most ulcers, not hidden anger at one's mother.

Dr. Gershon notes that symptoms stemming from the two brains get confused: "Just as the brain can upset the gut, the gut can upset the brain. If you were chained to the toilet with cramps, you'd be upset, too."

## Panic Attacks and Caffeine

Those specializing in the study of the belly–brain connection are called *neurogastroenterologists*. You do not have to be a neuroscientist, however, to make a cause-and-effect assumption about something you ate and its influence on your thinking and behavior, whether it is caused by the brain in your belly or in your head.

A good example is a person who suffers from panic attacks. The condition, which is believed to have a combined physical and emotional cause, produces a feeling of impending doom where there is no real danger. Medical specialists who treat such patients report that invariably, on their own, the patients had stopped drinking beverages containing caffeine because they recognized the association between their ingestion of caffeine and their symptoms. As discussed in Chapter 6, caffeine can trigger panic attacks.

## The Drunken Brain

Alcohol consumption offers another obvious example of the effects of ingested substances on brain function. Depending on the amount, the alcohol you ingest affects or damages your brain cells. When ingested by a pregnant woman, alcohol can cripple the brain of her unborn child. But most of the time, the effects of food and drink on brain function are subtle and occur over a long period of time.

## What Foods Will Keep the Belly Brain Happy?

Dr. Gershon points out that the brain in the gut figures out your diet, whether you are a meat eater or a vegetarian, and copes with it. If you eat protein, for example, it will tell your enzymes to process it. Your belly brain, however, can be affected by drugs such as the tranquilizer, Prozac, which may make you nauseated, or by contaminated foods. He emphasizes the major cause today of emergency room visits is food poisoning, not chest pain, as in prior years.

"The *heart healthy diet*—lots of fruits and vegetables—recommended today," Dr. Gershon says, "may be healthy for the heart but *hell on the gut*. Produce now in our markets and restaurants is often loaded with germs."

What does he eat?

"I don't eat seafood—I know, for example, how oysters feed on excrement in the water," nor does he eat chicken or pork products. Eighty percent of the former is contaminated with campylobacter and half the swineherd has toxoplasmosis—both germs can cause intestinal upsets.

He does like steaks and well-washed lettuce and he takes a multivitamin and vitamin E because his wife insists upon it. He says he eats most of his meals at home because his wife is a great cook!

## Belly-Brain Messages Need More Translation

Summing it up, scientists in the subspecialty of neurogastroenterology, as Dr. Gershon points out, sometimes refer to the enteric nervous system as a "microcomputer" and the brain as "the mainframe." The "brain in the belly" is not protected by the bony skull as the brain in the head is even though it contains many important circuits similar to the mainframe's. The "belly brain" produces or uses neurotransmitters and its own tranquilizers but it is still without a really good manual to understand its inner workings.

In the following chapters, you will learn more about how food, supplements, and other substances we ingest affect our central nervous system and its control over our behavior, intellect, and memory. Our brains consume a whopping 50 percent of our bodies' fuel, glucose, which is obtained from food. Since our brains are the most important part of our nervous systems, all of our other organs will undergo sacrifice to keep our brains going when we are under severe stress or when we are eating an energy-deficient, nutritionally poor diet.

In the next chapter, you will learn more about the messenger chemicals you make in your belly and brain that affect your mind.

# 2

# Food and Medicines of the Mind

The line between foods and drugs in prevention and/or cure of human maladies is fading. You consume foods, which are composed of a variety of chemicals, in relatively large amounts to supply your body with energy, regulate its processes, and repair its tissues. You take drugs, which are chemicals, in small quantities for a specific purpose, such as to kill pain or to soothe anxiety. Thanks to new research capabilities, it is becoming increasingly clear that there is something to the old idea that "food is your best medicine."

Today there are three major areas in which the disciplines of nutrition and pharmacology interact and are of vital importance to your brain's functioning:

1. Vitamins and minerals, in the prevention or treatment of conditions or diseases;
2. Drug–nutrient interactions, in which food can enhance or retard the effects of drugs and vice versa;
3. Foods that act as drugs on the brain. The raw materials for those self-produced brain "drugs" are proteins in the diet. Modern neuroscientists are proving in the laboratory what the ancients only surmised—that certain foods do affect the brain.

Take bananas, for example. In ancient India, bananas were called "the fruit of wise men." There is even a legend that claims it was the banana, not the apple, that was the forbidden fruit in the Garden of Eden. In any case, it was one of the first fruits cultivated by humans. The banana's botanical name, *Musa sapientum* (roughly translated as "smart herb"), is attributed to the Greek philosopher

Pliny, who noted, "sages reposed beneath its shade and ate of its fruit." What did the wise men of the past know that modern scientists are only now confirming in their laboratories about the effect of this particular food on the human brain? An average small banana contains about 81 calories, 1 gram of protein, 21.1 grams of carbohydrate, 8 milligrams of calcium, 25 milligrams of phosphorus, 352 milligrams of potassium, and 1 milligram of sodium. It is 99.8 percent fat-free and has 180 international units of vitamin A, 10 milligrams of vitamin C, and two neurotransmitter materials: 15 micrograms per gram weight of serotonin and 1.62 milligrams of tryptophan.

Later in this book we will discuss in more detail many of the components in a banana, but just briefly one banana provides the following benefits:

- Carbohydrates (sugars and starches), the material from which glucose, the major fuel for your brain, is derived. Ingesting carbohydrates can also affect your mood and cravings.
- Potassium, vital to the transmission of messages between your nerves.
- Low sodium, a benefit for those with sodium-caused water retention due to high blood pressure or kidney problems. Water retention can produce symptoms ranging from irritability to coma.
- Vitamin A, which is necessary for keen eyesight. Through eyesight, of course, we gain most of the information we feed our brains. A deficiency of vitamin A has also been found, at least in laboratory animals, to affect balance and cause abnormalities in taste and smell, two senses intimately involved in eating.
- Vitamin C, which has been linked to the production of dopamine, another neurotransmitter in your brain and one that is necessary for coordinated movements, and to the production of tyrosine, another neurotransmitter. Tyrosine serves as a building block for epinephrine and norepinephrine, neurotransmitters involved in strong emotions and alertness. Vitamin C also participates in the processing of glucose, the brain's primary food.

- Phosphorus, essential in all energy-producing reactions of cells, including brain cells.
- Serotonin, a neurotransmitter that inhibits secretions in the digestive tract and stimulates smooth muscles. It is an important regulator of both mood and appetite. Low levels of serotonin have been linked to depression.
- Tryptophan, a raw material for brain chemicals involved in mood and sleep.

It may be smart to include bananas in your diet, but bananas alone will not make you smart. Even though many of the observations made by ancient sages and ordinary people about the impact of certain foods on brain function may prove well founded, the research today concerning diet and the brain is often complicated by other factors such as culture, heredity, and personal experience. The results of experiments to correlate diet and brain function, therefore, are often inconclusive and controversial.

## Neurotransmitters—Messengers of the Mind

Neurotransmitters—those brain messengers sent between nerve cells—are made from the raw materials in food by the nerve cell body. They then travel down the *axon*—the long part of the nerve that looks like a telephone pole—and are stored in tiny capsules at the end of the axon to await a signal to spurt information to another nerve cell across the gap between nerves.

Neurotransmitter messages are received at sites called *receptors.* Each neurotransmitter fits into its own receptor on a cell like a piece in a jigsaw puzzle. Then a neurotransmitter may cause its host nerve cell to fire off a message or it may stop it from doing so in a matter of milliseconds. Some neurotransmitters can even cause a long-lasting change in a host cell by switching on the cell's own genes to create new transmitters.

It has recently been discovered that a single nerve cell may release two or more neurotransmitters or may pull a switch and produce one neurotransmitter instead of another. Thus, a single nerve cell can send different messages at various times, depending on what is going on in your body and what you ingested. The impact goes well beyond the single nerve cell and can affect your entire

**SYNAPSIS**

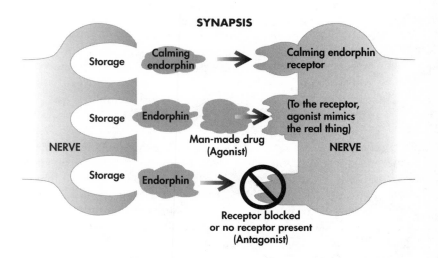

being. Consider the neurotransmitters called endorphins, for example. The most familiar of the self-made brain "drugs," their name derives from the Greek *endo* and morphine, meaning "morphine from within." Endorphins can sedate, cause euphoria, or kill pain, depending on where they are sent and where they are received. They are your self-made psychoactive drugs. You can increase their production by stress-relieving techniques such as meditation or by exercise. Haven't you heard of "Runner's High," the euphoria that occurs during vigorous exercise? This has been attributed to endorphins.

What happens when we ingest a substance that affects our central nervous system? Foreign chemicals—those that are not manufactured in the body and that act upon the brain, such as certain drugs and nutrients—exert their influence in two ways:

1. They may mimic your natural neurotransmitter and trigger a response by the nerve cell.
2. They may take up space on your host cell but fail to elicit a response.

When these substances mimic or take up space, they prevent the neurotransmitters you make yourself from binding to their own receptors. In the first case, drugs that mimic the real thing and turn on the cell are called *agonists*. In the second case, they are called *antagonists* or *blockers*. In fact, all drugs used to treat mental illness function by either mimicking or blocking the action of natural transmitters.

The long-term use of a psychoactive substance that mimics your body's self-made neurotransmitter may cause the shutdown of your body's production of the natural chemical. When the mimicry is then stopped, there may be an insufficient amount of your self-manufactured neurotransmitter available, and severe withdrawal symptoms may occur. This is the rationale behind such reactions as the D.T.s (delirium tremens) of alcoholics or the multiple mental and physical withdrawal symptoms of the heroin addict.

The same process is at work in people who suddenly stop drinking large quantities of coffee or colas containing caffeine. Their receptor sites for the caffeine molecules are empty, waiting for a jolt that never comes. As a result, they suffer headaches, malaise, and other symptoms. And if you wondered why it is so hard to stop smoking cigarettes, here's the answer. Nicotine is addicting because it attaches to specific receptors. When it is gone, those empty sites cry out for it until the body readjusts its chemistry.

The blocking or destruction of certain receptor sites is thought to play a major role in the mind-destroying Alzheimer's disease and even in the common memory problems of healthy people as they grow older. The neurons that produce and receive the neurotransmitter acetylcholine, which is vital to memory, are affected. It is believed that the loss or malfunctioning of these receptors may account for much of forgetfulness, in the same way that women who had "Twilight Sleep" while giving birth literally forgot the pain because the memory receptors in their brains were blocked by the drug scopolamine.

What if the receptors or the neurotransmitter is destroyed? This is believed to be the case with acetylcholine, the neurotransmitter vital to memory function. Researchers are studying acetylcholinesterase, the enzyme that destroys acetylcholine, in hope of stopping the destruction of this neurotransmitter and its receptors.[1] One of the avenues of research is the study of choline, a substance found in concentrated amounts in egg yolks and present in meat and some cereals. Choline serves as a raw material for acetylcholine as you will read later on in this book.

## The Need to Turn Off

Blocking or destroying a neurotransmitter is one problem, but once a neurotransmitter binds to a receptor, it must eventually be deactivated so that information transmission can resume. If not, we would have uncoordinated movements or paralysis. A general "turn off" for neurotransmission is believed to be a nerve messenger called *gamma aminobutyric acid (GABA)*. When GABA is released from a nerve cell and binds to the receptor of another, the host nerve cell is inhibited from firing its own message. A muscle relaxant such as Valium is thought to work by making GABA turn off nerves involved in spewing out such anxiety messages as "I am afraid of giving that speech" or "What if I can't make the grade?"

GABA is found in high concentrations in the brain but, oddly, seems to be absent from the rest of the body.[2] A number of food ingredients, as described later in this book, are believed to affect the amount of GABA in the brain.

Some neurotransmitters are not switched off by GABA but are deactivated by their own nerve cells which suck the transmitters back in. Drugs such as cocaine and amphetamines act by interfering with this reuptake mechanism.

Special enzymes also inactivate some neurotransmitters, as in the case of acetylcholinesterase and acetylcholine, mentioned above, and monoamine oxidase and various transmitters mentioned below.

## Dangerous Drug, Food, and Neurotransmitter Interactions

The interaction between neurotransmitters, foods and drugs can be serious—even fatal.

The neurotransmitters *dopamine, epinephrine,* and *norepinephrine,* which are involved in movement, blood pressure, and mood, are destroyed by the enzyme *monoamine oxidase (MAO)*. People taking MAO inhibitors (drugs for treating depression, including the herb St. John's-wort) are warned against eating foods like herring or drinking wine because these substances are high in tyramine, the raw material for epinephrine (*see* Glossary). The combination of high levels of epinephrine made by the body from the tyramine in ingested foods and the lack of epinephrine's turn-off enzyme, MAO, can send a person's blood pressure skyrocketing and cause a stroke.

Take the case of Charlie, a furrier, plagued by pickets in front of his store who wanted to prevent the slaughter of animals. A short, balding, fifty-three-year-old, Charlie didn't hunt or kill leopards or minks, he just sold coats, like his father before him. To make matters worse, his eldest daughter was getting a divorce and his youngest son was still "trying to find himself" at age twenty-five.

An internist, knowing that Charlie was having a hard time, prescribed an antidepressant. The medicine took effect, and about three weeks later Charlie was feeling so well that he decided to take out his wife, Lillian, for a celebration dinner. They went to their favorite restaurant. Charlie ordered pickled herring for an appetizer and calf's liver and onions for the main course, and he toasted Lillian with a glass of wine.

The furrier never made it home that night. He suffered a stroke. The tyramine in the herring, liver, and wine raised his blood pressure and the MAO inhibitor in his medication prevented the enzyme from breaking down the tyramine (the building block of the neurotransmitter, epinephrine). When tyramine builds up, serious symptoms may occur, including severe high blood pressure, excruciating headaches, nausea, and irregular heartbeat, within thirty to forty minutes after ingestion. In Charlie's case, the buildup of tyramine—and consequently the stimulating neurotransmitter, epinephrine—made his blood pressure shoot up. The increased pressure in his brain caused a weakened blood vessel to blow like a worn tire, and he suffered a stroke. Fortunately, he had no permanent disability. He recovered his appetite for life and no longer needs the antidepressant. Herring and liver are no longer on his menu, however. The former has too much salt and the latter too much cholesterol. Lillian won't let him drink wine, because she blames it for his illness. So Charlie's eating habits have really changed.

On the other hand, the tyramine food-drug combination that raises blood pressure can benefit people whose blood pressure drops too low when they stand up. Thirty-six-year-old Sandy, a homemaker and mother of three, suffered from positional hypotension. Every time she got out of bed or stood up from a chair, her blood pressure would suddenly drop; she would become dizzy and, on rare occasions, pass out. Her physician prescribed a monoamine oxidase inhibitor drug and told Sandy to eat 90 grams of cheddar cheese—equivalent to 28 milligrams of tyramine—per day. She was then able to rise from a lying or sitting position without discomfort.[3]

# Food and Drugs and Neurotransmitters

While Charlie's and Sandy's cases were rather dramatic, most drug-food interactions are subtler. Not every incompatibility is as obvious or as predictable. The seriousness and even the occurrence of food and drug interactions often depend on who you are: your heredity, weight, age, sex, and overall health. Some foods may clash directly with drugs; others lower, slow down, or magnify the amount of medication entering the bloodstream. In still other cases, the medication simply undercuts the normal nutrition. For example:

## The Butterfly and the Cabbage

The butterfly-shaped thyroid gland in your neck is the "governor" of metabolism, the regulator of the rate at which your body consumes oxygen. Thyroid hormone is required for normal growth and development of the brain and of muscles and bones. It indirectly affects the activity of your other glands of internal secretion. Too little thyroid hormone produces a slow metabolic rate and therefore slows down all of your body's chemical processing. For good thyroid function there must be normal pituitary gland function, sufficient iodine intake from food and water, and normal manufacture and release of thyroid hormone by the gland. In addition to lack of iodine in the diet, too little thyroid hormone can be due to diseases of the brain areas that regulate the thyroid gland or destruction of thyroid tissue by inflammation. Among the symptoms of a low thyroid output are slow speech, weight gain, general apathy and fatigue, emotional changes easily confused with depression or senility, and, in the extreme, coma. Treatment for the condition consists of taking supplemental thyroid hormone, which should be ingested before eating in the morning. If you were taking thyroid medication, it would be best to avoid excessive intake of kale, cabbage, carrots, peas, cauliflower, spinach, turnips, rutabagas, soybean products, peaches, beans, and Brussels sprouts. All of these vegetables contain substances that can inhibit the activity of the thyroid hormone and interfere with thyroid therapy.[4]

And while some foods, like the vegetables above, can interfere with medication, some medications can deplete nutrient absorption. Chronic ingestion of aspirin, for example, can deplete the body's store of B vitamins, particularly folic acid. Deficiencies of the B vitamins have been found to lead to pseudosenility among some elderly patients.[5] Aspirin and alcohol taken together can increase the risk of stomach irritation and internal bleeding. Diabetic patients who are taking tablets to lower their blood sugar may experience serious decreases in their blood sugar if they also take aspirin.

You can be sure alcohol, cabbage, and high-tyramine foods described in this chapter may involve interference with the brain's messenger system. Whatever food or drug you ingest, however, will in some way affect your neurotransmitters, those miraculous medicines of your mind.

Research into neurotransmitters and their activities is in its infancy. The following are neurotransmitters that have been identified thus far and their proven or believed functions:

| NEUROTRANSMITTER MAIN MENUS | |
| --- | --- |
| Neurotransmitter | Function (proven or believed) |
| Acetylcholine | Aids memory, transmits signals |
| Epinephrine (adrenaline) | Stimulates, prepares body for stress |
| Norepinephrine (noradrenaline) | Stimulates, promotes appetite |
| GABA | Turns off nerve signals |
| Glutamic acid | Catalyst |
| Glycine | Inhibits signals |
| Dopamine | Initiates movement |
| Substance P | Alerts to pain |
| Serotonin | Calms, affects appetite |
| Thyrotropin-releasing hormone (TRH) | Affects energy and mood |
| Luteinizing hormone-releasing hormone (LHRH) | Stimulates sexual appetite |
| Somatostatin (SRIF) | Affects growth and energy |

## NEUROTRANSMITTER MAIN MENUS (cont.)

| Neurotransmitter | Function (proven or believed) |
| --- | --- |
| Enkephalins and endorphins | Pain killers |
| Neuropeptide Y | Affects eating behavior |
| Vasoactive intestinal peptide (VIP) | Affects thirst, blood pressure |
| Cholecystokinin (CCK) | Affects appetite |
| Adrenocorticotropic hormone (ACTH) | Affects energy |
| Hypocretin 1 and 2 | Affect eating behavior |
| Insulin | Metabolism of carbohydrates |
| Vasopressin | Affects thirst, blood pressure |
| Oxytocin | Affects hunger, glucose |
| Angiotensin | Affects blood pressure |
| Glucagon | Affects hunger, glucose |
| Corticotropin-releasing factor | Affects appetite |
| Growth-hormone-releasing hormone | Affects sexual appetite |
| Calcium messenger system | Triggers changes in sending and receiving between nerve cells |
| Nerve growth factor | Promotes maintenance and repair in nervous system |
| Substance YY | Carbohydrate craving |
| CAST Peptide | Inhibits eating |
| Orexin-A | Believed to stimulate appetite |
| Orexin-B | Believed to stimulate appetite |
| Urocortin | Mimics stress hormone to suppress appetite |

The knowledge that there are receptors in the brain and through-out the body that recognize and bind specific neurotransmitters, hormones, and drugs is the foundation of much of the current search for new medications as well as efforts to increase the understanding of how food ingredients affect the brain.

Neurotransmitter-receptor interaction directly influences your mood, appetite, blood pressure, pain perception, coordination, and every other function of your brain. Conversely, what you eat and drink affects the production and function of your brain's neuro-transmitters. There is an exquisite balance in your brain's nervous system—a network of chemical keys and locks and switches that turns things on and off. These chemicals are both made from and influenced by diet. A nerve cell is like any other cell in your body in that it needs to receive oxygen and food and eliminate waste products. In the next chapter, we will describe some of the research now in progress involving amino acids, the very building blocks of the neurotransmitters that come from food, and how these bits of protein may affect your brain and your behavior.

# From Table to Able—Amino Acids

What family of chemicals in your foods will:

- Enhance your brain's ability to think and remember.
- Allow you to sleep and wake easily.
- Aid your coordination.

How much would you be willing to pay for them? You could fork over one hundred twenty dollars or more for a bottle of these magical substances—amino acids—or you could obtain the same witches' brew by paying a few dollars for a bowl of chili or for a pizza with cheese.

Actually, amino acids are as priceless as they are powerful. They are the body's building blocks from which proteins are constructed. Proteins not only create body tissues—muscles, bones, hair, and nails—they also transport oxygen and carry the genetic code of life to all of your cells. As if that weren't enough, proteins are used by your body to manufacture your antibodies (disease fighters), your hormones (gland messengers), and your neurotransmitters (nerve cell messengers).

Your brain is almost completely regulated by protein-derived amino acids. Their journey from your plate to your head depends on the content of your meals, your physical condition, your activity, and your environment.

When you eat a meal of meat, beans, or any other protein-containing food, digestive enzymes in your stomach and small intestines break apart the protein molecule into "free" amino acids. Your liver then controls the distribution of amino acids in your blood. As the amino acids move through your bloodstream, your body selects the particular amino acid building blocks it needs for its organs and its functions. That pizza you ate, therefore, may become part of your nails or the muscle of your big toe, or it may go to your brain to help get this information you are reading right now across your brain cells.

Your brain uses amino acids to build its nerve cell messengers, the neurotransmitters. Think of a neurotransmitter—such as dopamine to help you move or serotonin to calm you down—as a sentence. The amino acids are the "words" that are strung together in a certain order to form the "sentence." Each sentence, or neurotransmitter, carries a particular message between nerve cells in your brain. The neurotransmitter sentences are constructed in two ways:

1. Directly from the amino acids in the protein you eat.
2. Indirectly, by causing insulin to be released from your pancreas (the organ that controls the level of sugar in your blood), which then draws amino acids from your blood and tissues.

Amino acids are extremely powerful in small doses and are versatile in changing roles, depending on where they are used in the body. It is not surprising, therefore, that one of the hottest areas in pharmaceutical research today involves amino acids.

That they are essential to your brain and body and are derived from foods, however, does not mean amino acids are harmless and should be taken lightly. The amino acid levels in your body are exquisitely balanced. By overloading your system with one, you can affect the levels of others, which may produce serious adverse effects on your body and brain. For example, the *American Journal of Psychiatry* reported the case of a man who took up to 4 grams of L-glutamine, a form of the amino acid glutaric acid, every day for three weeks and wound up having grandiose delusions, total insomnia, and an uncontrollable sex drive.[1] These symptoms may appeal to some, but his psychiatrist reported that the patient was also psychotic and had hallucinations. Within a week after the patient was off the supplement, the symptoms cleared. Another man who took L-glutamine, which is easily accessible in health food stores, found himself losing sleep and experiencing hyperactivity and sharper mental activity. In general, he felt very uncomfortable.[2] When he stopped taking the amino acid, his symptoms subsided.

Long-term effects of taking L-glutamine as a supplement are of course unknown.

Serotonin, the brain messenger that regulates mood, is made from the amino acid tryptophan (see page 29). Fifteen women who had suffered recurrent episodes of major depression participated in an experiment in Oxford, England.[3] They had recovered from their last bout of blues and were no longer on medication. Researchers at Littlemore Hospital gave patients two amino acid mixtures. One potion was nutritionally balanced and contained the amino acid tryptophan, and the other was identical except it did not contain tryptophan. The women were tested for depression seven hours after drinking their mixtures. Blood samples were taken. The British investigators found that the tryptophan-free mixture produced a 75 percent reduction in the blood level of tryptophan and thus lowered brain serotonin. Objective tests and self-reporting showed the women deprived of tryptophan had "clinically significant depressive symptoms," while those who drank the mixture with tryptophan had "no mood changes."

This led the researchers to conclude that rapid lowering of brain serotonin function by lowering tryptophan can precipitate clinical depressive symptoms in well, untreated individuals who are vulnerable to major depressive disorders.

There are natural, daily fluctuations in amino acid levels in your blood. The content of your meals can cause major changes in blood.[4] Of the twenty amino acids your body needs, it cannot manufacture nine of them. Your body must get those nine—called *essential*—from your diet in order to sustain growth and health. In the following pages, individual amino acids, their known biological function, the foods that contain high levels of them, and certain product claims for them are described. A number of such claims for individual amino acid products have not yet been scientifically validated.

## Essential Amino Acids

1. **Histidine** (believed essential only for children). Necessary for nerve function and growth and blood vessel dilation. *Found in:* ham, veal, shredded wheat, beef round, chicken, egg noodles, cheddar cheese, dried milk (nonfat), gelatin, mustard seed, ginger, and basil.

*Promoted in products to:* supplement the diet and to treat arthritis symptoms, allergies, ulcers, anemia, or hearing loss.

2. **Isoleucine.** Necessary for growth. *Found in:* halibut, chicken, macaroni, processed cheese, beef, veal, salmon, milk, wheat germ, gelatin, eggs, and sesame seeds.
*Promoted in products to:* supplement the diet to increase energy and alertness.

3. **Leucine.** Necessary for liver function. It is used in the diagnosis of alcoholism and liver damage. Also employed as a dietary supplement but an overdose can cause imbalance in other amino acids and may affect immunity.
*Found in:* turkey, corn grits, beef, chuck, flank steak, cottage cheese, liver, processed cheese, milk, ham, oatmeal, rye bread, French bread, eggs, wheat germ, caviar, salmon, and fenugreek seed.
*Promoted in products to:* increase energy and alertness.

4. **Lysine.** Necessary for glucose metabolism, liver function, and antibody formation.
*Found in:* milk, turkey, legumes, salmon, beef, haddock, wheat germ, eggs, popovers, swordfish, tuna.
*Promoted in products to:* act as an antiviral medication, decrease irritability, bloodshot eyes; retard growth, hair loss, anemia, and reproductive problems.

5. **Methionine.** A principal supplier of sulfur to the body, an element found in every cell. Sulfur is essential for life and is necessary for cell structure and function. It is sometimes referred to as "nature's beauty mineral" because it is reputed to keep the hair glossy and the complexion clear and youthful. Methionine has been found to have antidepressant effects when metabolized with vitamin $B_{12}$ into a compound called S-adenosyl methionine (SAM). In several studies this compound was found to be as effective as some antidepressant drugs now widely used, ameliorating symptoms such as guilt, suicidal ideation, slowness of movement, work problems, and lack of interest. It was also reported to be more rapid in taking effect than conventional antidepressant drugs, with many patients showing

improvement after four to seven days as compared to the ten days to two weeks it usually takes with other medications.[5] Scientists at Massachusetts General Hospital gave 400 milligrams. of SAM to 195 depressed patients by injection. Depressive symptoms improved after both seven and fifteen days of treatment, and no serious adverse events were reported. The Massachusetts scientists concluded that SAM is a relatively safe and fast-acting antidepressant.[6] A short-term study was tried with SAM on patients with fibromyalgia, a group of common disorders characterized by achy pain, tenderness, and stiffness of muscles. The Danish scientists who conducted the study, however, found it to be of little benefit.[7] Still, there are many ongoing studies of this natural amino acid not only for its mood-elevating effects but for its affect on blood and immunity.

**Found in:** chips, soups, corn grits, bread stuffing, whole wheat, corn bread, wheat germ, egg yolk, caviar, hamburger, flank steak, liver, salad dressings.

**Products promoted to:** chelate heavy metals, fight depression, reduce bladder irritation, influence hair follicles and encourage hair growth. Used to give "fresh" potato flavoring for chips, soups, snacks, and salad dressing.

6. **Phenylalanine.** Along with another amino acid, tyrosine, it is a building block of the brain messenger norepinephrine, involved with memory function as well as with sex drive. An inborn metabolic defect in which there is an inability to process the phenylalanine in food (phenylketonuria, or PKU) leads to mental deterioration and eventually death if phenylalanine is not restricted in the diet. A deficiency of or an inability to utilize phenylalanine has also been linked to the destruction of nerve coverings. This condition then interferes with their transmission of messages, producing incoordination and other problems such as those seen in multiple sclerosis. A partner in the destruction of the nerve coverings, according to some theories, is an inability to utilize vitamin $B_{12}$. Therefore, phenylalanine and $B_{12}$ given together show promise in the treatment of multiple sclerosis and related diseases. In a four-year-study of patients with multiple sclerosis, D-

phenylalanine was given with B$_{12}$. In varying degrees, the patients experienced a reversal in bladder spasms and the return of muscle control.[8]

Phenylalanine has also been used as an antidepressant, and as an antispasmodic.

*Found in:* whole eggs, chicken, liver, milk, cottage and processed cheese, chocolate, pumpernickel bread, potato, brown rice, soy flour, noodles, whole wheat bread, hard rolls, wheat germ, caviar, tuna fish, swordfish, shrimp, steak, hamburger.

*Promoted in products to:* aid memory, reduce hunger pains, act as an antidepressant. The food industry is now injecting eight million pounds of phenylalanine into the food supply each year in the form of the sweetener aspartame (NutraSweet).

7. **Threonine.** The last essential amino acid, discovered in 1935. It prevents the buildup of fats in the liver.

*Found in:* whole eggs, gelatin, skim milk, turkey, hamburger, halibut, yeast, wheat germ, liver, flank steak, onion powder, ginger, flounder, haddock, herring.

*Promoted in products to:* aid digestion and assist metabolism.

8. **Tryptophan.** Of all the amino acids, tryptophan has perhaps most captured the interest of scientists and lay persons. A tremendous amount of scientific research is in progress with this amino acid, which is a building block for the calming neurotransmitter serotonin. Tryptophan was first isolated in milk in 1901. It is believed to work in partnership with tyrosine (see page 35) in producing not only serotonin but also the stimulating brain messengers dopamine and norepinephrine. Tryptophan is the least abundant essential amino acid present in the average diet.[9]

Laboratory and clinical findings suggest that tryptophan malnutrition and, consequently, tryptophan administration may have important roles in treating some brain and behavior problems.[10] A number of studies have been done on the use of tryptophan and its chemical relatives to treat depression and insomnia. Dr. Ernest Hartmann of the Tufts University School of Medicine, for example, has studied the effects of extra doses of tryptophan on groups of mild insomniacs and normal sleepers. Those who took tryptophan tablets fell asleep more quickly.[11]

Dr. Michael Yogman of the Children's Hospital Medical Center in Boston also showed the sleep-inducing effects of tryptophan. He reported that babies fell asleep faster when a solution of sugar and tryptophan was added to their bottles, but warned against mothers doing their own experimenting with tryptophan.[12] As we have pointed out, amino acids are not innocuous.

Dr. Richard Wurtman, an endocrinologist at MIT, showed that the levels of tryptophan in the brain directly control how much serotonin the brain will manufacture. Some types of depression are thought to be linked to abnormal serotonin levels. Thus, researchers have postulated that depression might be treated with increased levels of tryptophan, to help the body produce more serotonin. Some studies report benefits, others do not. The tryptophan is given as a pharmaceutical in doses of 2 to 12 grams daily. Even an amount as small as about 25 milligrams can significantly raise serotonin levels in the brain.[13]

Tryptophan has shown some promise as an alternative to stimulant drugs in children with learning disorders, according to researchers at the Ohio State University School of Medicine. Elaine D. Nemzer, M.D., and her colleagues tried one-week courses of tryptophan, tyrosine, amphetamine, and a placebo in fourteen children with attention problems. Amphetamine proved effective. Tryptophan showed promise. The placebo and tyrosine had no effect.[14]

The Ohio State investigators reported that children's parents said tryptophan worked very well in the home setting. Five of the parents even rated the amino acid higher than amphetamine. The teachers, however, did not see any significant difference in behavior with tryptophan. The researchers theorized that the difference in observations between parents and teachers may be that tryptophan can have a sedating effect that would be more noticeable at home than in school.

While indicating that additional studies would be

needed to determine various dosages and long-term effects, the Ohio researchers suggested three possible uses of tryptophan:

1. Where parents have trouble at home with children but schools do not.
2. During summer vacations, when a holiday from stimulation might be desirable.
3. As an evening supplement, when the morning stimulant dose wears off.

There is also a great deal of work in progress concerning tryptophan as an analgesic to reduce chronic pain.[15] Dr. Samuel Seltzer and his colleagues at nearby Temple University Health Science Center in Philadelphia experimented with tryptophan supplements to increase levels of serotonin in the brain as a means of dulling pain. A four-week double-blind study was conducted with thirty patients suffering chronic jaw pain radiating down one or more nerves. Half of the patients were given tryptophan, half were not. In a report in the *Journal of Psychiatric Research,* these researchers said that not only was there a reduction in pain among the tryptophan group, there was also a greater tolerance to experimental pain when applied to a tooth. Tryptophan, they concluded, reduced pain sensitivity.[16]

Recent reports postulate there may be a tryptophan gene associated with depression. Children who showed an altered response to tryptophan similar to children who already had manic depressive disorder later developed manic depressive disorder. The researchers who performed the study at the University of Pittsburgh concluded that tryptophan response abnormalities may serve as a trait marker for depression.[17] Similar results were found in women who had a family history of depression. When tryptophan was lowered in their system, their mood was lowered.[18]

***Found in:*** peanuts, oatmeal, banana, beef, flank steak, kidney, lamb, bouillon, Swiss cheese, almonds, milk, calf's liver, roast turkey, Parmesan cheese, egg yolk, peanut butter, egg noodles, string beans, flounder, herring, tuna, mustard seed, sesame seed, basil.

*Once promoted in products to:* calm, induce sleep, and relieve pain, its effects were presumably due to the production of serotonin. However, it was withdrawn from the market in 1989 and 1990 because more than 1,200 cases of eosinophilia myalgia syndrome (EMS) were reported to the Centers for Disease Control and the Department of Health Services. Three patients died. All patients reported use of L-tryptophan supplements before the onset of illness. The most commonly reported symptoms were muscle and joint pains followed by shortness of breath or cough and rash. The cause was found to be a contaminant in the tryptophan, not the amino acid itself, but over-the-counter sales of tryptophan are still, at this writing, banned.[19]

9. **Valine.** Necessary for growth and nitrogen balance. It is used as a dietary supplement.
   *Found in:* veal, liver, dried milk (nonfat), processed cheese, beef (round), lamb (leg), chicken, oats, corn cereal, cracked wheat bread, French bread, wheat germ, eggs, flounder, haddock, halibut, salmon, flank steak, hamburger.
   *Promoted in products to:* increase mental vigor, muscle coordination, and calm emotions.

# Nonessential Amino Acids

Nonessential amino acids can be obtained from your diet or manufactured in your intestines and liver. They are:

1. **Alanine.** Released by muscles to aid glucose production during fasting.
   *Found in:* the body.
   *Promoted in products to:* increase energy and muscle strength and to help the body utilize sugar.

2. **Arginine.** Plays an important part in the production of urine and is necessary for healing wounds, is the main component of some products touted as "overnight" diet pills. Arginine affects the secretion of growth hormone, which, in turn, supposedly affects appetite—the rationale

for its use in appetite-suppressant pills. In large doses it causes nausea, which may be another explanation for its appetite-suppressing quality. The FDA says that arginine is used in clinical settings to measure a patient's secretion of growth hormone, but the amount used is large and it is injected rather than taken orally. Because of its ability to stimulate growth hormone, clinical studies are now underway to see if arginine bolsters immunity in the injured, in patients recovering from operations, and in victims of infections or malignancies. In animal studies, it does stimulate the action of disease-fighting white blood cells.[20] Involved in the production of urine, growth hormone, and white blood cells. It has been reported patients with Alzheimer's disease have altered blood levels of arginine and another amino acid, ornithine, when compared to active or sedentary control populations.[21]

*Found in:* veal, peanuts, poultry, peanut butter, walnuts, milk.

*Promoted in products to:* improve immunity to bacteria, viruses, and tumors; promote wound healing and regeneration of the liver. It is said to increase the release of growth hormone aiding tissue repair.

3. **Asparagine.** Helps produce urine and is used as a diuretic.
*Found in:* soybean sprouts, asparagus and peas.
*Promoted in products to:* to help with fatigue and depression.

4. **Aspartic acid.** Used in nitrogen and energy metabolism and as a major substance for neurotransmitters. Aspartame (NutraSweet®) is derived from it.
*Found in:* sugar beets, sugar cane, molasses, and beef.
*Promoted in products to:* reduce fatigue, help expel ammonia, which is "harmful to the nervous system."

5. **Cystine.** Hair and skin are made up of 10 to 14 percent of this amino acid. It has been found to be important to wound healing and sugar metabolism.
*Found in:* chuck and round beef, leg of lamb, oatmeal, chicken, turkey, flour, milk, salmon, egg noodles, brown rice, eggs, poppy seeds, and fenugreek.

*Promoted in products as:* an antioxidant and to slow down the aging process, neutralize toxins, and to aid in the recovery from burns and surgical operations. Used in treatments for hair loss and brittle nails.

6. **Glutamic acid.** Involved in urine production, nitrogen and energy metabolism, and as a major neurotransmitter. MSG is made from it. Its magnesium salts are used in some tranquilizers.
   *Found in:* Oriental foods, seaweed, foods with MSG or aspartame.
   *Promoted in products to:* increase mental function; help speed the healing of ulcers; fight fatigue, alcoholism, schizophrenia, and the craving for sugar. A combination of the sugar, glucose, and the amino acid glutamic acid is being used to treat osteoarthritis or degenerative joint disease.

7. **Glutamine.** Aids urine production and may be involved in elasticity in cells.
   *Found in:* wheat flour and sugar beets.
   *Promoted in products to:* improve feed for chickens.

8. **Glycine.** Retards fat rancidity.
   *Found in:* gelatin and sugarcane.
   *Promoted in products to:* increase oxygen to cells and aid the production of hormones responsible for a strong immune system. It is also used as an antacid.

9. **Proline.** Found in collagen, an insoluble protein found in connective tissue, skin, bone, ligaments, and cartilage.
   *Found in:* wheat and gelatin.
   *Promoted in products to:* aid joint and tendon functions; and to maintain and strengthen heart muscles.

10. **Serine.** The nonessential amino acid *serine* is metabolized into choline, which is used to make acetylcholine, the very important neurotransmitter that sparks the sending of messages between cells (*see* page 230) and that is vital to the ability to remember. Helps produce the neurotransmitter involved in memory, acetylcholine.
    *Found in:* beef and gelatin.

*Promoted in products to:* aid in the body's use of sugar and help strengthen the immune system as well as protect nerve fibers.

11. **Taurine.** Found in almost every tissue of the body and at a high level in human milk. Most infant soy protein formulas are now supplemented with this amino acid because it is now believed it may be essential for fetal and infant brain and nervous system development. Taurine is almost absent from vegetarian diets. It is believed to be necessary for healthy eyes and is an antioxidant. It is also believed to be necessary for a regular heartbeat because it affects membrane excitability by normalizing potassium flux in and out of the heart muscle cells. Supplementation may prevent digitalis-induced irregular heartbeats. Aids digestion, scavenges free radicals (*see* Glossary), nerve stimulation. It is used in biochemical research and is in commercial emulsifying agents.
*Found in:* oysters, beef, liver, human milk, and mussels.
*Promoted in products to:* help control epileptic seizures and fight the signs of aging, particularly by acting against free radicals (*see* Glossary).

12. **Tyrosine.** Widely distributed in animal protein, is not considered an essential amino acid because it can be manufactured by the body from phenylalanine. When the enzyme that transforms phenylalanine into tyrosine is not active, the serious inherited disease PKU occurs. As mentioned earlier, PKU causes mental deficiency.

Tyrosine, in turn, is a building block for the nerve messengers epinephrine, norepinephrine, and dopamine, as well as for thyroid hormone and melanin, the dark brown and black skin and hair pigment. Norepinephrine and epinephrine are involved in the tendency toward strong emotions and alertness. Dopamine is involved in movement and mood. Thyroid hormone is necessary for normal metabolism of food and also strongly influences brain function and behavior. Mental retardation occurs in children and mental abnormalities in adults who have insufficient thyroid hormone.

Dr. Alan J. Gelenberg, a psychiatrist at Harvard Medical School, reported that some depressed patients who took tablets of tyrosine, in addition to their regular diet, improved. The tyrosine provided solely by a high-protein diet, however, did not have the same effect.[22]

In another study, this one done at the Massachusetts Institute of Technology (MIT), E. Melamed and his colleagues measured the amino acid levels in eleven healthy young men who consumed a diet containing 113 milligrams of protein per day and who took 100 milligrams per kilogram of body weight per day of L-tyrosine in three equal doses before meals.[23] The men's blood levels of tyrosine rose from .13 to .21 on the day they received the tyrosine. This led to the conclusion that ingesting supplemental tyrosine may increase the tyrosine levels in the brain, thus enabling the brain to manufacture its own neurotransmitters to combat conditions such as Parkinsonism, depression, and high blood pressure, in which neurotransmitter deficiencies play a part.

Is tyrosine a stress reliever? At the Naval Aerospace Medical Research Laboratory in Pensacola, Florida, D. F. Neri and his colleagues wanted to find out. Navy subjects were kept awake for twenty-four hours. Six hours after the experiment began, one-half of the subjects received 150 milligrams per kilogram of body weight in a split dose while the other half received a cornstarch placebo. Neither the researchers nor the subjects knew who received which one. The researchers found that those who received tyrosine had a significant "amelioration of the usual performance decline on psychomotor tasks" and were significantly more alert. The improvements lasted about three hours. The results of the study also suggested that tyrosine is a relatively benign treatment at this dose, they noted. The Naval researchers are continuing their studies, hoping that tyrosine may prove useful in counteracting performance decrements during episodes of sustained work coupled with sleep loss.[24]

**Found in:** peanuts, oatmeal, cheese, chicken, roast turkey, beef (round), leg of lamb, calf's liver, bouillon, bananas, milk, ham, egg noodles, egg yolks, almonds, sardines, sesame seeds, garlic powder, and shredded wheat.

**Promoted in products to:** act as a natural relaxant, to alleviate insomnia, reduce anxiety and depression, help in the treatment of migraines; helps the immune system, reduces the risk of artery and heart spasms and with lysine (*see* page 27) reduces cholesterol.

## Amino Competition

The U.S. Food and Drug Administration (FDA) believes that the ingestion of large amounts of individual amino acids can be harmful and in 1974 it removed amino acids from the agency's Generally Recognized As Safe (GRAS) list. However, the FDA has approved the addition of amino acids to foods for two purposes: fortifying protein-containing foods to improve food value, and treating metabolic disorders related to certain diseases. In the latter case, the FDA considers them "medical foods." These products have to be tested for safety and efficacy as if they were drugs.[25]

Megadoses of single amino acids, as pointed out before, can be dangerous. Tryptophan has produced fatty changes in the livers of rats. Because liver metabolism of tryptophan is similar in rats and humans, such findings raise serious questions about long-term supplementation to achieve positive effects as a drug.[26]

In liver cirrhosis (scarring due to disease or alcoholism), for example, there may be a buildup in the brain of tryptophan and, consequently, of serotonin. The brain then goes into the deep sleep known as *coma*. This scenario receives some support from clinical studies in which patients with liver coma were roused by administering amino acids that would counteract tryptophan by competing with it for entry into the brain.

This competition between amino acids to enter the brain explains why certain amino acids may enter the brain when a high-carbohydrate meal rather than a high-protein meal is eaten, even though amino acids are derived from protein. It has to do with the natural defense system called the *blood-brain barrier,* a collection of brain cells that act like Secret Service agents to protect a "head of state" against assassins and hecklers. Constantly on guard, the blood-brain barrier allows only a certain amount of particular types of amino acids to pass through at one time.[27]

There is competition within each type of amino acid to get past the barrier and into the brain tissue. Once there is "no more room," because its competitors got there first, the blood-brain barrier prevents other amino acids from entering. For example, high-protein meals fail to increase the level of tryptophan in the brain because the other amino acids are much more abundant in dietary proteins. The competition for access to the brain, then, becomes weighted against tryptophan.[28] Thus, whether an amino acid in your diet will get to your brain depends not only on the concentration of the amino acid in your diet and blood but also on the concentrations of its amino acid competitors.

## Protein and Parkinson's Disease

Recognition of this phenomenon has already shown promise in therapy with Parkinson's disease patients. More than one and a half million Americans suffer from this devastating nervous disorder, which is characterized by involuntary trembling of the limbs and facial muscles, extreme slowness of movement, and muscular rigidity that makes even simple activities like walking or picking up a book difficult. Levodopa, a drug that raises the level of dopamine in the brain, is a treatment that has freed many Parkinson's patients from the prison of the disease, but it often produces side effects that are as bad as the disease—rapid and unpredictable shifts in movement, ranging from excessive involuntary movements to almost no movements at all.

A number of Parkinson's patients have noted that hot, spicy meals result in violent movements, while meat products or other foods rich in protein make them stiffer and slower. These patients determined that a bland or vegetarian diet causes fewer or less severe symptoms.

The effects of protein on the absorption of levodopa was then studied, and it was discovered that some amino acids may block the absorption of the medication from the gut or block its entry into the brain.[29] On the other hand, many patients are unable to tolerate levodopa on an empty stomach and experience nausea and vomiting. Thus, patients must often compromise between getting levodopa's full effect by taking it on an empty stomach, and preventing nausea and vomiting by taking it with food.

A Yale Medical School physician, Jonathan H. Pincus, and his associates gave eleven Parkinson's patients a special diet regimen.[30] They were to eat carbohydrates all day and eat proteins only at night. From the time they woke up until 5:00 P.M., the patients ate no meat, poultry, dairy products, legumes, nuts, or baked goods (which contain milk and eggs). After a short time, nine of the patients "experienced a marked relief of Parkinsonian symptoms" as well as a lessening of the side effects often brought on by levodopa.[31] Moreover, eight of these patients were able to reduce their dosage of the medication by an average of 41 percent. Physicians in private practice who read about the results began trying the new therapy on their own patients and are reporting similar success.[32] But when the high-protein meal is eaten in the evening to make up for the lack of protein all day, "patients experience an exacerbation of Parkinsonian symptoms that can last up to three or four hours," Dr. Pincus and his colleagues pointed out. Nonetheless, the simple measure of avoiding protein during the daytime is allowing patients who suffer from the side effects of levodopa to enjoy hours of near-normal functioning and independence.[33]

So what should you eat to make sure your brain gets the amino acid building blocks it needs to manufacture neurotransmitters in your brain? Your first priority is a diet sufficient in protein. (The word *protein* itself means "of first importance.") Customary intake by Westerners is 100 grams of dietary protein. You contribute about 70 grams of self-made protein per day and you lose about 10 grams per day by elimination of waste. That means you have to process 160 grams of protein per day.

## Ingesting All the Amino Acids You Need

Proteins differ in nutritive value mainly due to their amino acid composition. If one essential amino acid is missing from the diet, a certain protein or proteins will not be formed, and an adult will enter a state of negative nitrogen balance while a child or infant will cease to grow.

In general, the proteins of animal origin provide the amino acids most humans need for maintenance and growth. The egg provides all of the essential amino acids. *High-quality proteins* contain the essential amino acids in an available form and in near-optimal proportions. Animal proteins—sometimes called "complete" proteins—such as eggs, meat, fish, poultry, and dairy products are high-quality proteins. Most plant proteins are deficient in one or more of the essential amino acids, and these amino acids may not be present in optimal proportions. The deficient amino acid is called the *limiting amino acid*. If a food with a limiting amino acid is combined with another food containing that limiting amino acid, protein quality is improved.

Plant foods often contain insufficient quantities of lysine, methionine and cystine, tryptophan, and/or threonine. Lysine is the limiting amino acid of many cereals, while methionine is the limiting amino acid of beans (legumes). Vegetarian diets, therefore, tend to lack one or another of the essential amino acids. For example, most rice is low in lysine, while some legumes are low in methionine but high in lysine. So a meal of rice and beans (legumes) provides a combination of food proteins. Nuts or seeds and legumes also provide complementary proteins. Soy is the one bean that meets almost all protein needs.

Some vegetable proteins can also be supplemented with a small amount of animal protein. The Chinese use small portions of meat or fish in stir-fried vegetables and rice dishes. Americans also use this technique with dishes such as macaroni and cheese, pizza, and even the common sandwich. Today you can buy foods that contain sufficient proteins so that, ostensibly, you will have an abundance of amino acids from which to build the neurotransmitters in your body. However, the way you cook your food has a significant effect on its amino acid value. For example, Cornell University researchers investigated the protein, amino acid, and nitrogen content of potatoes before and after cooking.[34] Fried potato skins have a decreased amino acid content of 45 percent. Frying the inside of the potato, as in french-frying, decreased its amino acid level by 36 percent. By contrast, baking the potato lowered the amino acid content of the skin by only 5 percent, and baking actually raised the amino acid content of the inside of the potato 13 percent. The skin of the potato has more amino acids than the inside, so you should bake your potatoes and eat the skin as well as the inside.

### ESTIMATED DAILY AMINO ACID REQUIREMENTS*

| Amino Acid | Children (10–12 Years) | Adults | Infants |
| --- | --- | --- | --- |
| Histidine | — | 8–12 | 28 |
| Isoleucine | 28 | 10 | 70 |
| Leucine | 42 | 14 | 161 |
| Lysine | 44 | 12 | 103 |
| Methionine + Cystine | 22 | 13 | 58 |
| Phenylalanine + Tyrosine | 22 | 14 | 125 |
| Threonine | 28 | 87 | 87 |
| Tryptophan | 3.3 | 3.5 | 17 |
| Valine | 25 | 10 | 93 |

*Given in milligrams per kilogram of body weight. Recommended Dietary Allowances, 10 ed. 1989—National Academy of Sciences, page 57.

Can you manipulate your amino acid intake to affect your brain? You certainly can, but it is best to do it through diet rather than to dose yourself with amino acids without medical supervision. If you want to calm yourself or fall asleep more easily, eat a meal high in carbohydrates and low in protein, which will raise your brain levels of tryptophan and the neurotransmitter serotonin.

Choices for a high-carbohydrate breakfast (not a balanced meal, but one weighted toward raising tryptophan) might include any of the following foods:

Pears
Pancakes with syrup
Pineapple juice
Bran muffin
Oat cereal
English muffin and jam
Decaffeinated coffee or tea

Choices for a high-carbohydrate lunch might include
any of the following:

Spaghetti
Macaroni
Fresh green beans
Whole wheat toast and tomatoes
Rye bread
Potato pancakes
Apple pie
Lemon meringue pie
Cranberry juice
Decaffeinated coffee or tea, or fruit juice

Choices for a high-carbohydrate dinner might include:

Fettuccine
Baked potato stuffed with vegetables
Barley
Eggplant
Vegetable casserole
Apricots
Cherries

If you want to be stimulated, be as sharp as possible, and use your
memory, or if you are going to participate in an athletic competition, you can stimulate your norepinephrine, dopamine, and acetylcholine levels by eating a diet rich in protein, especially tyrosine
and lecithin (to produce acetylcholine).

Choices for a high-protein breakfast might include any
of the following:

Eggs
Cottage cheese
Fish
Meat
Potatoes
Yogurt
Milk
Caffeinated coffee or tea

Choices for a high-protein lunch might include:
Egg salad
Sliced turkey
Sliced chicken
Cheese
Soybean products
Chili
Tuna
Caffeinated coffee or tea

Choices for a high-protein dinner might include:
Steak
Lamb chops
Pork chops
Veal chops
Halibut
Bluefish
Salmon steaks
Chef's salad
Pizza with cheese
Cheese soufflé
Milk
Caffeinated coffee or tea

The interaction in the brain among diet, amino acids, and neurotransmitters is very complicated and depends on many factors.
Psychologist Michael Trulson, for instance, questioned the immediate cause and effect of ingesting amino acids and changes in behavior at an annual meeting of the American Psychological
Association.[35] Dr. Trulson described experiments in which 10
grams of tryptophan per day were given alone or with noncom-
peting amino acids and brain waves were checked in the area
where dopamine receptors are most dense. He concluded that
there was no change in electrical activity or function.

Dr. Trulson suggested that there is no "simple relationship"
between diet and brain function, but that perhaps there is a "lag
time." He pointed out that it takes from ten days to two weeks
for antidepressant medication to take effect and that perhaps there

is also a delay in the effect of dietary amino acids on brain function.

As scientists continue their studies, more and more information will emerge. Next to water, protein is the most abundant substance in our bodies. All of our cells contain protein, and we could not think without the protein in our brains. Amino acids are the building blocks of protein and, thus, of our brains, our bodies, and our lives. Amino acids are extremely powerful in various combinations. If you are smart, your amino acids made you that way. Treat them with respect!

# 4

# Mood and Food: Brain and Blood Sugar

Are you often depressed or constantly procrastinating or irritable? As modern medical science has progressed, such moods are no longer attributed just to "personality" or "situations" but often to physiological causes. While there may be a number of medical reasons for any of the above, a mood may be diet-related and due to one of the following:

- Low blood sugar
- High blood sugar
- Food allergy
- Food sensitivity
- Food and drug interactions

In this and the next two chapters, we will describe how food may affect your mood.

First—and probably the most studied and controversial—concerns carbohydrates and behavior. Sugar and starches contain high levels of carbohydrates. Physiologists, medical doctors, and psychologists are constantly debating about how carbohydrates in the diet affect brain function and what is normal and what is not. For every report of experimental results testing carbohydrates and behavior, a spear is thrown by another expert criticizing the methods used and killing the conclusions.

The reason there is so much attention paid to carbohydrates is because of all the foods we eat, sugar apparently has the greatest detectable effect on our brains. Ingested carbohydrates are broken down into simple sugars and then converted into glucose—blood sugar—by our bodies. Our other tissues can burn fats and protein as well as carbohydrates, but our brains and nerves can use only blood sugar as fuel. In fact, the adult human brain uses 180 grams of glucose per day. When our blood sugar drops—and we all experience a drop when we are hungry—our brain function and consequently our mood changes. The big questions that need to be answered are:

- How much lowering of blood sugar does it take to cause behavioral alterations?
- Are some of us more sensitive to those alterations in blood-sugar levels?
- Is one carbohydrate better for our brains than others?

The following are case histories (the individuals' identities have been changed) gleaned from medical reports, concerning carbohydrate metabolism and behavior.

*Right before her monthly period and sometimes when she was depressed, Mary, a thirty-two-year-old schoolteacher, craved sweets. At such times, she could drink three ice-cream sodas at one sitting or down a whole box of chocolates. For the rest of the month, she was able to maintain a well-balanced diet.*

*Jack, a twenty-six-year-old college dropout, had a menial job, despite a high IQ. Periodic panic attacks and obsessive thoughts handicapped him. He constantly wanted to clean things—sterilize them—which was good for his job but bad for his family and social life.*

*Tommy, age five, was hyperactive in private school and under threat of expulsion, while his father, an advertising executive, seemingly had the opposite problem. About an hour after the traditional business lunch, Tommy's father would fall asleep during creative sessions at the agency.*

Do you recognize yourself or someone you know in any of the above cases? How does sugar affect you, personally?

In addition to the sugar and starches in foods on your plate, your body obtains blood sugar from the proteins (amino acids) and fats stored in your body under certain conditions such as vigorous exercise or lack of food. Making glucose from fats or proteins, however, is slower and more complex than making it from carbohydrates.

Carbohydrates come in many different shapes and forms as noted on pages 67–71. Unrefined or complex carbohydrates (unprocessed) found in beans and grains, for example, are made up of a long chain of molecules strung together like beads. During digestion, they slowly break down into blood sugar. Refined (processed) carbohydrates such as sucrose (table sugar) are made up of short chains of molecules that break down into blood sugar much faster. It takes about five minutes for table sugar to begin raising your blood-sugar levels. Complex carbohydrates are metabolized more slowly and do not cause the same quick rise and fall in blood sugar.

Your brain, your liver, your pancreas, and your thyroid, adrenal, and pituitary glands largely control the amount of glucose in your blood. If your blood-sugar level falls too low, your brain sends out an emergency order to your pituitary and thyroid glands to signal your liver to start turning up sugar production from body fat.

Since your brain can't store blood sugar, it is totally dependent on the glucose it receives from your bloodstream. When the glucose level in your blood is low, your brain may not receive enough energy and, therefore, you are unable to think clearly. In extreme cases, when the blood sugar drops too low, you brain may be severely affected and coma and death may result.

Too much sugar in the blood is known as *hyperglycemia*. Diabetics suffer from this. Too little sugar in the blood is known as *hypoglycemia*. Victims of low blood sugar suffer from this.

Results of studies have raised questions about the blood glucose effects of various carbohydrate sources. There are indications that foods with exactly the same carbohydrate content may have dramatically different effects on your blood sugar.[1]

No one argues about the fact that directly after a meal your blood-sugar level rises. Then, insulin is secreted by your pancreas to help move sugar into your cells, and then your glucose level drops. If your blood sugar falls to lower-than-normal levels following a meal, your brain will send out the distress signal. You may feel dizzy, fatigued, weak, and nervous, and your heart may pound—symptoms not unlike those of an acute anxiety attack. The symptoms are actually not the result of the fall in blood sugar but the stimulating hormone epinephrine sent out to signal the liver to make more glucose.

## Hypoglycemia—Low Blood Sugar

The level of sugar in your blood can vary from 50 to 110 milligrams per deciliter of blood if you are perfectly healthy. A blood-sugar level below 40 milligrams per deciliter is considered hypoglycemic. It is a condition that can be caused by several factors.

Many physicians say that true hypoglycemia is rare and that the diagnosis of "low blood sugar" is often given just because it is more acceptable than attributing symptoms to emotions. But can anxiety cause a drop in blood sugar? And can a drop in blood sugar cause anxiety in a healthy person? If you do not eat during the night, your body will normally release glucose from your liver stores. Even if you have been starving for days and your liver supply of glucose is exhausted, your body will sacrifice other organs to keep your brain supplied with blood sugar. However, in people with certain diseases (insulin-producing tumors, liver disease, alcoholism, and so forth) and in some with no discernible physical explanation, the blood sugar will gradually drop to abnormally low levels during fasting. Besides the symptoms mentioned earlier, headaches, an inability to concentrate, forgetfulness, and sleepiness will result. This state is known as *fasting hypoglycemia,* a condition that requires a careful search for its underlying cause.

Postprandial (after a meal) hypoglycemia, or *reactive hypoglycemia,* is the most common type. It occurs about two to four hours after eating. A very rapid absorption of glucose into the circulation and a subsequent outpouring of excess insulin causes symptoms such as dizziness, fatigue, weakness, nervousness, and heart palpitations.

### Glucose Tolerance Test

The standard test for diagnosing hypoglycemia is the glucose tolerance test. After an overnight fast, you are given a drink containing a highly concentrated sugar solution. Over the next three to five hours, blood sugars are measured periodically. After drinking the sugar, your blood glucose level will increase and then drop gradually to normal. But if you are hypoglycemic, your blood sugar will drop sharply several hours after the test and, at the same time, you will develop symptoms such as trembling and irritability. Since the oral glucose test is often stopped after three hours, the period of continued decline is often missed.[2]

Many doctors believe that the glucose tolerance tests are not really accurate. Dr. Dan Foster, professor of internal medicine at the University of Texas Health Science Center in Dallas and editor of *Diabetes,* says he doesn't use the test to diagnose hypoglycemia because he believes that low blood-sugar levels can develop in normal people following this test. Even after ordinary meals, 24 percent of normal people developed blood sugar levels lower than 50 milligrams per deciliter of blood, according to one study.[3] This is why many doctors advise those who suspect they have low blood sugar to have a measurement of blood sugar taken at the time when they experience symptoms or two hours after eating a normal meal.

Another reason the glucose tolerance test may not identify all those with an abnormal sugar metabolism is that insulin alone is not the only blood-sugar regulator. A hormone may play a part in blood-sugar swings that are not evident in the traditional glucose tolerance test.

In a major contribution to scientific understanding of carbohydrate metabolism, National Institute of Aging (NIA) investigators, in collaboration with University of British Columbia scientists, found that a hormone produced in the gut, *gastric inhibitory polypeptide (GIP),* may be critical for maintaining normal blood-sugar levels.[4] And still another recently discovered hormone, glucagon-like peptide 1 (GLP-1) has been shown to play a part in inhibiting the stomach emptying of liquid meals in type II diabetics.[5] These hormones may explain why current glucose tolerance tests may not be precise in all cases and that blood-sugar evaluation is more complicated than previously believed.

The higher incidence of diabetes among the elderly has spurred the NIA's Gerontology Research Clinical Physiology branch to study the phenomenon of declining glucose tolerance with age. A key issue is the degree to which tests of glucose tolerance can predict diabetes, a disease that involves blood vessel deterioration. As many as 50 percent—and some say 70 to 80 percent—of persons over the age of sixty show signs of impaired glucose metabolism.

Normally, the pancreas releases sufficient insulin to clear the blood of excess glucose within two hours. If the blood sugar is too high for the pancreas to clear, GIP comes into play. Hence, if you eat a meal containing a lot of sugar, you activate both insulin and GIP.

The NIA investigators also identified an unusual group of individuals whom they have labeled "disparate performers." These people cannot metabolize glucose given by vein, but they are normal performers on the oral test. They have been shown to overproduce GIP and thus to compensate for the primary trigger, glucose.[6]

GIP's part in providing blood sugar for the brain is not yet known, but what is certain is that insulin does have a profound effect on your brain and behavior. If you doubt the effect of insulin on your brain, consider that diabetics, in whom insulin is absent or inefficient, may become comatose if not supplied with an outside source of the hormone to process their blood sugar. And if you don't believe blood sugar affects mood, remember that "insulin shock" was once used to treat depression. When given a dose of insulin, the patient's blood-sugar level would fall rapidly and a comalike state would occur. Then the patient was given glucose to wake up. After awakening, many of the symptoms of depression and even schizophrenia were relieved.

Insulin shock is an exaggeration of the natural interaction between insulin, glucose, and the brain. Your intestines, liver, and endocrine glands constantly cooperate to ensure that your blood-sugar levels stay within a normal range. When you challenge these systems, either by excessive carbohydrate ingestion or by fasting, your organs' reactions to the challenge can be measured. If your blood-sugar level goes too high after carbohydrate ingestion, that's *hyperglycemia*. The most common cause of hyperglycemia is diabetes. If your blood-sugar level drops too low after carbohydrate ingestion, that's *hypoglycemia*.

Since the glucose tolerance test does not identify some people who do react adversely to refined sugar, Dr. Larry Christensen, of Texas A & M University, and his colleagues sought to develop a test that could identify these individuals. At a meeting of the American Psychological Association, Dr. Christensen pointed out: "Although most of the evidence has focused on the impact of carbohydrates in general as opposed to refined sucrose, we have, in our laboratory, obtained data suggesting that refined sucrose ingestion can produce symptoms such as depression, confusion, and fatigue in selected individuals."[7]

He emphasized *selected individuals,* since some people are unaffected. Dr. Christensen and his group studied a group of volunteers who answered newspaper ads calling for persons with the following symptoms: "depressed, tired, feeling bad most of the time."

After two series of studies, the Texas researchers developed the sixty-two-item Christensen Dietary Distress Inventory Scale, which contains cognitive, behavioral, and physiological items that can help identify those who are "dietary-mood responders." Dr. Christensen indicated that the scale could help diagnose those patients whose blood glucose tests are normal but who, indeed, are affected cognitively and emotionally by the ingestion of refined sugar.

Whether or not you are hypersensitive to refined sugar, you can still cause significant changes in your blood-sugar level by what you eat, and such changes can affect your brain function and behavior.

## Break the Fast

Did you eat a bowl of Kellogg's cereal for breakfast or graham crackers? If you did, you might have avoided "deterioration of mental functioning" and "animal passions." At least, that is what the creators of these products, John Harvey Kellogg and Sylvester Graham, maintained in the nineteenth century. Kellogg further concluded that the breakdown products of meat acted as dangerous toxins that, when absorbed from the colon, produced symptoms such as depression, fatigue, headache, aggression, and mental illness.[8]

Whether you swallow Kellogg's and Graham's ideas about meat, if you don't ingest their products or some other breakfast food, you may suffer a number of the symptoms they attributed to meat.

Breakfast—its very name says a lot about its effects on your body. The early part of the waking day is a period that is generally associated with the upward phase of the circadian rhythm, when there is a rapid increase in levels of alertness, arousal, and activation. It seems logical that breaking a fast would affect the level of sugar found in the brain and get the central processor revved up. Many of us cannot even communicate with others in our households until we have had our glass of orange juice or cup of coffee after awakening.

Dr. Ernesto Pollitt of the University of Texas had half a group of children skip breakfast while the another half ate a meal of waffles and syrup, milk, and orange juice. By late morning, those who had eaten breakfast made fewer errors solving problems than the children who had skipped breakfast.[9]

These results in short-term incidental memory and problem-solving accuracy were interpreted as being the result of attitude. That is, when the subjects missed breakfast, they were more likely to become fatigued. As a result, they were more excitable, had a harder time concentrating, and were not performing as well as they usually did.[10]

A Harvard University study conducted in Philadelphia and Baltimore public schools found that increased school breakfast participation correlated with less tardiness and absence, higher math grades, and reductions in problems like depression, anxiety and hyperactivity.[11]

The same is apparently true for adults. Researchers at the University of Health Sciences/Chicago Medical School tested 40 normal-weight adults, all of whom normally ate breakfast. Subjects fasted overnight and came to the laboratory in the early morning to perform baseline tests that measured reasoning, inference, and problem solving.[12]

While one-third of the subjects continued fasting, others ate one of two breakfasts containing 450 to 500 calories. In the high-fiber "balanced" breakfast, carbohydrates supplied 59 percent of calories and protein and fat each supplied roughly 20 percent of calories. In the low-fiber "unbalanced" breakfast 61 percent of calories came from carbohydrates, 35 percent were supplied by fat, and 4 percent were supplied by protein.

Participants were tested for cognitive performance thirty minutes after mealtime, and then two hours and four hours later. Results confirmed that eating breakfast of either nutritional composition was beneficial. Skipping breakfast consistently caused hunger and led to performance difficulties on tasks requiring concentration.

In terms of suppressing hunger, the balanced breakfast also was most effective. The unbalanced breakfast suppressed hunger only relative to fasting; but four hours later, those who ate the unbalanced breakfast were as hungry as those who fasted.

## Jack in a Box

*Jack, mentioned at the beginning of this chapter, is a dramatic example of the effect of breakfast on the brain. He was in a "box." He was chronically obsessive and, despite his high IQ, couldn't stop thinking about the presence of germs long enough to concentrate on his schoolwork. Neither psychological treatment nor medications had helped him.*

*A twenty-six-year-old university dropout, Jack had a fifteen-year history of psychotherapy and drug treatment for panic attacks and discomfort. He also suffered from acne, constipation, and hypertension. Hospitalization did not help him overcome his obsession. He reported that his panic attacks preceded a worsening of his obsessions, and that fluctuations in panic attack severity coincided with fluctuations in both his mood and his acne problem. These factors suggested a common, possibly dietary, cause.*

*He was skeptical about the ability of diet to help where so many previous orthodox treatments had failed, but Jack was willing to try anything. He felt he had nothing to lose. Jack was put on a hypoallergenic diet that eliminated such foods as cereal, grain, milk, eggs, chicken, chocolate, sugar, caffeine, pork, and chemical additives. He also was given a moderate course of nutritional supplements aimed at preventing obvious deficiencies. After several weeks on the hypoallergenic diet, a high-protein breakfast consisting of a normal-sized portion of meat, fish, or poultry, with or without a piece of low-carbohydrate fresh fruit, was added.*

*Jack has remained free of obsessions for twenty-three months. His prompt response to the addition of the high-protein breakfast to his regimen gave his doctors a clue that he might be suffering from reactive hypoglycemia. A two-hour glucose tolerance test confirmed their suspi-*

*cions. His blood glucose level dropped very low after the standard dose of glucose and, at the same time, he began to develop the mental discomfort that set off his former panic attacks.*

*It was Jack's lack of high-protein breakfast to regulate his blood-sugar level that caused his problems. Food sensitivity, his doctors believe, contributed to his difficulties, but he was gradually able to reintroduce the eliminated foods, with the exception of alcohol, without bringing back his symptoms.*[13]

## Tommy's Sugar High

*Tommy, mentioned at the beginning of this chapter, liked highly sugared, artificially colored cold cereals. He also loved the cookies his mother baked and the candy his grandmother gave him every time he visited her. His mother, on the advice of Tommy's pediatrician, gave her son warm oat cereal for breakfast and substituted fruit for cookies in his lunch. He was just as happy with frozen natural juice bars as he had been with candy as a treat. Tommy was not part of a controlled study and his improvement could be attributed to the attention he received from his parents about his food or to the fact that he had matured a little more. Nevertheless, his behavior in school was no longer a problem.*

*In millions of homes, children like Tommy are sent off to school after eating highly sugared cereals. Research by Betty Li and P. J. Schumann of the U.S. Department of Agriculture's Nutrient Composition Laboratory analyzed sixty-two ready-to-eat breakfast cereals for their sugar content. They found that only three of the sixty-two cereals apparently had no added sugar, two contained more than 50-percent sugar, and the sugar content of the rest fell between these two levels.*[14]

*Tommy's change in diet—from highly sugared foods to complex carbohydrates—not only made him feel better but also had a beneficial effect on the entire family. Seeing the improvement in his son's behavior, Tommy's father decided to change his own diet. Instead of his heavy, fat- and sugar-laden lunches, he ate a salad or broiled fish and skipped the traditional cocktail. He found that he had much more energy in the afternoon.*

## Breakfast Boosters

So what you eat or don't eat for your first meal of the day is important to your brain. In this rush-rush world, you may think you don't have time to eat breakfast but here are some helpful hints that nullifies that excuse:

***Ready to eat.*** Build a breakfast around foods that are ready to eat or take little preparation time. These include fresh and canned fruits, milk, yogurt, cheese, cottage cheese, ready-to-eat cold cereals, and instant breakfast mixes and bars.

***Ready to go.*** Try celery stuffed with peanut butter or meat or cheese spread, dried fruits or vegetable juices, a container of yogurt, and a low fat granola bar.

***Perk up cereals.*** Top cereals with fruit or stir chopped nuts such as peanuts, pecans, and walnuts into cooked cereals.

***Not hungry?*** Drink juice or milk. Something is better than nothing. Have some bread or crackers later in the morning, then drink some milk and eat some cheese, an egg, or peanut butter.

***Don't skip if you are on a diet.*** Skipping breakfast will not help you lose weight. In fact, studies show that most people who skip that meal tend to eat more later in the day. Some even select more calorie-laden foods than those who eat breakfast do.

# Timing of Meals

Tommy and his father are good examples of the effect of breakfast and lunch on behavior, although the carbohydrates affected them differently. It seems to have made Tommy more active and his father less active. The paradoxical effects could be due not only to their physiological reactions to carbohydrates but also to the time of day they were ingested.

The focus has been on the effects of carbohydrates on the brain and behavior associated with breakfast and lunch because these two meals are immediately relevant to efficiency during the working day. Particular attention has been paid to lunch because it has long been recognized that lunch produces the most obvious behavioral response to food intake.[15]

## Let's Lunch

Researchers have reported (and most of us have found it to be true) that there is a dip in alertness and efficiency at about 2:00 P.M., one or two hours after lunch. There are no such obvious efficiency changes in the morning after breakfast or later in the day following the evening meal.

Bonnie Spring, Ph.D., Harris Lieberman, Ph.D., and their colleagues at Texas Technical University, found in their studies that subjects who ate a high-carbohydrate lunch felt less alert than those who ate a high-protein lunch. The Texas group had expected just the opposite. They assumed that a high-carbohydrate breakfast would have more powerful effects than the same food eaten for lunch. The rationale was that at lunchtime one may still be digesting breakfast and may already have somewhat elevated levels of insulin; thus the effects of lunchtime carbohydrates would be blunted. In contrast, the investigators assumed, insulin levels and blood levels of amino acids would be low at breakfast, after having fasted for approximately twelve hours. Thus, the high-carbohydrate meal was expected to have its greatest impact at breakfast. Instead, most of the participants in their studies reported that after lunch, mental slump and feelings of fatigue were greater with a high-carbohydrate meal than with a high-protein one.[16]

The Texas Tech researchers are not sure about the interplay between regular circadian rhythms and the nutrient content of the meals, since it has been shown there are regular patterns of rises and falls in mental functions throughout the day. For example, perceptual search tasks may improve over the day, reaching a maximum at 8:00 P.M., while scores on tests that require short-term memory climb to a maximum at 11:00 A.M.

In an earlier study, Dr. Spring, formerly of Harvard University, found that adults had difficulty performing a simple speech test after eating a sherbet-like high-carbohydrate snack. The decline was especially marked for those over age forty. Her tests also showed differences in the way men and women felt after eating the sherbet: women had a more pronounced reaction and reported feeling lethargic and sleepy, while men simply reported feeling calmer.[17]

In a later study, Dr. Spring and her colleagues at the University of Chicago Medical School studied whether the fatiguing effects of eating lunch are greater for carbohydrate-rich meals than for other meals, and related the time course of behavioral change to blood sugar, insulin, and amino acids. On different occasions, normal women fasted overnight, ate a standard breakfast, and at lunch did one of the following:

- continued to fast.
- ate a high-carbohydrate, low-protein meal.
- ate a similar meal containing regular amounts of carbohydrate and protein.
- ate a high-protein, low-carbohydrate meal.

Meals were equal in calories and fat. Only the high-carbohydrate meal significantly increased fatigue, which could not be attributed to low blood sugar because blood sugar remained elevated. Fatigue began approximately when the high-carbohydrate meal elevated blood tryptophan but ended even though the tryptophan remained elevated. Tryptophan is an amino acid used by the body to make the calming neurotransmitter serotonin. Fatigue after a high-carbohydrate lunch could not be explained by reactive hypoglycemia or sweet taste, and could partially be explained by the idea that fatigue parallels an elevation of tryptophan.[18]

Angus Craig, Ph.D., of the University of Sussex in Brighton, England, wrote in *Nutrition Reviews* that the observed effects of eating a meal depend on the delay between ingesting the food and taking measurements. Observations made within one or two hours of starting a meal may differ considerably from those obtained after three hours. The effects also depend on the gap in time since the previous meal and on the time of day the test meal is eaten.[19]

Dr. Craig and his colleagues also found a dip in efficiency after lunch was eaten, but no change in performance when no lunch was consumed. This led the Sussex University investigators to conclude that, with some exceptions, lunch does have an adverse effect on performance for at least two hours afterward, whereupon the effect starts to wane.

Dr. Craig's group also discovered that accuracy on a simple test involving searching a page of type and crossing out all of the e's was significantly influenced after lunch. The test was affected both by the size of the test lunch eaten and by the size of the lunch ordinarily consumed. The effects on this "search-and-perceive" test of a heavy, three-course test meal seemed to be less for the person who normally consumed such a big meal than for one who normally ate a light lunch.

There are many debates about the association between high-carbohydrate and high-protein meals, time of day, cognition, and mood. None is more heated than the controversy over whether there is a correlation between high sugar intake and hyperactive behavior.

## Sugar, Attention Deficit, and Hyperactivity

The belief that sugar causes behavior and learning problems in children is widely held by the general public but is a subject that is highly controversial among some noted health professionals. Parents, grandparents, and teachers can testify that when children eat a lot of sweets they become hyperactive. Some research studies have concluded that sugar does adversely affect children's behavior and ability to learn, while others have said there is no correlation.

In a recent study, researchers examined the effect of eating sucrose (table sugar) on the behavior of children aged six to ten years.[20] The children were chosen for the study because their parents believed the children reacted negatively to sucrose. Preschool children were also studied. They are often considered sensitive to some foods. The researchers found no differences in the behavior of the children when they ate higher-than-normal amounts of sucrose compared to when they ate diets low in sucrose.

Actually, this and other research suggests sugars tend to calm both children and adults. The effect could go unnoticed due to other influences. For instance, the excitement of a birthday party or Halloween could override the calming effect of sugars.

In one study, Ronald Prinz, Ph.D., an associate professor of clinical psychology, and David Riddle, a doctoral candidate, under a grant from the National Institute of Child Health and Human Development, found a correlation between sucrose consumption and observed behavior in hyperactive and nonhyperactive four- to seven-year-old children. Mothers kept seven-day food records of the children's intake. At the end of the week, each child was videotaped while playing in a playroom. The trained observers who scored the videotapes were completely unaware of the children's characteristics and dietary intakes, and in fact were not even informed that dietary data had been collected. The observers were highly accurate in estimating the hyperactive group's estimated sucrose consumption. Dr. Prinz concluded that there "may be an association between diets characterized by a high sucrose component and reduced attentional performance in normal boys."[21]

In another experiment, further evidence was added that hyperactive children may be more susceptible than others to the effects of sugar on behavior. C. Keith Conners, Ph.D., and his colleagues at the George Washington University School of Medicine and the Children's Hospital National Medical Center reported at the August 1987 meeting of the American Psychological Association on the difference in reactions to sucrose between hyperactive and normal children.[22]

Hyperactive and normal children were assigned to receive one of three breakfasts—high-carbohydrate, high-protein, or fasting. On two separate days, each group received an aspartame challenge or a sucrose challenge at breakfast. Prior to eating breakfast, blood was withdrawn from a forearm vein by an indwelling catheter that was maintained throughout the testing day. Subsequent samples were drawn at 30, 60, 90, 120, 180, and 240 minutes. Samples were assayed for blood sugar, insulin, growth hormones, cortisol, lactate, glucagon, and fatty acids.

The children sat in a booth and performed a continuous task. This task was repeated in mid- and late morning. Errors of omission, commission, and reaction time were recorded. Results showed the same pattern of results across performance and hormonal measures. In each case, there was a difference between the hyperactive and normal children who had eaten the high-carbohydrate breakfast but not with the high-protein or fasting breakfast. Errors of omission were significantly worse for hyperactives when sugar was added to the high-carbohydrate breakfast but not when added to the high-protein or fasting breakfast.

Dr. Conners and his group believe the effect of the sugar-carbohydrate diet on behavioral changes was due to the increase in serotonin the combination caused. The researchers propose that either hyperactive children are more sensitive to a rise in serotonin or serotonin interferes with the regulation of dopamine and nor-epinephrine in the brain. "Sugar may not be harmful to normals but may interfere with cognitive function in hyperactives when they have a carbohydrate load prior to sugar ingestion," Dr. Conners concluded.[23]

Judith Rapoport, M.D., chief of the Child Psychiatry branch of the National Institute of Mental Health, conducted a study of children she described as "sugar responders." Twenty-one children were given behavioral tests after ingesting glucose, sucrose, saccharin, or a placebo. Dr. Rapoport concluded that the children were less active after having ingested the sugar than before, and that "it doesn't seem likely that any of these substances produce significant effects, even in a group of presumed sugar responders."[24]

## Carbohydrate Cravings

Among the unanswered questions about nutrition is why do all of us crave sweets? Dr. Bonnie Spring points out that carbohydrate craving is a recognized symptom that spans several diagnostic categories, positing difficulties for weight management. She says that studies indicate foods rich in carbohydrate but poor in protein induce drowsiness and impair concentration in healthy adult human subjects. Carbohydrate-rich foods induce greater fatigue and performance impairments than isocaloric (calorie-equal) foods that are high in protein. Yet, some individuals crave and selectively consume large quantities of carbohydrates, raising questions about the causes for this phenomenon. Carbohydrate cravers constitute a substantial subgroup of several clinical populations, including patients with bulimia, seasonal affective disorders, obesity, and smoking withdrawal. Recent findings suggest that carbohydrate cravers respond differently to carbohydrates than do more balanced eaters. Specifically, carbohydrates may have an antidepressant effect on the mood of individuals who crave them.[25]

## Carbohydrate Craving in Obesity

Judith Wurtman, Ph.D., of MIT's food and nutrition department, says she and her colleagues identified two groups of obese individuals who consume excessive calories primarily as snack foods: carbohydrate cravers, whose snacks consist mainly of carbohydrate-rich foods, and noncarbohydrate cravers, who consume about equal amounts of carbohydrate- and protein-rich foods as snacks.[26] In a study performed at the MIT Clinical Research Center, mood states were measured before and after the consumption of a carbohydrate-rich lunch by the two groups of obese snackers. After the meal, the moods of the two groups differed significantly. The *noncarbohydrate cravers* reported feeling considerably less vigorous, more fatigued, and sleepier than the *carbohydrate cravers*. Moreover, after the high-carbohydrate meal, they rated themselves more depressed, whereas the *carbohydrate cravers* reported themselves as less depressed. Thus some obese individuals may avoid consuming carbohydrate-rich foods because of the negative effects these foods have on their moods. In contrast, obese carbohydrate cravers may prefer to consume carbohydrate-rich snacks because of their positive effects on mood.

In another study, obese carbohydrate cravers were treated with a placebo or with fenfluramine, a drug that enhances the release of serotonin. Fenfluramine significantly reduced carbohydrate snacking.[27]

Conceivably, excessive carbohydrate cravings reflect inadequate serotonin levels in the obese craver's brain, and the craver learns to desire foods that enhance serotonin. For such individuals, carbohydrate intake may be reinforced by an improvement in mood.

***Sugar and Alcohol.*** Researchers at McGill University, Montréal, conducted two studies to examine the interaction between table sugar (sucrose) and ethanol in normal young fasting adult males. The first experiment was carried out with alcohol with sugar or alcohol with aspartame so all drinks were equally sweet. Subjects were tested for mood, memory, subjective intoxication, and psychomotor performance at baseline and at times up to 3.5 hours after ingestion of the drinks. Sugar attenuated alcohol intoxication but without influencing blood alcohol levels. Contrary to previous reports, the combination of alcohol and sugar failed to produce significant low blood sugar or any of the adverse behavioral effects associated with low blood sugar at later times after drink ingestions. The second experiment involved a simpler design in which the subject receiving no sugar did not get aspartame. This was to rule out the possibility that aspartame was exacerbating alcohol intoxication instead of sugar attenuating it. The second experiment also showed that sugar can attenuate alcohol intoxication in fasting humans without altering blood alcohol levels significantly.[28]

**Smoking, Weight Gain and Carbohydrates.** Many people are afraid to stop smoking because they fear they will gain weight. And many do—five to ten pounds on the average—but there is no unanimous opinion as to why.

Neil Grunberg, Ph.D., and Deborah Bowen report that recent human and animal studies indicate that body weight gains after smoking cessation or after chronic nicotine administration are partially a result of increased consumption of sweet-tasting carbohydrates.[29]

Nicotine affects the availability of glucose. Ex-smokers consume carbohydrates in order to alter the almost unbearable unpleasantness of tobacco abstinence. In effect, carbohydrates might be considered a self-administered tranquilizer. This theory is consistent with reported effects of carbohydrates on mood.

The good news is that most people who continue to eat a regular diet after giving up smoking will gain weight for three months, plateau for two months, and then lose the added weight after five months if they can forego bingeing on carbohydrates.[30]

**SAD-ness and Carbohydrate Craving.** Another recognized carbohydrate-associated problem is seasonal affective disorder (SAD). It is a condition in which people become depressed in fall and winter and are fine in the spring and summer. Most SAD victims are women whose symptoms began in their twenties or thirties. In addition to sadness and social withdrawal, these women suffer from overeating, carbohydrate craving, and weight gain.

Norman Rosenthal, M.D., of the National Institute of Mental Health's psychobiology section, was one of the first to identify SAD.[31] He reported that carbohydrate craving occurred in the winter months in 79 percent of SAD patients he and his colleagues studied. Carbohydrate craving is an early symptom, frequently beginning in September or October, generally before mood is affected. Some patients craved sweets and chocolates, whereas others preferred starches. Several patients used terms such as "compulsion," "craving," and "pressure to eat." Like the other symptoms, their cravings almost always subsided in the spring. Patients who have traveled during the winter months have reported feeling better when they are closer to the equator. Those who moved to more southern locations have reported an overall improvement in their symptoms.

These seasonal changes in mood and behavior resemble the annual rhythms found in a wide variety of animal behaviors, Dr. Rosenthal maintains. So-called circannual (yearly) rhythms are often synchronized in animals by day length, an effect generally mediated by the nocturnal secretion of melatonin by the pineal gland in the center of the brain. The pineal gland was thought to be the "third eye," and until the 1950s, it was thought to have no real purpose. It is now believed to be a sort of "biological clock" that sends out "ticks" to influence the activities of hormones.

In the 31 SAD patients studied by Dr. Rosenthal and his associates, exposing the patients to light reversed winter symptoms, carbohydrate cravings included. Symptoms were alleviated with the administration of five to six hours per day of bright, full-spectrum light of an intensity to suppress melatonin. When the patients were then given 2 milligrams per day of melatonin, their depressive symptoms did not recur but their carbohydrate craving became significantly worse. Luncheon meals containing different proportions of carbohydrates and protein were fed to 16 of the SAD patients. The effects of these meals on mood and performance were evaluated using self-report mood scales and a pencil-and-paper performance task. For comparison purposes, 16 normal volunteers matched for sex and mean age were given similar meals. Mood and performance data were analyzed. Plasma amino acid levels were also examined to confirm the experimental manipulation.

According to Dr. Rosenthal, it is conceivable that for patients with SAD, overeating—particularly of carbohydrates—may be part of a complex behavioral feedback loop involving efforts to keep the brain's neurochemicals in balance.

***Carbohydrates and the Brains of Bulimics.*** Researchers at NIH want to determine how the brain uses sugar in bulimia, depression, and obsessive-compulsive disorder. They used the PET scan, which pictures cerebral glucose use, in 11 patients with bulimia and 18 normal comparison subjects. All were women of comparable age and educational level. The bulimic patients were also tested for symptoms of major depression and obsessive-compulsive disorder. The patients with bulimia showed a correlation between blood flow in the front lobe of their brain and greater depressive symptoms. However, the changes in the use of glucose by the bulimic's brain have not been correlated with mood.[32]

June Chiodo, Ph.D., of Texas Technical University, links carbohydrate cravings to bulimic behavior.[33] The intake of high-carbohydrate foods by bulimics is characterized by extremes. Between binges, bulimics typically practice severely restrictive dieting, which may include avoidance of carbohydrates. In contrast, binges are characterized by the rapid intake of large quantities of foods, often involving high-calorie carbohydrates. Binges are usually triggered by feelings of tension, anxiety, or depression. The ingestion of food provides some relief from emotional distress, at least initially. By the end of the binge, however, bulimics report self-deprecating thoughts and typically vow never to binge again. They may also engage in purging behaviors.

The parallels between eating disturbance and emotional disturbance are impressive in bulimics, which suggests they might be interrelated. The first possibility is that dietary restrictions in the interval between binges play a role in perpetuating or exacerbating the affective disturbance. This hypothesis is supported by the evidence that depression increases in proportion to the number of meals skipped and by the finding that brain serotonin-depleting interventions—which include carbohydrate restriction—may induce depression.

The second possible relationship is that carbohydrate-rich dessert-type foods may have an antidepressant effect in bulimics. Data from Dr. Chiodo's laboratory suggest such an effect. It is believed that bingeing is an unwitting attempt to self-medicate uncomfortable mood states. Since the antidepressant effects of binge eating are short-lived, however, and since they may involve sweet foods that are high in protein as well as carbohydrates, it is doubtful that pharmacologic effects on brain serotonin represents a sufficient explanation. Dr. Chiodo purports that dessert foods are psychologically reinforcing. In our society, they represent "treats."

# Sugar Sense

John Bantle, M.D., of the University of Minnesota investigated the effects of different forms of sugar on the glucose levels in the blood of both normal and diabetic subjects.[34] He and his colleagues studied responses to five meals, each containing a different form of carbohydrate but all with nearly identical amounts of total carbohydrate, protein, and fat. The subjects were 10 healthy persons, 12 patients with Type I diabetes (requiring insulin injections), and 10 patients with Type II diabetes (adult-onset, requiring no insulin). The test carbohydrates were glucose, fructose, sucrose, potato starch, and wheat starch. In all three groups, the meal containing sucrose as the test carbohydrate did not produce significantly greater glucose peaks in the blood than did meals containing potato, wheat, or glucose as test carbohydrates. The meal with fructose as the test carbohydrate produced the smallest increments in blood-sugar levels.[35] Dr. Bantle concluded that fructose produces less post-meal blood sugar than do other common types of carbohydrate. But he cautioned that additional research is needed because the long-term effects of substantial amounts of fructose in the diet remain unknown. Until the mystery is solved, it makes sense to get your sugar as fructose from fruits, vegetables, and other items in which it is a natural part of the product.

Like sucrose, fructose contains no real nutritive value; however, it may be more effective than other forms of sugar in suppressing hunger. Since fructose does not cause the dip in blood sugar about two hours after it is eaten that sucrose does, it is not likely to cause the hunger sensation that occurs with the sucrose-caused blood-sugar drop. Therefore, symptoms also associated with low blood sugar—lethargy and/or irritability—may not be as likely to occur when fructose is substituted for sucrose. This, of course, has not been proven. The effects of extreme variations of blood-sugar levels on the brain are well known and accepted. The more subtle effects on the brain of sugar in the diet are the subject of many a debate.

## Sugar and Aging

Sugar is another element in our diets that is a candidate for being an aging factor. Anthony Cerami, Ph.D., who heads the Rockefeller University's Laboratory of Medical Biochemistry, believes that many of the breakdowns associated with age proceed from a single, fundamental chemical reaction between glucose and the proteins that comprise the body's metabolic machinery and structural framework.

"Until recently, glucose was generally considered a stable and innocuous molecule serving as a central source for energy. Scientists have since learned that it not only plays a part in metabolism—the body's use of energy—but also that this abundant and ubiquitous sugar is not always benign," says Dr. Cerami.[36]

Chemical catalysts called enzymes trigger most biological activities. Glucose, however, has the ability to react with proteins and with nucleic acids (the genetic material of cells) just by being next to them, a process called *nonenzymatic glycosylation.*

"A lot of complicated chemistry goes on," says Dr. Cerami, "and if the reaction is permitted to continue, eventually it produces a brownish yellow pigment that can bind two molecules together."

In other words, blood sugar can jumble protein and tangle molecules, leaving undisposed garbage in the cell. Dr. Cerami has named the resulting pigments "AGE," for advanced glycosylated end-products. The manufacture of these sugar-modified proteins is independent of the amount of sugar we consume. The body can produce glucose from starch and other foodstuffs, so the formation of AGE is a continuous, lifelong process whenever blood glucose is permitted to react with proteins.

One familiar manifestation of AGE is the browning of food. The skin of a roasted chicken turns brown because the dehydration that occurs during cooking accelerates the formation of AGE. The same thing happens when bread is toasted. The effects of AGE over time can be observed simply by comparing the brown, hard, dried apricots from a health food store with the artificially preserved supermarket variety, which are bright orange and soft. Pathologists have observed that the bones of older people are browner than the bones of younger people. "Like untreated apricots," says Dr. Cerami, "we're browning all the time." AGE does more than just discolor tissue. As Dr. Cerami explains, "AGE acts as a chemical glue to attach molecules to one another, forming what we call a cross-link. That is why overcooked meat is so difficult to slice and chew. You are literally sawing through cross-linked proteins with your knife and grinding them down with your teeth."

Dr. Cerami maintains that these same glucose-derived crosslinks have been traced to many physical manifestations of old age. While eating browned chicken and toast may not "age" you, understanding the process of why these foods turn brown may go far in helping scientists understand the process of human aging and thus how to slow it down.

## When the Label Says "Sugar"

Are there certain forms of sugar that are better for your brain than others? That question is under debate. The nutrition panel on a food label lists the total amount of sugars in a serving of the food. This amount includes sugars found naturally in foods, such as the sugars in grapes. It also includes added sugars. The ingredient list must name added sugars but you may not realize that corn syrup, for example, is a sugar, or that maltose is. There is no recommended level of intake or Percent Daily Value for sugar. There is no formal standard that says a certain amount of sugar in the diet is appropriate or inappropriate.

The FDA controls the use of terms on food labels. A "sugar-free" food must contain less than 0.5 grams of sugar per serving. A "reduced sugar" food must contain at least 25 percent less sugar per serving than the regular product—which may be very high in sugar.

Sugars may not be added to a food labeled "no added sugar," "without added sugar," or "no sugar added." Processing also must not increase the amount of sugars in the food.

The common sugars are described in the following pages:

*Sucrose.* White sugar (table sugar), powdered sugar, brown sugar, maple sugar, beet sugar, turbinado sugar, and raw sugar are all varieties of sucrose. The process used to refine sugar consists of pressing boiling sliced beets or shredded sugarcane to extract a liquid sugar, which is then purified in a series of steps including straining, heating, evaporation, boiling, centrifugation, dissolving, clarification (removal of suspended matter), filtration, crystallization, and drying.

As raw sugar is refined, its molasses content is rinsed away. The remaining sugar is dissolved in warm water to make syrup, which is filtered repeatedly to remove impurities and color. During this stage, the sugar is referred to as brown sugar, because it retains varying amounts of molasses, depending on the number of filtrations it has undergone. Thus, brown sugar varies in color from very dark brown to light brown. The flavor varies with the color: The lighter the color, the milder the flavor.

The mineral content of brown sugar is greater than that of the more refined product, white sugar. For example, 100 grams of brown sugar (about ½ cup) provides about 3.4 milligrams of iron as compares to the 0.1 milligrams in white sugar, and 385 calories as compared to 373 calories in white sugar.[37] So you get a slight bonus of nutrients and taste from brown sugar. A tablespoon of granulated sugar has 46 calories and 11 grams of carbohydrate. The same amount of powdered sugar has 30 calories and 8 grams of carbohydrate, while brown sugar has 50 calories and 13 grams of carbohydrate. It takes sucrose about five minutes to begin raising blood sugar.[38]

**Molasses.** Molasses is concentrated syrup from sugar-bearing plants, primarily sugarcane and sugar beets. It is a mixture of sucrose and other materials such as fat and protein and a small amount of minerals such as iron. One tablespoon of molasses has 50 calories and 13 grams of carbohydrate.

**Glucose.** A sugar that exists naturally in the blood and in grape and corn sugars, glucose is sweeter than sucrose. It is a source of energy for plants and animals. Glucose syrup is used to flavor sausage, hamburger, meat loaf, luncheon meat, and chopped or pressed ham. It is also used as an extender in maple syrup. Five glucose units strung together in a long sugar chain form the starch found in wheat, corn, potatoes, and rice. Glucose is two-thirds as sweet as sucrose. It takes two minutes for glucose to start raising blood sugar because no digestion is required. It moves directly through the stomach and intestinal walls into the bloodstream.[39]

***Fructose, levulose, or fruit sugar.*** Most fruits contain fructose. The claim that fructose is "natural" appears to be based on the fact that fructose is found naturally in fresh fruit. Table sugar is also natural, however, as it comes from cane sugar. Fresh fruit contains only 20 to 40 percent fructose; the rest of its sugar content is largely sucrose and glucose. Fructose can be up to twice as sweet as sucrose. It is used as a medicine, as a preservative, as a common sugar, and to prevent grittiness in ice cream.

Fructose and sucrose also differ in their ability to stimulate insulin secretion. Sucrose causes the pancreas to secrete a more immediate and probably larger spurt of insulin than does fructose. Scientists think that more insulin is needed to metabolize sucrose because the glucose half of the sucrose requires insulin to be absorbed into the cells or metabolized by the liver. Fructose requires no insulin for the initial stage of metabolism by the liver, but it does require insulin for the portion that is converted to glucose. Thus, fructose does simulate insulin secretion, but not as rapidly and probably not as much as does glucose. Fructose therefore causes less of a rise and fall in blood-sugar levels than sucrose. Fructose was used in the treatment of diabetes before the introduction of insulin therapy. It is still widely used in Europe in the diabetic diet.[40]

Fructose is about 70 percent sweeter than sucrose, so less is needed as a sweetener in recipes. There are about 48 calories in a tablespoon of fructose and 12 grams of carbohydrate. It takes fructose about twenty-five minutes to start raising your blood-sugar level.[41]

***High-fructose corn syrups.*** Increasingly popular as a sweetener in foods, high-fructose corn syrups are composed of a fifty–fifty mixture of fructose and glucose. It is made by either chemically splitting sucrose into its two component sugars and then separating out and purifying the fructose, or by treating corn syrup with enzymes to convert some of it glucose to fructose. High-fructose corn syrup contains anywhere from 10 to 58 percent glucose. One tablespoon of it has about 58 calories.

***Lactose.*** Also known as milk sugar, saccharum lactin, and D-lactose, lactose is a slightly sweet-tasting, colorless sugar composed of glucose and galactose. Galactose is called "brain sugar" because it is found in the covering of the nerves in the brain. Lactose is present in the milk of mammals—humans have 6.7 percent and cows 4.3 percent. It appears commercially as a white powder or crystalline mass, a byproduct of the cheese industry. Lactose is inexpensive and is widely used in the food industry as a culture medium, such as in souring milk, to maintain moisture, and as a nutrient in formulas for infants and debilitated patients. It is also used as a medical diuretic and a laxative. A number of people are intolerant of lactose, particularly as they grow older. Lactose intolerance results when the enzyme lactase is not secreted in sufficient quantities to digest the lactose that has been consumed. The result can be abdominal distention, cramps, and other digestive problems. Lactose has about 50 calories per fluid ounce.

**Maltose.** Comprised of two glucose units, maltose is found in starch and glycogen. Commercially, its colorless crystals derive from the action of enzymes of the malt extracted from barley on starch. It is soluble in water and is used as a nutrient, as a sweetener, and as a table-sugar substitute for diabetics. It is also used in making beer, maple syrup, and corn syrups and is an ingredient in bread and infant foods. Maltose is only one-third as sweet as sugar or about 126 calories per ½ cup.

**Honey.** Honey is a mixture of glucose, fructose, and water. Commonly thought of as pure fructose, honey actually contains as much glucose as fructose. Because of its taste and texture, some people feel that a smaller amount of honey satisfies the desire for sweetness better than table sugar, although there is no real nutritive advantage. Honey has about 65 calories per tablespoon.

**Corn syrup.** Also known as corn sugar or dextrose, corn syrup is the most common form of dextrose. It consists primarily of glucose. It is used in maple, nut, and root-beer flavorings for beverages; ice cream; ices; candies; and baked goods. Corn syrup is also used on envelopes, stamps, and sticker tapes; in ale, aspirin, bacon, baking mixes, powders, beer, bourbon, breads, breakfast cereals, pastries, candy, carbonated beverages, catsup, cheeses, cereals, chop suey, chow mein, confectioners' sugar, cream puffs, fish products, ginger ale, ham, jellies, processed meats, peanut butter, canned peas, plastic food wraps, sherbet, whiskey, and American wines. It is a common allergen. A tablespoon of corn syrup contains about 58 calories and 14.5 grams of carbohydrate.

**Starch.** Starch is stored by plants and is taken from grains of wheat, potatoes, rice, corn, beans, and many other vegetable foods. Such foods are also rich in fiber and various other nutrients. In many foods, however, the starch is not digestible until it is cooked or processed in some other way. Starches vary in calorie content, but cornstarch has about 40 calories and 33 grams of carbohydrate per tablespoon. Starch takes about ten minutes to begin raising blood-sugar levels.[42]

**Modified starch.** Modified starch is ordinary starch that has been altered chemically to modify such properties as thickening or jelling. Babies have difficulty digesting starch in its original form. Modified starch is used in baby food on the theory that it is easier to digest. Questions about safety have arisen because babies do not have the resistance that adults do to chemicals. Among the chemicals used to modify starch are propylene oxide, aluminum sulfate, and sodium hydroxide (lye).[43]

## Sugar Sense and Maintaining Blood-Sugar Levels

**Eat hard fiber.** Diets that are high in fiber and carbohydrates are associated with lower blood glucose and serum lipid levels. There is no significant difference in the blood-sugar response between whole-meal bread and white bread or between white and brown spaghetti. But when white flour is given in the form of spaghetti, blood glucose levels rise much less than they do when the same amount of white flour is given in the form of bread, which suggests that food form rather than fiber content may be important in determining the blood-sugar response. It has been suggested that the hard form (pasta) reduces the starch's accessibility to digestive enzymes.[44]

**Eat more raw foods.** The way a food is cooked can also result in alterations in the blood-sugar response to a food. Studies have indicated that ingestion of raw starches such as purified amylopectin or cornstarch causes a much flatter blood sugar and insulin response as compared to cooked forms of these starches. Increasing the percentage of raw food in the diet has been suggested in the past as an aid to controlling blood glucose.

***Total your carbohydrates each day.*** The carbohydrates in one meal affect the assimilation of carbohydrates in the next meal. Studies of carbohydrates given in a slowly digested form indicate that they have physical effects not only during and immediately following the time the carbohydrate is ingested but also at the time of subsequent standard meals, where they seem to improve the body's carbohydrate tolerance. Breakfasts containing lentils, which are associated with flattened glycemic and insulin responses, are followed by significantly flatter blood-sugar responses to a standard lunch as compared to breakfasts containing identical amounts of carbohydrate in the form of bread.

***Give carbohydrates time to reach your brain.*** By eating slowly, you can mimic the effects of a slow-release carbohydrate. Thus, bread eaten continuously at an even rate—small portions eaten over four hours—results in a blood-sugar pattern similar to that of a relative portion of lentils eaten within fifteen to twenty minutes. Similar effects are seen when a comparative amount of glucose is sipped slowly over a four-hour period.

***Don't drink liquids with your sugary foods.*** It has been demonstrated that ingestion of a sugar in the liquid part of a meal results in a different metabolic response than when the sugar is ingested in the solid part of a meal. This may be due to the fact that liquids make the contents of your stomach pass through more rapidly; sugar may then be absorbed more quickly into the bloodstream through the small intestine.[45]

***Time your carbohydrates.*** Since studies have shown that some people are adversely affected by eating a high-carbohydrate lunch and, conversely, may be positively affected by eating a high-carbohydrate dinner, if you find you are so affected, create and time your meals accordingly.

***Exercise if you crave sweets.*** Gerald Reaven of the Stanford University School of Medicine questions whether we have gone too far on high-carbohydrate diets. The low-fat diets currently in vogue are also high in carbohydrates. Says Reaven, "Anyone who consumes more carbohydrates has to dispose of the load by secreting more insulin."[46] A slim, physically fit person is already very sensitive to insulin and secretes only a small amount in response to carbohydrates. But diabetics and hypertensives secrete much more insulin because their tissues are relatively insensitive to insulin. People with hypertension have higher blood sugar and insulin than people who don't have hypertension.[47]

**Don't have sodas and other empty calories in the house.** Candy, pastries, sugar-containing soft drinks (some colas have as much as ten teaspoons of sugar in each glass), and alcoholic beverages should be avoided because they cause a rebound drop in blood sugar. If you don't have them at hand, you won't be as tempted and your intake will be cut way down.

**Sugar and alcohol may not mix.** Sugar makes alcohol more potent so don't drink and drive and don't drink and eat sweets.

**Try all-fruit butters and jams.** Naturally sweetened fruit butters and jams in place of sugar-sweetened jellies and jams may not reduce your sugar intake by much, but they do have more nutrients than the regular kinds.

**Keep fresh fruits handy.** The body, as we have seen, more easily metabolizes fructose. You will take in a lot of nutrients with it if you opt for fruit.

**Eat six to seven small meals per day.** If you feel that you may have the symptoms of low blood sugar described in this chapter, consult your physician. If he or she okays it, try eating small meals more frequently. In that way, you can keep your blood-sugar level more even.

We Westerners do ingest a tremendous amount of refined carbohydrates. The U.S. Department of Agriculture estimates that in 1996, about 67 pounds of sugar (cane or beet); 85 pounds of corn sweeteners; and 1 pound of other sweeteners (honey, maple syrup) per capita were delivered into the food supply. That adds up to a total nutritive sweetener usage of about 153 pounds per capita. The sugar industry organization hastens to add that these numbers do not account for waste sugars used up in fermentation as in bread baking, or use in pet food. They claim the FDA estimates that the amount of added sweeteners (sugar, corn sweeteners and others) amount to 43 pounds per person—about 11 percent of total calories.[48]

If you use your brain, which uses glucose, you can cut down on refined, highly sugared, empty-calorie foods. You can achieve the following benefits:

1. You'll be less hungry. Robert E. Hodges and W. H. Krehl pointed out in the *American Journal of Clinical Nutrition* that participants in experiments complained of hunger on high-sugar diets but said they felt "stuffed" on sugar-free diets containing complex carbohydrates.[49]

2. Your cholesterol level will drop. A diet high in refined sugars and carbohydrates raises blood cholesterol and other fats, while a diet high in complex carbohydrates lowers blood fats. Research has also established that cholesterol drops if sugar in the diet is replaced with green leafy vegetables, whole grains, and the carbohydrates from legumes.[50]

3. You will avoid wide mood swings and improve your energy level and intellectual ability.

# 5

# Food Allergies, Your Brain, Body, and Behavior

After a meal, do you become restless? Anxious? Irritable? Hyperactive?

Could it be something you ate?

Although modern medical scientists have been reluctant to attribute mood swings to allergy or intolerance to foods, the early Greek physician and philosopher Hippocrates was not. He was one of the first to note that cow's milk could cause health problems for some people. The actual number who are allergic to cow's milk today or any other food is unknown. The effect of food allergy on the brain is even more difficult to determine.

Some immunologists and psychiatrists are convinced that allergy plays a part in a number of brain disorders, including depression, schizophrenia, Alzheimer's disease, hyperactivity, and autism. There are even more experts who believe that allergies have nothing to do with these disorders. A great deal has yet to be learned about how food allergy or sensitivity affects the brain, but with increased understanding of brain chemistry and more sophisticated diagnostic tests, there is increasing evidence that, indeed, a relationship exists between "offending foods" and brain function.

In a very interesting study performed by Australian researchers, the brain waves of 15 children suffering from food-induced attention deficit hyperkinetic syndrome (hyperactive kids with learning problems) were mapped.[1] The EEG (electroencephalograph) mapping of the electrical activity of their brains was done before and after ingestion of previously identified provoking foods. The investigators conducting the mapping did not know if a child had eaten an innocuous food or one to which that child was allergic.

When a youngster did eat the provoking food, the researchers could clearly see that the youngster's brain wave activity increased significantly in the front and side areas of the brain. The study's conductors at the Institute for Child Health Research, Clinical Sciences Division, said the investigation was "the first to show an association between brain electrical activity and intake of provoking foods in children with food-induced attention deficit."

No one knows for certain just how much food allergy or sensitivity can directly affect brain function. One thing no one can deny, however, is that if you suffer from an allergy of any sort, the discomfort can affect your mood, and behavior.

An *adverse reaction* or sensitivity to a food means *any abnormal reaction* to a food or food additive that is eaten, whether caused by allergic or nonallergic mechanisms. The following are descriptions of the different adverse reactions to food:

**Food intolerance.** Does not involve the immune system. It is an adverse reaction to food due to such factors as enzyme deficiencies, contaminants or toxins, drug use, heredity, psychological disorder, or underlying disease. If you get indigestion from eating beans, that's an *intolerance*. The adverse reaction is usually caused by factors in the diet other than protein. One of the more common food intolerance reactions may be the result of the body's inability to digest lactose (milk sugar). Many people, particularly as they grow older, have this "lactose intolerance." They are deficient in the enzyme needed to process lactose.

**Pharmacologic food reaction.** An adverse reaction to a chemical found in a food or food additive that produces a druglike effect, such as caffeine in coffee causing the "jitters" or the amines in cheese causing a headache. The "Chinese restaurant syndrome," manifested by anxiety, flushed face, and pressure in the chest, has been shown to be caused by eating large amounts of the flavor enhancer MSG. Sulfite preservatives are now known to have the potential to cause a serious attack of asthma and even death.

**Food poisoning.** An adverse reaction caused by a food or food additive without your immune system being involved. Toxins (poisons or bacteria) may be either contained within the food or released by microorganisms or parasites contaminating the food.

**Food allergy.** Involves the immune system. If you are allergic to a food or food additive, your body's immune system overreacts to it. The food or food additive may be harmless to others, but you suffer irritating, uncomfortable symptoms because you are hypersensitive to it. The word *allergy* is derived from two Greek words that can be roughly translated as "altered response."

The National Institute of Allergy and Infectious Diseases estimates that there are 35 million people in this country who have allergic reactions to substances that, in similar amounts, are apparently completely harmless to most people. The number of ailments diagnosed as allergies is undoubtedly going to rise as more and more is discovered about this group of diseases and as our environment becomes more and more complex.

A turning point in the field of allergy occurred in 1967 at the Children's Asthma Research Institute and Hospital in Denver. Drs. Kimishige and Teruko Ishizaka—a husband-and-wife team of scientists supported by the National Institute of Allergy and Infectious Diseases—discovered the antibody now known as *immunoglobulin E (IgE)*, which is responsible for most allergic reactions. The substances that cause allergic reactions are *allergens* and *antigens*. If you are allergic, the first time you encountered an allergen, your body made millions of IgE antibodies against it. When you again encountered the same allergen, again IgE leads to the release of *histamine*, which comes from cells in the connective tissues, especially beneath the mucous membranes and the skin, and *bradykinin*, which is found in blood plasma. Histamine can cause swelling of the mucous membranes in the nose and itching of the eyes. Bradykinin can contract the smooth muscle of the walls of the small tubes in the lungs. This sequence of events does not necessarily occur when something you eat "doesn't agree with you." It is very difficult to recognize a food allergy because:

- Allergic reactions may be delayed from several hours to days after ingestion of the offending food.
- You may eat the food only once in a while.
- There may be hidden additives and contaminants in the food.
- You may be allergic to that food only at certain times.
- There may be an interaction between a food and a drug you are taking.
- The quantity of food eaten may influence the reaction.
- The cooking method may influence the reaction.

Symptoms of delayed allergy may include anything from muscle aches to mental symptoms, drowsiness, and confusion, all of which are also symptoms of many other, nonallergic ailments. There is no doubt, however, about a food allergy when an anaphylactic attack occurs. It is an immediate, dramatic, life-threatening, generalized allergic reaction. It may involve any system of the body but usually affects the skin, nose, throat, lungs, stomach, heart, and blood vessels. The first signs may be a red, itchy rash and a feeling of warmth. These may be followed by light-headedness, shortness of breath or sneezing, a feeling of anxiety, stomach or uterine cramps, and/or vomiting and diarrhea.

Almost any food can be an allergen. Also, some people can become sensitive to the artificial coloring agents, vegetable gums, and other substances widely used in prepared foods. There are eight foods that cause 90 percent of all food allergic reactions.[2]

1. Milk
2. Eggs
3. Wheat
4. Peanuts
5. Soy
6. Tree nuts
7. Fish
8. Shellfish

Anaphylaxis is a sudden severe potentially life-threatening allergic reaction. As little as half a peanut can cause a fatal reaction for severely allergic individuals. Some schools have stopped serving peanut butter because of the danger to some allergic children. Some very allergic children can have a severe reaction if they are kissed by someone who has eaten peanuts or if milk is splashed on their skin.

It is also important to avoid cross-contact with foods that may cause food allergy. A child who can eat plain chocolate brownies, for example, served with a spatula that was used to serve a cake containing peanuts may suffer a severe reaction.

Sometimes an allergen is a food that has been eaten for many years without any ill effect. Unknown to the victim, the allergy has been developing slowly. If symptoms of a food allergy appear quickly—during a meal or just after a specific food has been eaten—it is usually fairly easy to discover the responsible allergen. But if the reaction is delayed, then it is necessary to investigate by the process of elimination, excluding a few foods at a time from the diet to see whether symptoms are relieved; or by the technique of challenge—that is, by initially giving a limited diet to which other foods are gradually added, one at a time, until symptoms appear. If the allergy is mild, it may never be possible to pinpoint the food allergen.

The prick skin test or a blood test such as the RAST, or radioallergosorbent test, are commonly used to determine if an allergy exists. A prick skin test is usually cheaper and can be done in the doctor's office. The doctor places a drop of the substance being tested on the patient's forearm or back and pricks the skin with a needle allowing a tiny amount to enter the skin. If the patient is allergic to the substance, a wheal (bump) is formed at the site within a few minutes. A RAST requires a blood sample. The sample is sent to a medical laboratory where tests are done with specific foods to determine whether the patient has IgE antibodies to that food. The results are usually received within one week.

Although both tests are reliable, many doctors use the RAST for young children or for patients who have skin problems that would make it difficult to read results of a prick test. The result of either test must be combined with other information, such as a history of symptoms and a food challenge, to determine if a food allergy exists.

Other conditions in the stomach and intestines that may be quite serious can cause symptoms that mimic food allergy. A careful history is the best diagnostic tool. You could help your physician and yourself detect a food allergy, if it exists, by using the chart on page 88.

In some food groups, especially legumes and seafood, an allergy to one member of the food group may result in your being allergic to some other member in the same group. This is known as *cross-reactivity*. Persons allergic to peanuts, for example, are more likely to be allergic to soybeans, peas, and other legumes than to walnuts or pecans. However, a number of people may be allergic to both peanuts and walnuts. These allergies are called *coincidental allergies*.

Some children's specific food allergies may disappear completely as they mature. If a food causes an allergic reaction in an adult, however, it must usually be dropped from the diet permanently. This means all forms of the allergen—for example, a person allergic to eggs may have to avoid eating prepared foods that contain eggs, such as cakes, custards, and waffles. He may also have to forego certain protective immunizations, like the influenza vaccine.

## Food Allergens and Neurotransmitters

Food allergens are usually proteins. The fact that neurotransmitters in the brain are made from proteins suggests that brain allergies may exist. Cooking can reduce the effect of some protein allergens but may increase the effect of others.[3] Most of the allergens can still cause reactions even after they have undergone digestion.

Since we are concerned with food and the brain, let's get to the most commonly accepted food/brain/allergy connection: the headache. When you have a headache, it is not actually your brain that aches but rather it is the blood vessels in and around your brain that are producing the pain. However, when your head aches, you can't use your brain efficiently.

### Can Headaches Be Due to a Food Allergy?

Headaches are often caused by allergies.

One particular form of headache is the *migraine* (literally, "half the skull"), which some surveys say affects 10 percent of all Americans. It is generally agreed now that migraines are often allergic in origin and a hypersensitive reaction to food protein may trigger an attack.

### The Miserable Migraine

A migraine headache usually starts out as a pain located on one side of the head which may spread to the opposite side. Any movement often aggravates the pulsating, throbbing ache. The migraine may be accompanied by a number of other symptoms. The most common are nausea and vomiting. Other manifestations include dizziness, pallor, increased sensitivity to light, sound and smells, scalp tenderness, malaise, and diarrhea and weakness. It usually lasts from 4 to 72 hours but may continue for days.

About 10 to 20 percent of people who suffer from migraine have a visual warning called an "aura" before the head pain strikes. These sufferers may see colors, flashing lights, zigzag lines, or bright spots, or may experience loss of vision and numbness. There may be a transient inability to speak, or thick speech.

Migraine afflicts both men and women, although women tend to experience migraine more commonly than men do by a ratio of three to one. Peak prevalence for migraine in both genders is between the ages of 25 and 44.

Children's migraines may be similar to that in adults. However, stomach complaints and mental changes may be more characteristic of childhood migraines. Youngsters may have symptoms such as nausea and vomiting, diarrhea, anxiety, loss of balance, sudden irritability, intolerance of noise or light. Children may experience migraine without accompanying headaches. This is "abdominal migraine."

A cousin of migraine is *cluster headache*. It usually occurs in men in early to midlife and may be episodic or chronic. The episodic presents as a cluster of attacks over the course of weeks or months, followed by a headache-free period. The chronic form occurs without an interim and bouts of headache clusters may persist for years. The location and severity of cluster headache pain can resemble that of migraine. However, important differences exist between the two headache types.

The pain of cluster headache is severe and primarily localized to the eye, temple forehead, or cheek. Frequently the cluster headache is an excruciating, boring pain located behind or around one eye spreading over the affected side. Stuffy nose, flushing, and red eyes may accompany it. The attacks of headache are of great intensity but brief duration—usually 15 to 90 minutes. Attacks can occur about five times a day for two or three weeks at a time and then disappear for six months.

During the late 1960s, British and Danish physicians pinpointed two major abnormalities that underlie migraine headaches.[4]

1. A decrease in blood flow through the brain before the headache
2. An increase in blood flow through the brain during the headache

Although there is still much to be learned, many scientists now believe that migraine is the result of a sequence of events that results in increased activity of pain fibers. This causes the blood vessels in the brain to dilate resulting in more stimulation of painful nerve endings and then the throbbing agony of a migraine hits. These changes are postulated to be related to a self-produced brain chemical, serotonin (5-HT). Serotonin has a wide range of activity in the body. The changes it causes depend upon the type of receptor for it on a cell. Receptors are like "docks" on the surface of a cell to which a cruising serotonin ties up. Several types of serotonin "docks" have been identified. During a migraine attack, it is believed that the serotonin level decreases, allowing the blood vessels to dilate. The key to many of the new migraine medications on the market or in clinical testing is serotonin mimics—that is, they simulate some of its action.

It is not clear why there are changes in serotonin or what initiates those changes in some people and not in others. It is known, however, that in a susceptible person, one or more of a range of factors can "trigger" a migraine attack.

### FOODS AND THE SUBSTANCES THEY CONTAIN THAT MAY CAUSE HEADACHES

| Foods | Culprit |
| --- | --- |
| Cheese | Tryptophan and tyramine |
| Chocolate and cocoa | Dopamine and phenylethylamine |
| Ale, wine, especially red wine | Tyramine |
| Herring | Tyramine and salt |
| Alcohol | Histamine |
| Tomatoes | Histamine |
| Coffee | Caffeine |
| Chocolate | Theobromine |
| Colas | Caffeine |
| Tea | Caffeine and theobromine |
| Oranges and other citrus fruits | Histamine |
| Cured meats | Nitrates and nitrites |
| Flavor enhancers | MSG and salt |
| Preserved foods | Nitrates or MSG |

| FOODS AND THE SUBSTANCES THEY CONTAIN THAT MAY CAUSE HEADACHES *(cont.)* | |
| --- | --- |
| **Foods** | **Culprit** |
| Aged cheeses | Mold, tyramine |
| Artificial sweeteners | Glutamate |
| Shellfish | Pen *a* 1 (isolated allergen) |
| Fish | Gad *c* 1 (isolated allergen) |

Other common allergy-inducing foods include licorice, meat tenderizers, milk, mushrooms, nuts, onions, (pickled, canned, or jarred), pork, salad dressing, sauerkraut, some types of beans (including broad, Italian, lima, fava, soy), soy sauce, and yeast breads and yogurt.

By avoiding these foods, you may experience complete or marked relief from migraine.

## Tension–Fatigue Syndrome

The term *tension–fatigue syndrome* refers to alternating periods of anxiety and listlessness associated with allergic diseases. As early as 1922, W. R. Shannon described the cases of eight children suffering from a variety of behavior complaints such as extreme nervousness, irritability, unruliness, insomnia, decreased appetite, and poor school performance. He believed that these complaints were due to irritation of the nervous system by allergic reactions. Because marked improvement in seven of the eight patients was reported upon the elimination of certain foods from the diet, he suggested that food proteins were common triggers of such reactions.[5] In 1954, Dr. F. Speer enlarged on the observations and said that the behavior of affected children seemed to have two contributing facets:

1. Hyperactivity, restlessness, emotional instability, and insomnia manifested tension.
2. Fatigue was evidenced by listlessness and constant tiredness that was not made better by resting.

## Hyperactivity by Any Other Name and Diet

Hyperactivity, attention deficit disorder, or tension–fatigue syndrome—depending on who is referring to the constellation of behavior—may be caused by anxiety, a physical ailment, or the environment, or it may be strictly in the eyes of the beholder. The prevalence of the syndrome is not clear, but it has been estimated to involve between 5 and 10 percent of American schoolchildren. Benjamin Feingold, a California physician, in 1973 presented the possible relationship between attention deficit disorder with hyperactivity and natural salicylates as well as other food additives. On the basis of experience in treating adult patients with aspirin intolerance, Dr. Feingold promoted a theory that hyperactive behavior and learning disorders in children might be the result of a reaction to natural salicylates in certain foods. Later, because of the known cross-reactivity between aspirin and tartrazine, Food, Drug and Cosmetic Act (FD & C) Yellow Dye No. 5, all food colorings were suspected as offenders. Still later, the preservatives sodium benzoate and BHA/BHT were incriminated. A regimen called the Kaiser Permanente Diet or Feingold Diet was popularized by Dr. Feingold in a book on the subject. The special diet, devoid of foods suspected of having not only significant levels of natural salicylates but also food coloring and preservatives, was alleged to produce improvement in 50 percent of the patients with hyperactivity and attention deficits. For more information about the Feingold Diet, see Chapter 7.

The controversy concerning the link between food allergies and hyperactive behavior continues, as do debates over a number of other brain/behavior/allergy links.

## The Depression/Allergy Connection

What role does allergy play in the "blues"? In tests of depressed patients the percentage of those with allergies ranged from 33 to 70 percent, compared to 2 percent in controls.[6]

The apparently high incidence of "allergy" in depression requires further study, according to John W. Crayton, M.D., associate professor of psychiatry at the University of Chicago. He points out that the medications widely used to treat depression today, tricyclic antidepressants, are potent antihistamines, and that the same histamine-controlled reactions in allergy might also be involved in certain depressions. An observation that adds evidence to the allergy/depression connection is that the gene associated with depression lies on chromosome 6, near the genes involved in the immune response. The clinical significance of this finding in relation to adverse reactions to foods remains to be determined.

## The Schizophrenia/Allergy Connection

The link between schizophrenia, the most common type of psychosis, and allergy may be even more intangible than that of allergy and depression, and yet there are some intriguing connections. The prime suspect has been a common allergen, wheat. The first clue emanates from epidemiological studies. It has been noticed that in populations that do not have wheat in their diet, schizophrenia is also absent. The second clue is that patients with schizophrenia seem to have more allergies than people who are not schizophrenic but are suffering from other mental disorders.

Experts of the Schizophrenia Association of Great Britain emphasize milk allergy in their literature. A gluten protein, *alpha gliadin,* which is purified from wheat flour, is active against nerve tissue. The same amino acid sequence found in alpha gliadin also has been found in casein, the major protein in milk. The clinical significance, if any, of these findings is unknown.[7]

## Autism and Allergy

Researchers in Israel in 1982 reported a study of autistic children at the Geha Psychiatric Hospital in Petah Tiqva. The investigators found that the brains of these youngsters may be misperceiving a basic brain protein as a foreign body and, as a result, systematically destroying it through an allergic reaction. The resulting brain damage, although undetectable, may be responsible for the constellation of emotional, intellectual, and social handicaps that characterize the disorder.[8] Autistic children have an inability to form meaningful interpersonal relationships.

A study reported in 1995 at the American College of Allergy, Asthma and Immunology in Dallas added evidence to the earlier finding. Sudhir Gupta, M.D., chief of the division of basic and clinical immunology at the University of California, who made the report, studied 25 autistic children, ages 3 to 10 years. He found 10 of the autistic patients had antibody "deficiencies or dysfunctions." The autistic children were injected with immunoglobulin—serum containing antibodies from nonautistic children. Dr. Gupta reported improvement, to varying degrees, in almost all of the autistic patients treated. "Some of the important changes we noticed," he said, "were that the children were much calmer, had better eye contact, improved attention span and speech, increased verbal expression, and were more aware of their surroundings. One of these patients is now attending regular school."[9]

## Alzheimer's and Allergy

Alzheimer's disease, that brain-degenerating, memory-destroying condition afflicting mostly older adults, is also suspected of being linked to a brain allergy. Autopsies on its victims show that there are "dead spots" on the nerves in their brains composed of tangles of nerve fibers and deposits of waste material. Researchers at Albert Einstein Medical Center in New York took material from the brains of Alzheimer's victims at autopsy and extracted antigens from it. They found that the antigens reacted with brain tissue from other Alzheimer's victims but not with that from people who had died from other causes. This led Einstein investigators to conclude that there is an "antigen-antibody" reaction involved in Alzheimer's, since the brain tissue from Alzheimer's victims was highly selective for that of other Alzheimer's patients.[10]

Such research reports are intriguing, but the question of whether a brain allergy exists still has no definitive answer. Since allergic reactions can damage other organs, such as the lung and the skin, there is reason to believe that they may also injure the brain, despite the barriers nature has erected to protect it. The effects may be as devastating as Alzheimer's or as mild as an irritable mood.

## Mood and Food Allergy

Dr. John Crayton of the University of Chicago is one researcher who has found a possible link between food and mood, but he is quick to point out the limitations of such findings.[11] In his study, a group of 35 volunteers—some with complaints of food sensitivity—were fed capsules of powdered wheat, milk, or choco-late, foods often associated with allergies. He found that changes in mood, coincidental with changes in the immune system, did occur in this group. He theorizes that food-induced reactions may cause local swelling in the brain that leads to mood swings, but cautions that this is early work and not yet understood.

Dr. Crayton points out that because of the widespread reports of food sensitivity producing behavioral effects, the question has been raised as to whether food could produce effects on the brain and behavior in the absence of effects on other body systems. He said a review of the case histories of several workers in this field suggest that individuals with food sensitivity with only brain and behavioral dysfunction must be extremely rare. In most studies, all of the subjects had both physical and mental symptoms.

The real problem, he said, is defining whether the allergic con-dition actually causes the behavioral symptoms on a physical basis or whether the emotional or behavioral symptoms are primarily psychological reactions to being physically ill.

Summing it up, the debate about food allergy has experts on one side explaining the commonly reported links between food al-lergy and behavior as:

1. Coincidental, because behavioral symptoms and al-lergy are both so common that they can often coexist in the same person.
2. Any chronic condition such as allergy can create emo-tional problems both in the victim and the victim's family and result in tension and fatigue.
3. Allergy may cause symptoms of wheezing, sneezing, itching, coughing, and shortness of breath which, in turn, may make you so uncomfortable or so upset that you are irritable and can't concentrate.

The experts on the other side say that brain allergy does exist and that it causes all sorts of emotional, behavioral, and physical problems.

There is no scientific proof of primary brain allergy, other than so-called anecdotal reports based mostly on the observations of family members, psychologists, and physicians. That does not mean that it doesn't exist, however, and it is certainly possible that a definitive link between food allergy and the brain will be uncovered.

In the meantime, there is only one way to "cure" a food allergy: avoid the offending substance. Here are some hints:

**Keep a diary.** You can help yourself and your physician identify the allergen by keeping a diary of *everything* you eat and drink for a week or two—that includes snacks, gum, and candy.

**Keep a record of your symptoms.** If you record your well-being or distress about an hour after you have eaten the meals and recorded the food in your diary, you will probably begin to make

---

### FOOD DIARY

Whether you are allergic or intolerant to a food that makes you feel bad, there is only one sure way at this time to cure the problem— avoid the food. You are the best judge of your response. And the most effective way to identify your problem food is to keep a record. The following is a simple method of doing so.

*Instructions:* List each food once down the left side of the chart. Use a *B* for breakfast, an *L* for lunch, a *D* for dinner, and an *O* for other to indicate when you ate the food. If symptoms occurred, put an *X* over the letter. For example, if you ate tuna for lunch on Wednesday, you'd list tuna, mark an *L* under Wednesday, and, if symptoms occurred, put an *X* over the *L*. In the diary at the bottom of the chart, record the food that caused the symptom, the date the symptom occurred, and under what circumstance, and a description of the symptoms. For example, Wednesday, week 1, write: Tuna. Lunch at a restaurant. Developed a headache.

| WEEK 1 | WEEK 2 |
|---|---|
| DATE: | DATE: |
| FOOD:    S / M / T / W / T / F / S | FOOD:    S / M / T / W / T / F / S |
| _____ | _____ |
| _____ | _____ |
| _____ | _____ |
| _____ | _____ |

DATE: _____ FOOD EATEN: _____

CIRCUMSTANCES: _____

SYMPTOMS: _____

an association between something you ingested and your mental and physical symptoms of distress.

***Buy foods without the offenders.*** Whether you have an allergy or a sensitivity, once you have identified the substances that bother you, you can obtain foods that are made without it. They may be more expensive, but you may like certain dishes and think them worth the extra cost.

## For More Information

Food allergies and intolerance are important to your general health and to your brain. Certainly, if you don't feel well physically, you are going to be in a bad mood. If you fear for your life because of a potential severe allergic reaction, you are going to be anxious. There is still much to be learned about the actual effect on your brain of a food allergy or intolerance. In the meantime, if you want to learn more about food allergies, you may contact the following organizations:

American Academy of Allergy, Asthma & Immunology
Phone: 1-800-822-ASMA (2762)
website: www.aaaai.org

American Academy of Pediatrics
Phone: 1-847-228-5005
website: www.aap.org

Food Allergy Network
Phone: 1-800-929-4040
website: www.foodallergy.org

Allergy and Asthma Network: Mothers of Asthmatics
     Inc.
Phone: 1-800-878-4403
website: www.aanma.org

# 6

# Protecting Yourself from Brain Toxins

The Great Wall of China is nothing compared to the barrier with which you were born to protect your brain. Your *blood-brain barrier* is constructed of closely packed cells to prevent passage of harmful substances from your bloodstream. There are, however, certain "hacker" chemicals that can sneak through and cause glitches in your central "computer." These troublemakers might be natural ingredients, or deliberate or inadvertent additives in your food.

While detection of cancer-causing agents in our diets may be imperfect, little if any testing is being done to determine if food additives may be toxic to the brain and nerves. A number of scientists believe that neurotoxins are even more of a problem in food than carcinogens.[1]

Charles Vorhees, Ph.D., associate professor of pediatrics and developmental biology at the University of Cincinnati, points out: "The fact that food can produce adverse effects on behavior has long been known but efforts to systematically evaluate foods and other chemicals for such effects are a more recent pursuit."[2] The fields that have evolved to assess these effects have come to be termed:

- *Behavioral toxicology:* The study of chemical effects on mature organisms.
- *Behavioral teratology:* The part of behavioral toxicology that focuses on the unborn and the newborn and the consequences for later life of exposure during these key periods of brain development. The young organism is more susceptible to many chemicals and the aftermath of exposure is more likely to be permanent in children than in adults.[3]

The relatively young discipline of behavioral toxicology came into existence in 1975, when Dr. Bernard Weiss and his colleague, Dr. V. G. Laties, at the University of Rochester, pointed out brain function deficits can be as disabling as tissue damage. Dr. Weiss, a professor of biophysics expressed frustration at trying to test neurotoxicity in foods.[4] He noted there was little funding to study neurotoxins in foods, even though there is a great need to do so. On the other hand, there is a lot of money to fight any bad publicity about multibillion-dollar food ingredients. The same is true today. Out of more than 300 research projects in FDA laboratories in 1998, fewer than 12 concerned neurotoxicity, and most of those concerned attempts to develop standardized tests to show behavioral changes in animals exposed to neurotoxins.[5] (At this writing, there is a political move afoot to close all FDA research laboratories.)

The U.S. Food and Drug Administration's (FDA) Thomas J. Sobotka, Ph.D., said the public has become alarmed and has demanded some assurances that appropriate and effective measures are being taken to minimize the environmental presence of neurotoxic substances, particularly in the daily food supply. The fact that some chemicals can adversely affect the nervous system is not a new concept in regulatory toxicology. In the process of evaluating the safety of proposed food chemicals, he notes the traditional concept of neurotoxicity focused on obvious pathological changes in the structure of the brain and nerves.

This view, however, does not reflect the full spectrum of adverse effects that a neurotoxicant may exert on the nervous system. Dr. Sobotka says, "In humans, neurotoxicants can adversely affect a broad spectrum of behavioral functions, including the ability to learn, to interact appropriately with others, and to perceive and respond to environmental stimuli; basically these represent everyday functions that enable people to live productive lives. The focus placed on neurotoxicity will encourage the development of more relevant information about the potential adverse effects of chemicals on the structural and functional integrity of the nervous system, and should help obtain the information needed for a reasonable assessment of potential neurotoxic hazard."[6]

What can you do about the conflicting information? You have to pay attention to the source, study the literature, and make up your own mind. When possible, you can bypass unnecessary, potentially harmful food additives and do your best to avoid potentially destructive natural ingredients and environmental contaminants. While whole volumes could be written about neurotoxins in the diet, the following are some of the most common:

- Pesticides, particularly the organophosphate bug killers, which are related to nerve gas developed during World War II.
- Ergot, a fungus found on rye, barley, oats, and triticale that is toxic at certain levels and medicinal at others. When toxic it can cause convulsions, itching, blood vessel and tissue damage, and gangrene. When beneficial, it can alleviate migraine headaches and control bleeding.
- Mycotoxins, poisons produced by certain molds, including the aflatoxins. Contaminated foods can produce toxic compounds on virtually any edible that will support mold growth.
- Mercury, an element used in herbicides and fungicides, that can cause severe neurological damage.
- Polybrominated biphenyls (PBBs), a fire retardant which may cause cancer and neurological symptoms when a contaminant in the food supply.
- Polychlorinated biphenyls (PCBs), industrial chemicals, they are chlorinated hydrocarbons which may cause cancer and nerve damage when ingested in food. They have been found directly and indirectly in animal feed and animal food products through water, paints, sealants, heat-transfer products, plastics, and cardboard in food packaging materials. In the 1980s, the Environmental Protection Agency estimated that 91 percent of us carry a measurable quantity of PCBs in our fatty tissue.[7]
- Tin is used in cans that hold acid fruits and vegetables. The acids in such foods as citrus fruits and tomato products can leach tin from the inside of the can. The tin, if methylated by the body, becomes a neurotoxin that attacks the central nervous system. Cans lined with enamel or other materials can prevent this leaching.[8]

- Food additives such as glutamate, aspartate, and cysteine-S-sulfonic acid (see below) and the coloring FD & C no. 3 are examples cited as potential neurotoxins.

Below are some specific examples of common substances—both intentional and unintentional—in our food that may affect the brain and behavior.

## Lead in the Head

One neurotoxin that has been well studied but that is still with us, despite regulations and massive efforts to get rid of it, is lead. According to the American Academy of Pediatrics, exposure to lead is widespread and causes serious impairments to children at relatively low levels of exposure—the effects of which are largely irreversible.

Lead can cause mental deficiency in children. Lead can contaminate acidic foods and beverages (fruits, fruit juices, cola drinks, tomatoes, tomato juice, wine, and cider) by storage in improperly lead-glazed ceramic ware. Commercial canning can also create problems. Freshly opened cans of grapefruit juice and orange juice have lead concentrations that exceed the Environmental Protection Agency (EPA) standard for drinking water, which is 0.05 micrograms per milliliter, says Dennis Bourcier of East Carolina University, Greenville. "Lead-soldered cans account for about 14 percent of total human lead ingestion," he adds. Although this solder makes good can seals, children are sensitive to lead and canned juices reach critical lead levels of five times the EPA standard within five days after opening. Juices should be put in nonmetallic containers as soon as they are opened.[9]

## Seeing Red About Red No. 3

One of the most suspect food additives, as far as the brain is concerned, however, is FD & C Red No. 3 (erythrosin). A coal-tar derivative, it is used in canned fruit cocktail, fruit and cherry pie mix (up to .01 percent), maraschino cherries, gelatin desserts, ice cream, sherbet, candy, confectionery products, bakery products, cereal, and pudding. When erythrosin was applied to isolated nerves in the muscles of frogs, it increased the release of the neurotransmitter acetylcholine. The University of Maryland researchers, George J. Augustine, Jr., and Herbert Levitan of the zoology department, who performed this study, said the results suggested that erythrosine might prove useful as a tool for studying the process of neurotransmitter release but that its use as a food additive should be reexamined.

"Our observation that a widely used food coloring agent, such as erythrosin, could dramatically and irreversibly alter synaptic transmission [messages across the gap between nerves] at low doses is consistent with previous studies suggesting that this and other food additives can alter behavior," they noted. "While it may be tempting to use these in vitro findings to support claims that these substances would cause behavioral changes when ingested by laboratory animals or humans, such conclusions are premature until it can be determined whether this and other additives have access to the central nervous system. It is not yet known how much of the ingested dye—it was estimated in 1968 that the maximum daily ingestion was 2 milligrams per person—is free in the blood or how readily it crosses the blood-brain barrier."[10]

In 1990, the FDA banned erythrosin in cosmetics and externally applied drugs but not yet in food.

## Aluminum and Alzheimer's

Is there a connection between aluminum, the third-most-abundant element on earth, and Alzheimer's, the devastating brain-degenerating disease that affects 2.5 million middle-aged and older Americans?

Alzheimer's disease was first described in 1906 when Alois Alzheimer, M.D., a German physician, told his colleagues of a fifty-one-year-old woman who had severe atrophy of the brain and an unusual clumping and distortion of fibers in the nerve cells of the cerebral cortex, or outer layer of the brain. The patient's problems began with memory loss and disorientation, progressed to depression and hallucination, and eventually resulted in severe dementia and death.

Dr. Alzheimer did not know what caused the tangles and no one has come up with a verifiable answer as yet. The National Institutes of Health scientists list three risk factors: family history of the disorder, head trauma, and environmental toxins, particularly aluminum.[11]

The aluminum-intoxication hypothesis got its start when some scientists found brain changes similar to those of Alzheimer's disease in animals that had been injected with aluminum. Other researchers found an excess accumulation of aluminum within the neurofibrillary tangles in the brains of Alzheimer's patients.

Aluminum has also been implicated in dialysis dementia, a frequent side effect of long-term kidney dialysis. However, the brain changes in dialysis patients are not the same as those in Alzheimer's patients. Rochester's Dr. Weiss says the case against aluminum is not proven, except in dialysis, in which there is a breakdown of the blood-brain barrier and aluminum can get in.

The connection between aluminum and Alzheimer's, however, is hotly debated among researchers working in the field. You ingest aluminum primarily through foods and drugs, such as antacids and buffered aspirin, although small amounts can come from foods and beverages you store in aluminum cans or cook in aluminum utensils. (The aluminum manufacturers suggest that the questions about aluminum cookware were raised by competitors promoting other types of utensils.) But can aluminum leave your intestines and penetrate the blood-brain barrier?

The prestigious British medical journal *Lancet* published a publically funded study that concluded drinking water with aluminum can increase the risk of contracting Alzheimer's by 50 percent. The Medical Research Council's epidemiology unit conducted the study over a ten-year period. It concluded that people under seventy years living in areas where the concentrations of the mineral in drinking water is higher than 0.11 mg per liter had the increased risk.[12]

Scientists at the National Institutes of Health, using sophisticated computer-driven electron beam X-ray microprobes, discovered a surprising correlation between certain elements and nerve-damaged brains. They found silicon, which is derived from silica and used as an anticaking agent in foods, and the mineral calcium in nerve tangles in certain areas of the brains of victims with the degenerating nerve disorder Lou Gehrig's disease (amyotrophic lateral sclerosis) and in those with Parkinsonism with dementia. Silicon, like aluminum, may interfere with the transmission of nerve messages.[13]

FDA officials, however, maintain that no direct causative effect between aluminum and Alzheimer's disease has been shown to date.[14] Nevertheless, if you want to cut down your ingestion of aluminum, you can follow these simple precautions:

- Avoid digestion tablets containing aluminum.
- Avoid underarm deodorant sprays containing aluminum (sprays are easily inhaled).
- Avoid aluminum saucepans when cooking acidic foods.
- Avoid processed foods with aluminum food additives listed on the label.

## Excitotoxins

We have two basic types of neurotransmitters in our brains—one type stimulates the release of messages between cells and the other inhibits the release. While we need so-called excitatory neurotransmitters, if we have an overabundance, they can turn into what is now called *excitotoxins*. Three popular food additives—monosodium glutamate (MSG) to enhance taste, the artificial sweetener aspartame (NutraSweet®), and hydrolyzed vegetable protein—contain potential excitatory nerve stimulants. The products are worth billions on the worldwide market but there is a great deal of controversy concerning their effects on the brain.

Russell L. Blaylock, M.D., a neurosurgeon and an assistant clinical professor of neurosurgery at the University of Mississippi Medical Center, is the author of *Excitotoxins, the Taste That Kills*. He says excitotoxins in food might aggravate or even precipitate many of the neurodegenerative brain diseases, such as Parkinson's disease, Huntington's disease, ALS (amyolateral sclerosis), and Alzheimer's disease.

"What all these diseases have in common is a slow destruction of brain cells that are specifically sensitive to excitotoxin damage," Dr. Blaylock says. "Neurons that use glutamate for transmitter are destroyed by high concentration of glutamate, while other neurons that use other transmitters are spared."

Dr. Blaylock says the cause of tangled nerve formations in Alzheimer's is still not understood, but the fact that such tangles are in the brain cells involved with processing glutamate raises interesting questions. Why are glutamate nerve cells susceptible to tangle formations? Is it a genetic abnormality, or do viruses invade this particular cell type? Both possibilities are intriguing. What if these neurons are producing abnormally high levels of glutamate, which could then act as a toxin? If this is true, the nerve degeneration associated with Alzheimer's disease might be halted with drugs that inhibit the effects of excess glutamate.[15]

## Glutamate and MSG

MSG is the sodium salt of glutamate and is glutamate, water, and sodium. In the early 1900s scientists isolated the ingredient—glutamate—in plants that is the essential taste component responsible for greatly enhancing flavor.[16] In the early part of this century, MSG was extracted from seaweed and other plant sources. The FDA has been evaluating MSG's safety since 1970.[17] While some people admittedly have adverse reactions to MSG, the FDA maintains that the additive is safe.[18] Indeed, the European Communities' Scientific Committee for Food and the Joint Expert Committee of Food Additives of the United Nations Food and Agricultural Organization and the World Health Organization have also placed MSG in the safest category of food additives.[19]

The producers of MSG point to research that shows it has potential to enhance food intake in older individuals. Over the years, research has shown that losses in taste and smell are major contributors to poor nutritional status among older persons. A study found moderate levels of added MSG in certain foods, such as mushroom soup and mashed potatoes, increased food intake in an institutionalized older population.[20]

Dr. Blaylock says both glutamate and aspartate are involved in activating a number of brain systems concerned with sensory perception, memory orientation in time and space, cognition, and motor skills. It is important to note, he says, that the brain depends on a delicate balance of excitatory and inhibitory systems, that is positive and negative impulses. Disruption of this balance can lead to anything from a minor tremor of the hand to uncontrollable forms of seizures. The producers of monosodium glutamate, on the other hand, maintain studies show the human body processes the glutamate added to food in the same way it does the glutamate found naturally in food.[21] Dr. Blaylock is not alone in his suspicions about glutamate. John Olney, M.D., professor of psychiatry, Washington University, St. Louis, Missouri, has long been a critic of glutamate, especially where it may affect the brains of children. He says it is sometimes argued that glutamic acid and aspartic acid (another amino acid used in artificial sweeteners) are safe food additives because humans have been exposed to these compounds in one form or another for many years without sustaining harm. This argument overlooks the fact that brain and retinal damage from glutamic acid or aspartic acid is a silent phenomenon. When infant animals are given neurotoxic doses of glutamate (the salt of glutamic acid) or aspartame (aspartic acid combined with the amino acid phenylalanine) they fail to manifest overt signs of distress while nerves in the brain and eye are actually degenerating. Indeed, there are no obvious changes in the animal's appearance or behavior until it is approaching adulthood. Thus, if glutamate or aspartame were to damage the hypothalamus of a human infant or child, delayed sequelae such as obesity and subtle disturbances in neuroendocrine status of the individual are the types of effects to be expected, and it would not be until adolescence or perhaps early adulthood that such effects would become clearly evident.[22]

The hypothalamus is the brain control area involved in emotions, movement, and eating. Less than the size of a peanut and weighing a quarter of an ounce, this small area deep within the brain also oversees appetite, blood pressure, sexual behavior, sleep, and emotions, and sends orders to the pituitary gland.

Hydrolyzed vegetable protein (HVP) is added to many of the same foods seasoned with MSG. It is made by adding an acid to a vegetable protein such as soy. This breaks up the protein into free amino acids. There are actually two types of this flavor enhancer: light, which is used primarily in cream soups and sauces, and dark, which goes into meat soups and stew. Both are high in monosodium glutamate. HVP, which can be listed on labels just as "natural flavoring" also may contain aspartate and cysteine. HVP, therefore, can be very high in excitatory amino acids. What about sensitivity to HVP? Some scientists believe, however, that persons who report a sensitivity to hydrolyzed proteins may be sensitive to the soy, wheat, or other protein source used to produce the hydrolysate, rather than to glutamate itself. Thus, reactions could be due to ingestion of soy, wheat or other proteins that are not completely hydrolyzed.[23]

## How Sweet Is It?

Glutamic acid (glutamate is its salt) derives its flavor-enhancing effects from its excitatory action on taste buds. Aspartame, when combined with phenylalanine, also interacts with the taste receptors, resulting in the perceived sweet taste. The FDA approved aspartame in 1974 but objections that it might cause brain damage led to a stay, or legal postponement, of that approval. Another problem arose: an FDA investigation of records of animal studies conducted for Searle drug approvals and for aspartame raised questions. The FDA arranged for an independent audit, which took more than two years and concluded that the aspartame studies and results were authentic. The agency then organized an expert board of inquiry, whose members concluded that the evidence did not support the charge that aspartame might kill clusters of brain cells or cause other damage. However, persons with an inborn error of metabolism, phenylketonuria, must avoid protein foods such as meat that contains phenylalanine—one of the two compounds of aspartame. The board did, however, recommend that aspartame not be approved until further long-term animal testing could be conducted to rule out the possibility that aspartame might cause brain tumors. The FDA's Bureau of Foods viewed the study data then available and concluded that the board's concern was unfounded. Aspartame was approved for use as a tabletop sweetener in certain dry foods in 1981 and in soft drinks two years later.

In 1984 news reports, fueled by the announcement that the Arizona Department of Health Services was testing soft drinks containing aspartame to see if it deteriorated into toxic levels of methyl alcohol under storage conditions, created alarm. The Arizona health department acted after the director of the Food Sciences and Research Laboratory at Arizona State University submitted a study alleging that higher-than-normal temperatures could lead to a dangerous breakdown in the chemical composition.[24] The authors checked with representatives of the FDA, which said there are higher levels of methyl alcohol in regular fruit juices, and so as far as the agency was concerned, the fears about decomposition were unfounded.

Questions also were raised about whether glutamic acid in combination with aspartame might contribute to brain damage, mental retardation, or hormone problems. The American Medical Association's Council on Scientific Affairs and the FDA have concluded that there is no evidence that aspartame, either alone or in combination with glutamate, can contribute to brain damage, mental retardation, or endocrine dysfunction. The AMA Council statement said: "Available evidence suggests that consumption of aspartame by normal humans is safe and is not associated with serious adverse health effects. Individuals who need to control their phenylalanine intake should handle aspartame like any other source of phenylalanine."[25]

Anecdotal reports of difficulties attributed to the sweetener include painful menstruation, spotting between menstrual periods, severe depression, dizziness, headaches, seizures, and birth defects. In 1986, the FDA refused to hold public hearings on the safety of aspartame. The FDA says it investigated 2,000 cases of alleged adverse effects from aspartame including 85 alleged epileptic seizures. The agency concluded that of those complaints, 17 might possibly have been related to aspartame but that 5 of those 17 patients had a history of epilepsy.[26]

Richard Wurtman, M.D., a professor of neuroendocrine regulation at MIT, has conducted laboratory studies showing that aspartame, given alone, nearly doubled central nervous system levels of phenylalanine in rats and quadrupled brain phenylalanine concentrations when administered with glucose. The excess phenylalanine was converted to tyrosine.

Phenylalanine and tyrosine compete with other amino acids for transport across the blood-brain barrier, so the amino acid tryptophan was significantly lower in the brains of rats that received glucose and aspartame than in those of control animals. Moreover, the calming neurotransmitter serotonin, manufactured from tryptophan, was similarly decreased. Dr. Wurtman infers that people who ingest aspartame, especially in combination with carbohydrate snacks, may be in danger of altering neurotransmission with unknown effects on emotion.

He says his studies show that the effect of the phenylalanine in the brain doubles when aspartame and carbohydrates are combined. Forty percent of the compound is comprised of the excitotoxin aspartame. Like glutamate, aspartate is a powerful brain toxin that can produce similar neuron damage. NutraSweet® is used in many diet foods and beverages. It is well recognized that liquid forms of the excitotoxins are much more toxic to the brain than dry forms, as they are absorbed faster and produce higher blood levels than when mixed with solid foods. No one knows what is a safe amount. There are several groups of people that might be especially susceptible to such high doses. These include people who are taking drugs that act on the brain (such as medications for high blood pressure), people with a history of seizures, youngsters, and pregnant women. For adults who do not fall into the above categories, Dr. Wurtman suggested that moderate amounts of aspartame a day should not be hazardous.[27]

## What About Children?

Is there a problem with MSG and children? Dr. Blaylock believes the younger the children, the greater the dangers from these excitotoxins. Babies exposed to excess glutamate and aspartate are at particularly high risk. We know that infant animals fed MSG have higher blood levels of glutamate than those who have not consumed MSG and these levels stay higher longer than in adults. It has been pointed out for twenty years that prior to 1969 the amount of glutamate added to a single 4½-ounce jar of baby food contained up to twenty-five times more free glutamate than could be found in the same amount of mothers' milk.[28]

The MSG producers say there is no problem with their product. They deny that children metabolize oral MSG more slowly than adults. They cite research at the University of Iowa that concluded children as young as one year old process glutamate as effectively as adults.[29]

Youngsters, however, born with certain brain disorders, such as homocystinuria, Rett's Syndrome, and incidents of low blood flow and oxygen to the brain, have been found to be more sensitive to overstimulation by aspartate and glutamate.[30] Children with migraine headaches may also be more sensitive to these compounds. Italian researchers reported recently that they evaluated glutamate and aspartate metabolism in 15 children with migraine headaches and compared them to 16 healthy children who did not suffer from migraines. The investigators from the University of Rome La Sapienza found that there was an "imbalance of the excitatory amino acids in the blood of children with migraine and might reflect a similar alteration in the nerve cells in their brains."[31]

In a recent study to determine the effects of leptin, a protein that acts on the hypothalamus' appetite center in the brain, newborn mice were given MSG.[32] The result was that the baby animals had damage to the area of the brain in which leptin is active. Leptin could not suppress weight gain in these MSG-treated mice as it could in the untreated mice. In another experiment MSG-treated mice had twofold higher percentage of body fat than untreated controls.[33]

## Pregnant and Breast-feeding Women

To facilitate fetal growth and development, most amino acids are actively transported across the placenta. Research indicates that amino acid concentrations are higher in the fetus, regardless of what the mother consumes.[34] The MSG producers cite a study that showed when glutamate was injected directly into the bloodstream in pregnant monkeys, no increase in glutamate levels were found in the fetus and the research concluded that the placenta is "virtually impermeable to glutamate."[35] That research was performed in 1979 but in 1997 investigators at Xian Medical University, People's Republic of China, found that oral administration of monosodium glutamate at a late stage of pregnancy did, indeed penetrate the placental barrier. The uptake in the fetal brain of mice was twice as great as that in the maternal brain. The results also indicated that the threshold for convulsions was lowered in the litter and the ability to learn to go through a maze was significantly impaired.[36]

The MSG producers also like to cite research that shows MSG ingestion has no effect on breast milk. They say breast milk has ten times the amount of free glutamate as cow's milk[37] and women who consumed MSG at 100 milligrams per kilogram body weight had no notable increase of glutamate in their milk, and there was no effect on the infant's intake of glutamate.[38]

## MSG and Food Intolerances

In 1968, Robert Ho Man Kwok, M.D., described a collection of symptoms he allegedly experienced after eating Chinese food. He coined the phrase "Chinese Restaurant Syndrome" (CRS) to describe these symptoms, which included numbness at the back of the neck and a feeling of pressure in the face and upper chest muscles.[39]

As a consequence of Dr. Kwok's account, G. R. Kerr and colleagues developed a subjective questionnaire to assess the prevalence of CRS in the population. The survey employed listed 18 adverse symptoms related to food, of which 3 were related to CRS. Of the 3,222 general households that responded to the survey, 43 percent reported food-related adverse reactions, but only 1.8 percent reported possible CRS symptoms.[40]

Adding to this, data from the Centers for Disease Control (now Centers for Disease Control and Prevention) in Atlanta showed that reported reactions to MSG accounted for less than one percent of food related complaints between 1975 and 1987.[41] In 1995, the Federation of American Societies for Experimental Biology (FASEB) report stated its discomfort with the use of the term CRS because of its pejorative tone and the inherent limitations of the implied circumstances of exposure.[42]

Richard Kenney, M.D., of George Washington University conducted a double-blind placebo-controlled investigation of subjects who believed they reacted adversely to MSG. Subjects were given a soft drink solution for four days, and on two of the days the solution contained 6 grams of MSG. Two of the six subjects reacted to both solutions and the other subjects reacted to neither solution. Kenney further noted that while a reaction may occur to an extremely large ingestion of MSG, the reaction is usually transient and benign.[43]

Nonetheless, anecdotal reports suggest that a small percentage of the population may be sensitive to MSG. However, these reactions are mild and transitory.[44, 45]

## MSG and Sodium Reduction

The MSG producers claim that contrary to popular belief, MSG is not high in sodium. MSG contains only one-third the amount of sodium as table salt, sodium chloride (12 percent versus 39 percent sodium). When small quantities of MSG are used in combination with a reduced amount of table salt during food preparation, the flavor-enhancing properties of MSG allow for far less salt to be used during and after cooking.[46] It would be hard to deny that if HVP and MSG are used in the same meal, the amount of sodium would be high.

## How Safe Is "Safe"?

Many organizations, including the Joint Expert Committee on Food Additives of the United Nations Food and Agriculture Organization and World Health Organization, the American Medical Association, and The National Academy of Sciences have all declared MSG safe at its current use level.[47]

Glutamate, a salt of the amino acid glutamic acid, is a remarkably potent, rapidly acting nerve toxin in laboratory cell cultures. It causes swelling of the nerve after only ninety seconds of contact.

Why glutamate causes nerve injury is unknown. More than a decade ago it was believed that glutamate neurotoxicity is a direct consequence of overexciting nerves. More recently it has been thought that a calcium influx triggered by glutamate exposure might be involved in glutamate toxicity. Under normal circumstances, the brain appears well equipped to handle large amounts of glutamate in harmless fashion, rapidly removing it and sequestering it away inside cells where it is nontoxic. In recent years, however, a number of disease states have been linked to glutamate neurotoxicity— among them, Huntington's disease, a hereditary brain-degenerating condition, and nerve loss associated with acute brain or spinal cord injury due to stroke or trauma, where injured nervous tissue may be unable to safely absorb glutamate and may, in addition, release glutamate from storage, leading to extension of the original injury. It is now suspected that glutamate and related neurotransmitters may also be involved in the nerve tangles that form the brain cell

degeneration found in Alzheimer's disease victims. Some researchers have demonstrated that in Alzheimer's disease there is a
decrease in the brain receptors to which glutamate binds.
It is believed responsible for the so-called Chinese Restaurant
Syndrome, in which diners suffered from chest pain, headache, and
numbness after eating a Chinese meal. Dr. Blaylock says some reacted at doses as low as 1 to 2 grams, while others required doses
as high as 12 grams to produce the same reaction. Overall about 10
to 25 percent of people eating a meal containing MSG developed
these adverse physical reactions first described by Dr. Kwok. Yet
when human volunteers fasted overnight and then were fed MSG
alone, virtually all developed full-blown symptoms of the Chinese
Restaurant Syndrome. So even moderate low blood sugar plays a
major role in magnifying the toxicity of these excitotoxins.[48]
    Some researchers believe that the Chinese Restaurant Syndrome
is caused by a sudden elevation of glutamate in the blood which
produces a blood vessel response. Another theory holds that some
individuals have glutamate-sensitive receptors in the esophagus
that can cause a heartburnlike reaction to MSG.
    Researchers at the University of Ottawa, Ontario, Canada, in-
trigued by the debate that swirls about the validity of symptoms
described by many people after ingestion of MSG, decided to challenge the studies. They gave 5 grams of MSG or placebo to 61 subjects in a random sequence. Neither the subjects nor the
researchers knew who was receiving the MSG and who the
placebo. Subjects who reacted to the 5 grams then underwent
rechallenge again with a placebo and with 1.25, 2.5, or 5 grams of
MSG. The results were that 18 did not respond to either the MSG
or placebo, 6 did to both, 15 to the placebo, and 22 to MSG. Total
and average severity of symptoms after ingestion of MSG were
greater for the 22 reactors than those who reacted to the placebo.
Rechallenge of the 22 revealed an apparent threshold dose for re-
activity of 2.5 grams MSG. The reactors suffered headache, muscle
tightness, numbness/tingling, general weakness, and flushing. The
Canadian investigators admitted they do not know what causes the
characteristic symptoms but do not think it is an allergic reaction.
They said the FDA recommends that instead of calling it the Chinese Restaurant Syndrome, it should be referred to as the "MSG
Symptom Complex."[49]

MSG has been found to cause brain damage in young rodents and brain damage effects in rabbits, chicks, and monkeys. Baby-food processors removed MSG from their products. MSG is on the FDA list of additives that need further study for mutagenic, teratogenic, subacute, and reproductive effects. The final report in 1980 to the FDA of the Select Committee on Generally Recognized as Safe substances stated that while no evidence in the available information on MSG demonstrated a hazard to the public at current use levels, the uncertainties that exist require that additional studies be conducted. GRAS status continues while tests are being completed and evaluated. But MSG is an unnecessary addition to food and, therefore, is not worth even the slightest risk.

Dr. Blaylock says that one reason it is so difficult to convince the FDA of the connection between MSG and delayed brain damage in humans is because it may take ten years before clinical signs of neurological damage show up. This damage is slow and cumulative, with each dose of MSG or aspartame.

There are many conditions in which the blood-brain barrier is not protective. Among them: heat stroke, brain trauma, encephalitis, strokes, high blood pressure, severe low blood sugar. He says Parkinson's may be because of a lifetime of insults to the blood-brain barrier. The barrier may become more porous as we age. Some areas of the brain have no or insufficient blood-brain barrier. Blaylock says, "I believe that there is enough research evidence to demonstrate the harmful effects of excitotoxins in food additives that all persons having a history of sensitivity to MSG or a strong family history of one of the neurodegenerative diseases should avoid all foods and beverages containing these excitotoxin 'taste' additives. Doing so could mean the difference between a normal life and one spent suffering from a crippling disease."[50]

The FDA does not place regulatory restriction on the use of glutamic acid, nor does it have a program for monitoring how or in what amount glutamate is used. Although glutamate is no longer being added to baby foods as it once was, young children are exposed to large loads of it through commercially available soups (1,300 milligrams) and in everything from bubble gum to soda. Since this artificial sweetener is not vital to well-being—except, perhaps, for some diabetics who have sweet cravings—you should ask yourself if it is really a necessity in your diet. It would certainly be smart to avoid giving artificially sweetened products to your children. The same is true of MSG.

It is up to you to decide for yourself about MSG safety based on the above. Ask yourself if MSG is a necessary additive.

The fact is also that neurotoxins are not necessarily chemicals that are hidden in our food or drink or that are put there against our will. They may be substances that we take by choice because they make us feel better or because we prefer the taste or look when they are in a dish or glass.

# The Hangover Brain

Two of the most common psychoactive substances ingested—alcohol and caffeine—can have an adverse effect on nerves. If you have ever had a hangover or staggered around after one too many cocktails, your brain has experienced the obvious neurotoxicity of alcohol. What actually happens when you down that glass of beer or wine or shot of liquor?

Alcohol speeds through your body. It doesn't have to be digested. It can be absorbed into your bloodstream directly from your stomach wall and small intestine. Its effects always are determined by the amount in your blood. When you finish an average drink—wine, beer, or a cocktail—the alcohol is carried by your bloodstream to every cell in your body.

The most visible damage is to your central nervous system. If you are moderately intoxicated, you may experience a "loosening of the tongue" and a lowering of your inhibitions, because the part of your brain that controls your reason and judgment is affected first. As the level of alcohol in your blood rises, the drug becomes a depressant, causing your mood to change and your sexual performance, especially if you are male, to be impaired. Alcohol then affects your coordination, depth perception, and reflex actions. Alcohol can dilate the blood vessels in your brain and put you into the characteristic morning-after-the-night-before state.

This "hangover" can muddle your thinking and coordination long after the headache and malaise are not obvious. Stanford University researchers reported in the *American Journal of Psychiatry* on alcohol-impaired pilots' cockpit performances fourteen hours after the flyers had their last drink. The study showed that a hang-over can harm a pilot's cockpit performance even when alcohol is no longer detectable in his bloodstream. Furthermore, the pilot may not be aware of the impairment.[51]

Dr. John Brick, laboratory director of the Alcohol Behavior Research Laboratory at Rutgers University, said there are several possible explanations for alcohol affecting performance, as in the case of the pilots, after the substance had disappeared from the blood. The most likely explanation involves changes in the central nervous system caused by intoxication. Nerve signals may not come back to their original states immediately upon the removal of alcohol but instead may take some time to readjust.

This newly recognized time lag for the neurological effects of alcohol to dissipate has led the Federal Aviation Administration to reevaluate the eight-hour requirement for pilot alcohol abstinence before flights. This long delay in getting alcohol out of the system should not be that surprising. It has long been known that alcohol withdrawal symptoms usually occur between twenty-five and forty-eight hours after the last drink and that delirium tremens occur three or four days later. Such a delay often complicates care.

The D.T.s are associated with chronic drinking. But what about people who just overdo it occasionally? In most states, you are considered legally drunk when one of every thousand parts of your blood (0.1 percent) is composed of pure alcohol. In some people this can occur when any more than two drinks are ingested within an hour. At 0.2 percent alcohol (five or more drinks in a short time) the midbrain is affected and you stagger, perhaps dropping off to sleep. At 0.3 percent you are very drunk and in a confused stupor. At 0.4 percent you might become comatose and require hospitalization.

If you raise your blood levels to over 0.3 percent alcohol, the activity of your lungs, heart, breathing, and circulation are greatly depressed. The expression "dead drunk" comes from the fact that alcohol has the potential to completely paralyze breathing and cause death. This tragedy has happened a number of times during fraternity pledging when candidates were forced to drink a lot of alcohol in a short period of time.

More commonly, alcohol takes a longer time to do its damage. The link between heavy alcohol consumption and loss of gray matter has long been suspected but now has been precisely measured. Heavy drinking shrinks the brain, according to a report in the *British Medical Journal*.[52] The brains of the alcoholics studied weighed an average 105 grams less than those of teetotalers or moderate drinkers. The brains of 44 people who died at an average age of 58 years were examined. Half had been drinking heavily for at least 30 or 40 years and their brains weighed an average of 1,315 grams. The other half, who were either teetotalers or who drank well within the safety limits of alcohol intake, had brains weighing 1,420 grams.

Charles J. Golden and his colleagues at the University of Nebraska Medical Center reported that computerized X-rays, or CAT scans, of the brains of 11 chronic alcoholics averaging just over 29 years of age revealed reductions in density in their left hemispheres but not in their right. These results suggest that the logical-thinking left hemisphere is more sensitive than the right hemisphere to the effect of alcohol, and that significant brain changes can occur at a fairly early age among alcoholics.[53]

## Alcohol and Stroke

As with many chemicals that affect the brain, a little can be beneficial and too much can be harmful. Alcohol has long been considered a pernicious drug that increases the risk of liver, heart, and lung disease, as well as the risk of involvement in a serious automobile accident. Now stroke can be added to that list, according to researchers from the National Heart, Lung and Blood Institute. Although alcohol consumption has been cited as a risk factor for stroke, its role was thought to be tied to high blood pressure, since alcohol consumption has been documented to increase blood pressure. A study from the Honolulu Heart Program, however, found that alcohol intake is a factor independent of hypertension for increasing the risk of stroke. The study followed more than 8,000 men over 12 years to ascertain the variables associated with the subjects who developed various forms of cerebral vascular accidents. Careful follow-up of all subjects demonstrated that 190 of the original sample experienced a brain hemorrhage, 90 had a blood clot in the brain, and 24 had a stroke of unknown cause. In 1997, however, it was reported at the American Heart Association Meeting in Orlando, Florida, that a study of physicians showed that moderate drinking—about one drink a day—could stave off deadly second heart attacks and strokes by from 20 to 30 percent.[54]

On the other hand, researchers report that heavy drinkers of alcohol differ from the general population in several respects. Poor nutrition may be a confounding factor as well as an inherited tendency toward alcohol use. Both of these variables may predispose individuals to a brain hemorrhage, but no one is yet sure why.

People who switch from hard liquor to wine or beer in an effort to protect their brains and bodies from alcohol toxicity aren't helping themselves, says psychiatrist William Hazle, M.D., the medical director of the Stanford Alcohol and Drug Treatment Center in Palo Alto, California. "Alcohol is alcohol, and it offers the same potential for addiction in whatever form it's consumed. For example, a standard twelve-ounce bottle or can of beer, a four-ounce glass of wine, or a shot of liquor all provide the same alcohol content."[55]

## How Much Alcohol Is Too Much?

A drink or two can raise your spirits and make you friendlier and more relaxed. But some people can't stop at two drinks, and it may be the inborn way they send messages between their brain cells rather than circumstances that keeps them drinking.

At the National Institutes of Health's Clinical Research Center, 150 participating outpatient alcoholics are receiving a chemical that is converted in the brain to dopamine. Others will receive one that is converted to serotonin. These two neurotransmitters are found in decreased levels in the brains of some alcoholics. Researchers hope that by increasing either serotonin or dopamine, the craving for alcohol may be reduced in alcoholics.[56]

Dr. Daniel Goldman, the principal investigator in the National Institutes of Health genetics study, says that when alcohol contacts nerve cell membranes, which are composed of proteins and fatty substances called lipids, it makes the normally viscous membranes more fluid. These altered membranes may cause faulty nerve signal transmission, leading to abnormal brain functioning and scrambled brain messages. Such alcohol-related nerve cell changes may even alter the individual's tolerance to alcohol and perhaps lead to physical dependence and other brain and drinking problems.

Many of the studies today are highlighting brain chemistry as well as life experiences as a factor in alcohol abuse. For example,

Conrad M. Swartz, Ph.D., M.D., of the University of Chicago Pritzker School of Medicine, reported in 1986 that children and grandchildren of alcoholics who had been adopted at birth and raised by others release much less of the stress neurotransmitter epinephrine in response to mental stress or alcohol than do adopted children who did not have alcoholic biological relatives.[57] The effects of alcohol consumption might be perceived as similar to a state of stress, because both are accompanied by an elevated release of neurotransmitters involved in emotion.

## Caffeine "Nerves"

Americans consume about a third of the world's coffee beans. Caffeine is a potent stimulant that acts on the central nervous system and is the most widely used psychoactive substance.

Caffeine is thought to produce its effect by blocking the action of a brain chemical known as *adenosine,* a self-made sedative. Clinical investigators have found that many people with panic attacks avoid caffeine after noticing that it causes attacks.

The effect caffeine has on the brain's neurotransmitters is probably why even moderate amounts of caffeine can trigger and magnify phobias and panic attacks in the estimated two to six million Americans afflicted with these disorders. Dr. Thomas Uhde of the National Institute of Mental Health (NIMH) studies panic disorders and reports that people who suffer from these attacks were given caffeine—about four cups' worth of coffee—and then their blood was tested. The NIMH researchers found that the panickers experienced a sharp rise in blood levels of the brain hormone cortisol and lactate, a substance known to produce panic attacks. The normal participants who served as comparisons in the tests had no rise in these substances after ingestion of caffeine. Because of the association between caffeine and panic attacks, Dr. Uhde said, some 60 percent of people with disorders will stop drinking coffee before they see a doctor or therapist because they have discovered its exacerbating effect on their illness.[58]

W. Leigh Thompson, M.D., Ph.D., co-director of clinical pharmacology and critical care medicine at Case Western Reserve University, says the effects of caffeine on your brain have a lot to do with whether or not you regularly consume it. If you normally don't drink it, you will feel stimulated after drinking one cup of coffee or tea. You may undergo a slight increase in blood pressure, your kidneys will be stimulated to produce more urine, your body's smooth muscles will be relaxed, and, most noticeably, you will feel awake and alert. If, however, you habitually consume either beverage, you will probably get little caffeine effect. If you ingest about 400 to 500 milligrams (four to five cups) of caffeine a day and show no effects from this large intake, you may have become physically dependent on caffeine. This is due to tolerance: your body's becoming accustomed to a substance.[59]

Since there is such a wide variation in caffeine sensitivity among individuals, caffeine may or may not affect your ability to sleep. Israeli researchers examined rates of clearance of caffeine from plasma in caffeine-sensitive individuals and found them to be an average of some 30 percent lower than in control subjects. Caffeine-sensitive individuals also drank less than average amounts of coffee.[60] Whether differences in rates of clearance are inherited, the product of differential exposure to caffeine, or both, remains to be explored.

Vanderbilt University School of Medicine researchers in Nashville, Tennessee, reported that upon consumption of caffeine 30 to 60 minutes before sleep, some individuals showed delayed sleep onset, a decrease in total sleep time, and reduced subjective estimation of the quality of sleep. However, the researchers noted that tolerance to the effects of caffeine on sleep also occurs. More non-coffee drinkers reported an increase in delayed sleep onset than did habitual heavy coffee drinkers, and non-drinkers showed a greater decrease in sleep quality after coffee consumption.[61] Therefore, if you find that caffeine affects your ability to sleep, you should avoid caffeine for at least five hours before bedtime.

If you decide that you are ingesting too much caffeine daily, don't stop all at once. You can become drowsy, depressed, and develop a headache due to sudden withdrawal. in fact, an article in the *New York State Journal of Medicine* by a physician and a rabbi reported the High Holy Day headaches that some religious patients suffered on Yom Kippur, the Day of Atonement, when a twenty-four fast is customary. Those heavy coffee drinkers in the congregation reported that caffeine-withdrawal headaches began about twelve to sixteen hours after their last dose of caffeine. Therefore, if you decide to cut down your caffeine intake, do it gradually over a week or two.[62]

## HIGH-CAFFEINE PRODUCTS

| Product | Caffeine Content |
| --- | --- |
| Coffee, caffeinated (6-oz. cup) | About 75 to 125 mg |
| Coffee, decaffeinated (6-oz. cup) | About 3 to 5 mg |
| Tea (6-oz. cup) | 30 to 65 mg |
| Cocoa (6-oz. cup) | 5 mg |
| Bittersweet chocolate (1-oz. piece) | 35 mg |
| Soft drinks (12-oz. glass) | |
|   Cola | Up to 70 mg |
|   7-Up, Sprite | 0 mg |
| Over-the-counter drugs, such as antihistamines to fight drowsiness, weight-loss drugs and stay-awake pills | up to 200 mg |
| Prescription drugs, such as the painkillers Darvon and Cafergot | 32 to 100 mg |

# What Is Being Done to Protect Us from Neurotoxins?

Dr. Thomas J. Sobotka, Ph.D., of the Neurobehavioral Toxicology Team, Center for Food Safety and Applied Nutrition of the FDA, says the agency acknowledges that brain dysfunction is an important aspect of neurotoxicology but there is no universal agreement as to how to incorporate this concern into the process of safety assessment. Some toxicologists question the very need for such tests. Other scientists feel that there is an inherent need to consider brain and behavior changes as well as conventional toxicology criteria. Dr. Sobotka says this attitude is based on the concern that, for some chemicals, nerve function changes may still occur at dose levels below which other signs of toxicity are evident.[63]

He also points out that the FDA does not require specific neurobehavioral testing as part of its routine screen. However, the agency does have the authority to require such special neurobehavioral testing for any chemical substance if there is any evidence

of nervous system involvement. The only time, then, that neurotoxicity is taken into account is when there is neuropathology or
any obvious clinical sign of nerve damage, such as paralysis,
tremor, or convulsion.

Hugh Tilson, Ph.D., head of the neurobehavioral section of the
National Institute of Environmental Health Sciences Laboratory of
Behavioral and Neurological Toxicology, in North Carolina, maintains that routine tests for nerve toxins should be included when
screening for food additives. Such tests would involve performance
of reflex tests, measures of muscle strength. The cost of the testing
equipment would be several thousand dollars per laboratory.
When weighing costs, he says, we must ask: What is the cost of
treating a single individual whose brain has been damaged by a
neurotoxin?[64]

# What To Do in the Meantime

- If you suspect you or a family member may be react-
  ing adversely to food colorings, salicylates, or other
  food additives, try to eliminate those foods with which
  you associate your symptoms. It can't hurt and it may
  help.
- Do not store acidic foods and beverages in lead-
  glazed ceramic ware or in cans. Consider storing such
  foods in glass containers especially if you have young
  children.
- Do not use aluminum cookware, if you have a choice,
  and do not use underarm deodorant sprays containing aluminum. Do not swallow digestion tablets containing the metal. Ration your intake of processed
  foods with aluminum.
- Avoid alcohol when you need your brain to work at
  its optimum, such as when driving, studying, or operating machinery. Even a little bit can dampen your intellect.
- Avoid alcohol and liquor in medications if you are
  pregnant or are taking any psychopharmaceuticals
  such as tranquilizers or antidepressants.

- Control your intake of caffeine, especially if you are pregnant or if you suffer from a great deal of anxiety.
- Skip the artificial sweeteners. There are troubling questions about aspartame and other artificial sugar substitutes. They are unnecessary except perhaps for diabetics—sweeteners do not really help with weight reduction. Pregnant women and children, especially, should avoid ingesting aspartame.
- Do not add the flavor enhancer MSG to your foods. It is an unnecessary and questionable ingredient, especially when the meal also contains aspartame.
- Write to your legislators and insist that additives be tested for neurotoxicity prior to being added to our food. Foods that may be contaminated with neurotoxic pollutants should be identified and removed from the market.

# 7

# Smart Food for Smart Children

Thirty-two-year-old Kathy, in her twenty-ninth week of pregnancy, was admitted to the hospital in Baltimore for observation of a skin rash and hives that developed after she had eaten steamed crabs and cherries. Her blood pressure was low and she was having contractions every two to three minutes. Her baby's heartbeat was slow and irregular.

Once the physicians determined that the baby's distress was secondary to Kathy's food allergy, the doctors gave Kathy oxygen, intravenous fluids, and a standard dose of antihistamines to fight the allergic attack. Kathy's labor contractions stopped and her baby's heartbeat returned to normal within two hours. Eleven and a half uneventful weeks later, she delivered a healthy boy whose intelligence and reflexes were normal.[1]

This case illustrates that what a pregnant woman eats can directly affect her unborn child.

A human unborn baby presumably can taste and smell the food it is offered,[2] but what can it do if it doesn't like the menu in the uterus? It can't get up and go out to the supermarket and select its own diet. And yet, there is no time in human life when the brain is more vulnerable to the effects of food than in the womb. Interference with the orderly sequence of brain development can not only cause physical changes in the brain but also affect behavior and intellect. A great deal of experimentation with animals and observation of children who are undernourished indicate that the consequences of poor nutrition before and soon after birth in intellectual ability and behavior are dependent upon:

- The nature.
- Severity.

- Time during development.
- Duration of the nutritional deprivation.[3]

Nutritional insults can be devastating if they occur during the brain growth spurt, which in human babies extends from the second trimester of pregnancy to the age of two years. The rapid increase in cells and the formation of the connections between brain cells makes the baby's brain most vulnerable to diet during this period. While nerve cells are forming according to a complex schedule of events, insults inflicted at a particular time may interfere with nerve cell types. An example of how such an "insult" can be prevented involves the B vitamin, folic acid.

## The Importance of Folic Acid

Folic acid can prevent neural tube defect (NTD), a malformation of the brain or spinal cord (neurological system) during embryonic development. Infants born with spina bifida, in which the spinal cord is exposed, can grow to adulthood. They usually suffer from paralysis or other disabilities. Babies born with anencephaly, where most or all of the brain is missing, usually die shortly after birth. These NTDs make up 5 percent of all U.S. birth defects each year.

In 1991, the British Medical Research Trial reported that women with a previously NTD-affected child, who took folic acid or multivitamins with folic acid before and during early pregnancy, had a reduced risk of having other NTD-affected children than those who took multivitamins without folate or no vitamins at all. Based on this and other findings, the U.S. Public Health Service recommended that all women of childbearing age take 0.4 milligrams of folic acid per day.[4]

"Folic acid is the sleeping giant of preventive medicine," said Godfrey P. Oakley, Jr., M.D., M.P.H., director of the Birth Defects and Developmental Disabilities Division of the U.S. Centers for Disease Control and Prevention (CDC). Speaking at a Ceres Forum program cosponsored by the American Institute of Nutrition, Oakley described neural tube defects as an "unchecked epidemic" that adversely affects six pregnancies every day.[5]

If all women of childbearing age consumed sufficient folic acid,

50 to 70 percent of birth defects of the brain and spinal cord could be prevented, according to the CDC. Yet, only 15 percent of women aged 18 to 45 are aware of the fact according to a survey conducted by the Gallup Organization for the March of Dimes Birth Defects Foundation.[6]

## Timing Is Everything

The challenge is getting women to take folic acid when it can do the most good to prevent neural tube defects. Folic acid is critical in the first four to six weeks of pregnancy when the neural tube is formed. This means vitamin use should begin before pregnancy occurs. In the survey, 93 percent of women who've had a child in the past two years or are now pregnant reported they took multivitamins during pregnancy, but only 21 percent did so before pregnancy began. To complicate matters further, since as many as one-half of all pregnancies are unplanned, according to the March of Dimes, the critical stage of neural tube formation will likely occur before many pregnancies are detected. For this reason, all women capable of becoming pregnant are advised to eat a balanced diet and take daily multivitamins containing folic acid.

Good dietary sources of folate include leafy, dark green vegetables, legumes, citrus fruits and juices, peanuts, whole grains, and fortified breakfast cereals.

## The Fortification Debate

In addition to the recommendation that women take multivitamins, current policy discussion is focusing on potential fortification of cereal grains with folic acid. Proponents of fortification, including CDC and the American Academy of Pediatrics, claim fortification is critical to bolster intakes of women who for various reasons do not consume sufficient folate from food or vitamin supplements. In particular, minority and low socioeconomic populations have lower intakes of folic acid and greater incidence of neural tube defects.

The Food and Drug Administration has proposed fortifying the food supply with 140 micrograms of folic acid per 100 grams of grain, including pasta, rice, cornmeal, flour, and other grain products. This is estimated to prevent up to one-half or 2,000 NTDs annually. But there's been considerable debate on both sides of the proposal, including from the Centers for Disease Control, which is advocating a higher level of fortification. One argument against such higher levels is that those at increased risk due to poor diets are likely to get the least amount of supplementation from food, while those who don't need it at all are going to consume the largest amounts. Furthermore, folic acid can mask pernicious anemia, a condition resulting from vitamin $B_{12}$ deficiency. If this condition is not properly treated, it can cause permanent neurological damage.

Some physicians argue that the number of people at risk for pernicious anemia and for neurological damage is much higher than the anticipated number of NTD cases to be prevented. At this point, no one seems sure of what upper level of fortification is safe, and we'd be exposing some 260 million people through the food supply. If a problem does occur, how will it be discovered? Everyone in the country will have been exposed, so there will be no control or comparison groups. It'll also be difficult to quantify the exact benefits of folate fortification, because the NTD rate has been declining due to prenatal diagnosis and termination of such pregnancies. On the other hand, reports of folic acid being able to prevent neural tube defects in babies had been reported as early as 1983 but it took more than a dozen years for it to be put into medical and governmental practice. Thousands of babies were born, in the meantime, with NTD at a tremendous emotional and financial cost to their families.

## Protein for Young Brains

Protein, of course, is just as important to a child's brain as folic acid. When babies are undernourished from the second trimester of pregnancy to the age of two—the time of the greatest brain growth—their brains are lighter in weight. They have a decrease in the number and size of their brain cells and in the thickness of their cerebral cortex—the brain area most involved in learning, language, and reasoning. If the nutritional deprivation occurs early in life, the deficit is permanent. A later insult reduces brain cell size but the deficit may be reversible.

The amount of *myelin* deposited is reduced in undernourished babies. The myelin sheath functions as an insulator for the electrical impulses conducted along nerves. If it is deficient, "static" occurs when nerve messages are sent and such brain functions as movements, speech, and thinking are affected.[7] For the brain to function normally not only must there be an appropriate number of brain cells with well-placed connections, but brain nerve cells must be able to manufacture and release neurotransmitters to relay impulses between nerve cells. Nutrition, as we have pointed out again and again in this book, affects neurotransmitter production.

Protein malnutrition can impair behavior by reducing the ability to think clearly and by affecting motivation and social characteristics. Some researchers believe that malnutrition in children does not need to produce obvious lesions in the brain to affect intellect, behavior, and learning. The action may be indirect. Undernutrition may interfere with the ability to concentrate during critical periods of development and lead to motivational and personality changes, any one of which may impair learning *performance* rather than learning *capacity*.[8]

## Mineral Musts

In nutrition, the term *mineral* denotes certain chemical elements which are found in the ash that remains after a food or a body tissue is burned. Some of these elements are essential to the proper functioning of the body—hence they must be regularly supplied by the diet. Other elements are not known to be essential, yet they may get into the body by various means.[9]

The following are some of the minerals scientists believed may be missing from pregnant women's diets.

***Iodine.*** This deficiency is believed to be the factor most responsible worldwide for brain damage in children. Iodine is needed for the function of the thyroid gland. In early pregnancy, the fetus is apparently dependent on its mother's thyroid hormone. After the fetal thyroid develops, the baby makes its own. A lack of thyroid hormone during brain development impairs cell division, growth, and the formation of synapses between nerve cells, and suppresses the myelination (covering) of nerves. A woman's iodine-deficient diet during pregnancy can result in severe retardation of her child or a milder syndrome of physical incoordination, with or without some deficit in intelligence. The most severe illness is known as cretinism, in which there is mental retardation, physical incoordination, deafness, and, in some cases, dwarfism.[10] The similarity of these abnormalities to those that occur in zinc deficiency supports the concept that deficiency of any nutrient critical for brain development can disrupt the well-ordered maturation of the brain.

*Zinc.* This mineral is essential for the activity of many enzymes. Hence, various investigators support the association of zinc deficiency as a factor in birth defects of the brain. When a mother does not have enough zinc in her diet, it has been shown in animal experiments in the United States and Europe, there is an adverse effect on the behavior of the offspring after birth.[11] It is believed that this effect is due to the zinc deficiency causing changes in the levels of serotonin and other brain neurotransmitters.[12] Development of the "smell" center of the brain is abnormal in many zinc-deficient animal fetuses, and the fetuses frequently have hydrocephalus (water on the brain). A statistical difference has also been found between zinc levels in the blood of babies born with small brains compared to those of normal babies.[13] Furthermore, in children, insufficient levels of zinc have been associated with lower learning ability, apathy, lethargy, and mental retardation.

*Manganese.* A diet deficient in this mineral in pregnant mice and guinea pigs has shown that this micronutrient may be essential for the brains of unborn human babies. When animal mothers had a diet deficient in manganese, their babies staggered after they were born. This condition was due to impaired formation of the inner-ear mechanisms involved in balance. The problem can be prevented by feeding pregnant rats and guinea pigs one milligram of manganese per gram of diet. In addition to impairing inner-ear development, manganese deficiency has also been reported to lower the neurotransmitter content of the brain. Although manganese deficiency–induced behavioral abnormalities in humans have not been described, behavioral effects of manganese overdoses are well known. Manganese poisoning in miners has resulted in Parkinson's disease, a common disorder of the part of the brain that controls movement, and demented behavior due to accumulation of the element in the brain.[14]

## The Drink That Goes Right to an Unborn Baby's Head

Alcoholic beverages are the most common cause in the Western world of damage to the brains of unborn children from something their mothers consume. It is estimated that as many as 2 percent of all live births may show effects of alcohol exposure on the fetus. Prenatal exposure to alcohol affects the development of various systems, including those of the muscles, skeleton, and nerves. Many infants with fetal alcohol syndrome have symptoms that point to abnormal development of the brain, particularly of the areas that control movement and speech. Such abnormalities include muscle weakness, incoordination, and difficulties with language and thinking. Anatomical studies of the brains of mature humans who had been exposed to alcohol before birth show that their brains are smaller and that the organization of their brains' nerve cells is abnormal.[15]

As little as one alcoholic drink a day in early pregnancy can adversely affect an unborn child's growth.[16] The well-documented effects of mothers' excessive drinking on their offspring include growth deficiencies, specific facial deformities, and brain dysfunction that may be related to abnormal brain development. And although alcohol can be harmful to the fetus at any time during pregnancy, researchers believe that the most toxic effect on the development of the human nervous system is relatively late in pregnancy, particularly during the final three months.[17]

Incidentally, alcohol is present in more than seven hundred prescribed liquid medications including decongestants and cough medicines. So read labels carefully if you are pregnant or if you want to give even an over-the-counter medication to your child. Ethanol affects children's bodies more rapidly than it does adults, and children are more susceptible to its effects, which include central nervous system impairment, decreased reaction time, muscle incoordination, and behavioral changes.[18]

## Take the Milk and Skip the Coffee, Tea, and Colas

Caffeine is another common ingredient in drinks and medicine that, when ingested by a pregnant woman, can go right to her unborn child's head. Its effect, however, is highly controversial. In order to study the effects of caffeine ingested by the pregnant mother on the development of her offspring, scientists at the Hebrew University in Rehovot, Israel, administered caffeine to pregnant rats by mixing it with drinking water during the last seven days of pregnancy.[19] This is a period of rapid development, roughly equivalent to the rapid development during mid-pregnancy in humans. Three groups of pregnant rats were treated with varying doses of caffeine. One group was given a dose roughly equivalent to 4 cups of coffee per day for seven days. The second group was given 8 cups per day and the third about 12 cups per day. The pups born to these three groups of rats were followed from birth well into adulthood and were compared on various measures of physical and behavioral development to the pups born to rat mothers that did not receive caffeine.

The results showed that the lowest dose of caffeine (equal to about 4 cups of coffee daily) caused hyperactivity in the offspring but no serious learning problems. However, the animals whose mothers were treated with the two higher doses (equal to about 8 and 12 cups of coffee daily) showed learning deficits on complex learning tasks. In addition to learning deficits, the animals exposed to the two higher doses of caffeine before birth were significantly more obese in adulthood than those in the low-dose group or the non-caffeine–treated control group. Both the obesity and the learning disability became more severe with increasing age.

Two of the later reports in Europe found similar effects in humans. Researchers at Belgrade University, Yugoslavia, studied 1,011 women their first three days after delivery. The investigators discovered non-smoking mothers who had an average intake of 71 milligrams of caffeine a day had babies with lower-than-average birth weight.[20] Scientists in the Netherlands evaluated the outcome of ten mothers carrying twins. Five women were examined before and after drinking coffee. Blood flow of the mother and umbilical blood flow, fetal heart rate, and twin behavior were documented and found to increase after coffee intake. Swallowing and breathing also showed "significant" changes.[21]

Researchers at U.S. National Institute of Child Health and Development, on the other hand, say their studies show no adverse pregnancy outcome with moderate caffeine consumption. The Americans monitored 431 women and the amount of caffeine they consumed from conception to birth. After accounting for nausea, smoking, alcohol use, and maternal age, the researchers found no relationship between caffeine consumption of up to 300 milligrams per day and adverse pregnancy outcomes, including miscarriage. A follow-up of 500 of these offspring seven years later found the children showed no effects on IQ and attention tests.[22]

## What to Eat and What Not to Eat If You Are Pregnant

It would be best for your baby's brain if you avoided ingestion of all alcoholic and caffeinated beverages. Such libations are unnecessary, and while a minimum amount may do no harm, why take any risk at all? Remember that colas, chocolate, and medicines may contain caffeine. Medicines may also have alcohol.

A pregnant woman should, of course, have medical supervision during gestation. Those who have a family history of diabetes or high blood pressure must follow a carefully monitored diet. Diabetes and high blood pressure often make their first appearance during the physical stress of pregnancy. However, for healthy women without medical problems, there are still special needs, particularly for calcium, iodine, and certain vitamins. Chapters 3, 8, 11 provide information about specific nutrients.

Folic acid, as pointed out previously, is vital in helping to prevent spinal and brain birth defects. Vitamin $B_6$ is also important. It is a coenzyme in the body's manufacture of the neurotransmitters GABA, dopamine, and serotonin and therefore is required for a baby's development of the central nervous system. In severely deficient human infants, seizures, behavioral problems, and movement disorders occur. Researchers say that while it is not yet possible to define the exact amount of vitamin $B_6$ required to support optimal brain development, pregnant and lactating women should be encouraged to consume a diet that is rich in vitamin $B_6$.[23]

## Good Nutrition for a Newborn

In recent years, scientists have discovered that nerve regulation systems are organized differently in the young than in the adult. Additionally, there may be two or three transitional stages *after* birth. The interaction of a mother and her baby has been found to regulate certain aspects of the infant's nervous system development. For example, it has been found in rats that the rate and quality of milk provided by the mother regulates autonomic nervous system development in the infant. There is also evidence that touch and smell stimulation may serve to regulate the behavior responses of the infant by affecting the accumulation of brain neurotransmitters.[24] These are additional reasons that a human child should be breast-fed if at all possible. If not, then a mother should hold and cuddle her baby during bottle-feeding.

There have been limited opportunities to perform formal randomized studies on the effect of early nutrition in humans. In a study of preterm infants begun in 1982 and carried on until the children were eight years old, researchers at The Institute of Child Health in London were able to compare the effect of a variety of diets. Their findings suggest that the youngsters fed a nutrient-supplemented preterm formula performed better than those fed standard formula milk. They also concluded that human milk may contain factors which promote brain growth or development. Outcome data from the study showed that a very brief period of dietary manipulation (on average for the first four weeks of life) influences later development.[25]

The protein content of human breast milk is particularly suited to a baby's metabolism, and the fat content is more easily absorbed and digested than that in cow's milk. Because it contains antibodies from the mother, breast milk can also provide immunity against certain infections and allergies. There is more vitamin A and vitamin E and twice as much iron in human milk, which may protect against anemia in the baby and thus protect the red blood cells that carry oxygen to the baby's brain. Zinc and taurine, an amino acid that not only aids in digestion but also is thought to be important in brain and nervous system development, are also more available in breast milk.[26]

Remember: what a mother ingests may be passed through the

breast milk to the baby, affecting the baby's brain and body. Alcohol, for example, passes easily into breast milk. Large amounts of beer or wine can make your baby drunk, affect his coordination and emotions, and lead to dehydration. Caffeine reaches the breast milk in smaller amounts, but if you ingest enough caffeine, your baby may become irritable and have trouble sleeping.

Recreational drugs, of course, should not be taken at all. Prescription drugs and over-the-counter medications, even such common ones as antihistamines and painkillers, should not be taken unless prescribed by a doctor. If a medicine works, it has a systemic effect—that is, it affects your entire body. If it has a systemic effect, it may affect the unborn child.

## The Undernourished Brain, Intelligence, and Behavior

Human studies have shown that even a mildly undernourished child can affect a mother-child relationship. The malnourished child who is apathetic and unresponsive to the mother's attentions elicits less response or stimulation from the mother. This, in turn, can affect the child's behavior and learning ability.

It is difficult to separate direct effects of malnutrition on the brain and the effect of malnutrition on the ability to receive information. Malnourished children show decreased motivation, concentration, and attentiveness, which may impair successful learning. Undernutrition, therefore, is a significant nongenetic factor influencing the development of the brain in unborn and young children. Severe malnutrition, not only in the first few months of life but any time within the first two years, has long-lasting consequences on cognitive development. Jamaican boys who were severely malnourished during the first two years of life had lower intelligence scores and decreased intellectual ability compared with their brothers, sisters, and classmates.[27]

A short exposure to malnutrition in a previously well-nourished population may not have lasting effects. This was shown in males born during the Dutch famine of 1944–45, who at eighteen years of age had scores on intelligence tests similar to controls from non-famine areas.[28, 29] To achieve this rehabilitation, nurture as well as nutrition is necessary according to the Research of Joaquin Cravioto, M.D., professor of pediatrics and scientific director of the National Institute for Children's Health Sciences and Technology, Mexico City. A world-famous expert on the effects of malnutrition on children's brains, he maintains a good mother-child interaction after a child has been nutritionally rehabilitated can bring the majority of such children back to normal age levels of performance.[30]

Dr. Cravioto and his colleagues measured the mental performance of children who had suffered from malnutrition and were then well nourished. The results showed that children who recovered from malnutrition had significantly lower intellectual quotients than their brothers, sisters, and other healthy children of the same social class. The children who had received stimulation during the period of hospitalization, however, had higher levels of performance than the group without stimulation, which proved the importance of nonnutritional variables such as cuddling and playing.

Dr. Cravioto says that the disappearance of the developmental lag in the survivors points to the strong association among nutrition, stimulation available at home, and brain function. Nutrition plays a major role in some brain functions and stimulation may influence another set of brain functions.

## Food for the Growing Brain

A child has special dietary requirements because of rapid growth. A reduced version of an adult diet is not sufficient. Youngsters have an increased need for calories and for all nutrients, one of the most important of which is iron. Iron-deficiency anemia is the most common nutritional deficiency problem in the United States.[31]

Folic acid, vitamin $B_{12}$, and copper are also important in making red blood cells. Protein is necessary for bone and cell growth, including nerve cells in the brain, and calcium is vital for building strong bones and teeth during childhood and adolescence. Some experts believe the RDA's for calcium should be increased to 1,000 to 1,200 milligrams per day for children. The new recommendations for children's diets, however, are controversial, even among such illustrious groups as the American Heart Association, the American Cancer Society, and the American Academy of Pediatrics. The National Institutes of Health, the American Heart Association, and the American Cancer Society recommend lowering the amount of fat in children's diet. Some believe the pendulum, especially concerning fat, has swung too far.

## A Question of Fat

The American Academy of Pediatrics finds "no compelling new evidence" that current diets should be modified. The pediatricians set the acceptable upper limits of fat intake in children at 40 percent of total calories. The pediatricians questioned whether diets such as those recommended by the National Institutes of Health would adequately support growth, especially during the adolescent growth spurt:

> *The safety of diets designed to decrease intake of refined sugars, decrease consumption of fat and cholesterol, and limit sodium intake has not been established in growing children and pregnant women. An increase in cereal grains at the expense of animal protein with a decrease in the density of essential nutrients without further dietary advice might result in a decrease of some protective micronutrients such as vitamins and minerals that might pose health risks to children.*[32]

Many experts disagree with the American Academy of Pediatrics dietary recommendations and point out that hardening of the arteries, which affects not only the heart but also the brain, begins in childhood. In a study reported in the *New England Journal of Medicine,* researchers at Louisiana State University Medical Center reported that the earliest stages of heart disease were found in teenagers who had high total cholesterol levels in their blood and high levels of the dangerous LDL cholesterol. The study was done on thirty-five youngsters, with an average age of 18 years, who died unexpectedly and who had been tested previously for cholesterol. All but six of them had "fatty streaks," thought to be precursors of fibrous cholesterol lesions, in their aortas, the artery that carries blood from the heart to the brain and the rest of the body.[33]

Still, the pendulum seems to be swinging toward fat and cholesterol in the diet of young children. Indeed, a study of seven infants referred to North Shore University Hospital in Manhasset, New York, carried a caution to parents who are "overly concerned" about their infants' diets. These children of college-educated parents failed to thrive. The babies had decreased growth and poor weight gain. The researchers, Michael Pugliese, M.D., and Fima Lifshitz, M.D., said in the study that the parents perceived those children as being similar to themselves—that is, obese, prone to atherosclerosis, and chronically dieting to reduce weight. The restrictive diets, however, typically including lean meats, low-fat dairy foods, and complex carbohydrates—foods already present in the parents' diets—caused the infants to experience inadequate weight gain and have a decreased linear growth rate. The infants were consuming only 60 to 94 percent of the recommended calories intake for age and sex. Whether this study stands the test of time or whether the slower growth and weight gain may not be as undesirable as the pediatricians believe is yet to be determined.[34]

Evidence is building. Researchers at Purdue University go even further in their cautions about low-fat diets for children. Bruce Watkins, Ph.D., professor of lipid chemistry and metabolism at Purdue University, and Bernhard Hennig, Ph.D., professor of cell nutrition at the University of Kentucky, say that children under age 5—especially infants—are getting too little fat in their diets. At least that's true for many infants and toddlers, and even children as old as 5 years, all of whom may need more fat in their diets than adults, the two nutritionists say.[35] "The scientific community is focused in one direction, and that is reducing dietary fat in all individuals," Watkins says. "But trying to adapt fat recommendations from adults to infants and toddlers is not the best way."

Dr. Hennig agrees. "There's little information that restricting fat before two years of age could be beneficial, but there's plenty of evidence that this could be dangerous," he says. "One of the main reasons is that it may retard growth and development."

According to the researchers, restricted fat intake in children reduces growth and visual acuity and limits mental development. "For example, omega-3 fatty acids—which come from fish and certain plant oils—are crucial for brain development and for development of the retina," Watkins says.

The researchers conducted a scientific review of available information and concluded that dietary fat recommendations for adults have been inappropriately applied to children, who have a different physiology and different growth needs than adults. The federal government's 1995 Dietary Guidelines, produced by the U.S. Department of Agriculture and the U.S. Department of Health and Human Services, recommend that fat intake be restricted in children beginning at age 2.

Drs. Watkins and Hennig, however, suggest that we should *not* restrict fat until 5 years of age, and then reduce it gradually throughout childhood and teen years. They say that limiting dietary fat to less than 30 percent of total calories in young children may reduce growth and lead to nutritional shortages.

The relative low-fat nature of infant formula is a special concern for these researchers. "Certain fatty acids are found only in human milk. They are not found in sufficient amounts in infant formulas," Dr. Hennig says. "The companies that make the formula should mimic human milk as closely as possible. These companies are aware, at least, that this is important, and they are working on this."

Dr. Hennig points out: "We don't know the essential fatty acids that are needed for bone and cartilage development. For example, omega-3 fatty acids are found in breast milk, but are not in infant formulas in this country. We know that these fatty acids are important for normal growth development and appear to have an increasing role in preventing disease later in life."

In addition to the need for fat in early development, Dr. Hennig says there is a theory that offers another reason infants should have comparatively high-fat diets: These diets may lower their cholesterol when they become adults.

"Blood cholesterol can come from diet, or we can produce it in our bodies through internal synthesis," Dr. Hennig says. "There may be a reason that human mother's milk is very high in fat. There is a provocative theory that high fat content in breast milk may suppress the enzyme that causes the body to synthesize cholesterol early in life. The reason would be that if dietary fat is high enough, then the body would not need to produce more of its own. But if the fat isn't there early in life, the body begins producing excess cholesterol, and this may continue even later in life."

The researchers recognize that childhood obesity is an increasing and persistent problem in the United States, but they maintain: "Instead of restricting fat, we need to encourage physical activity in children. The problem is that kids today spend too much time in front of the television."

## The Trouble with TV

They are not the first to cite TV as a cause of obesity in today's children. William Dietz, M.D., Ph.D., formerly with the New England Medical Center Hospitals in Boston, reports that his studies have led him to this conclusion: "There was a strong, significant relationship between television viewing and obesity that persisted even when we introduced control after control."[36]

Dr. Dietz, who is now the director of the Division of Nutrition and Physical Activity of the CDC, maintains, "Children eat more while they are watching TV and they eat more of the foods advertised on TV." Dietz says, "The message that TV conveys is that you will be thin no matter what you eat. Nearly everyone on television is thin. In addition, children who are watching television are inactive."

Dr. Dietz says when he studied the metabolic rate of a 12-year-old boy watching TV, the child had a basal metabolic rate that dropped by 200 calories an hour while he watched cartoons, as though he was in a trance or stupor. In a recent study, Dietz and his colleagues found that those children who watched more than 5 hours of television per day compared to those watching for 2 hours or less had an 8.3 times greater incidence of obesity. In fact, they concluded, "sixty percent of overweight incidence in children ten to fifteen years of age can be attributed to excess television viewing time and that reducing viewing time could help prevent this increasingly common chronic health condition."[37]

It is not just the inactivity, evidently, that causes the obesity. It's the commercials that contribute. A. W. Logue, Ph.D., associate professor in the psychology department at the State University of New York at Stony Brook, says in her text *The Psychology of Eating and Drinking* that television is one of the clearest examples of the indirect influence of one organism on the food preferences of another.

"Children living in the United States view an average of some 22,000 commercials a year, and more than fifty percent of these advertised foods that are low in nutrition. . . . Several experiments have shown that when children are exposed to commercials for low-nutrition foods, their reported preference for those foods as well as their tendency to buy or eat those foods increases. On the other hand, when children are exposed to commercials that present nutritional information, their preference for nutritive foods is not affected. To some extent these differential results may be due to the greater amount of effort and money that is put into producing low-nutrition food commercials, compared with commercials carrying nutritional information. Nevertheless, the implications of this research are alarming. Most of the commercials that are seen by children appear to be teaching the children to prefer low-nutrition foods."[38]

**Discourage eating meals or snacks while watching TV.** Try to eat only in designated areas of your home, such as the dining room or kitchen. Eating in front of the TV may make it difficult to pay attention to feelings of fullness, and may lead to overeating.

# What About Sugar?

One of the major objections regarding television and diet as far as children are concerned is that the commercials urge youngsters to eat highly sugared foods, particularly breakfast cereals and candy. Here are the results of Dr. Bette Li's testing of the sugar content of breakfast cereals, including granola cereals touted as "natural and healthy." Dr. Li and her colleagues Priscilla Schuhmann and Joanne Holden are with the Nutrient Composition Laboratory of the U.S. Department of Agriculture, Beltsville, Maryland.

Human and animal experiments have linked sugar and unruly behavior in children. A study found significant correlations between carbohydrate-protein ratios and directly observed aggressive and restless behavior in a sample of 28 hyperactive children. An estimation of sugar intake based on large categories of food also was associated with the same behaviors in the hyperactive group. Among the normal control children, the dietary carbohydrate-protein ratio correlated only with restless behavior. However, the study did not prove that sugar caused the hyperactivity or aggressiveness. It could be that active or aggressive children simply crave more sugar.

One way to study causal effects is with a challenge study. Two investigators have carried out such experiments. The National Institutes of Health researchers conducted studies with 21 children whose families had responded to an advertisement seeking children with adverse behavior patterns that supposedly worsened following sugar ingestion. The children received challenges of sucrose, glucose, or a sweet-tasting placebo.[39] By adding saccharin to all three challenges, having the tests at least two days apart, and administering the substances as a lemon-flavored ice slurry, a double-blind study was maintained. This study found none of the behavioral changes that had been observed by the mothers. Furthermore, children with no psychiatric diagnosis as well as those with one or more psychiatric diagnoses were found to be significantly less active on sugar.

In contrast, at Children's Hospital in Washington, D.C., investigators gave regular orange juice or juice sweetened with sucrose or fructose to 13 emotionally ill children. Compared to the control group, the children who received sugar showed an increase in total activity.[40]

In the 1970s, anecdotal reports suggested sugars cause hyperactivity in children. Research, however, failed to confirm this theory. Hyperactivity was not seen in children after consistent high intakes or single large doses of sugars. In a recent study, researchers examined the effect of eating sucrose (table sugar) on the behavior of children aged 6 to 10 years.[41] The children were chosen for the study because their parents believed the children reacted negatively to sucrose. Preschool children were also studied. They are often considered sensitive to some foods. The researchers found no differences in the behavior of the children when they ate higher-than-normal amounts of sucrose compared to when they ate diets low in sucrose.

Actually, this and other research suggests sugars tend to calm both children and adults. This effect could go unnoticed due to other influences. For instance, the excitement of a birthday party or Halloween could override the calming effect of sugars. But try to convince parents and grandparents who deal with sugar–fired-up kids whirling around the place. We, ourselves, have witnessed it with one of our grandchildren.

## Caffeine and Kids

Cola drinks are popular among youngsters. How much does their caffeine affect the brainpower of kids?

A study was done in which 30 high-caffeine consumers were found among 800 schoolchildren. The high-caffeine consumers were matched against children (controls) who reported low caffeine consumption.

High consumers were more likely than low consumers to be rated hyperactive by their teachers, and one-third of the high caffeine-consuming group—9 out of 30—met the criterion for clinical hyperactivity based on their teacher rating scale scores.

Nineteen of the high-caffeine group and 19 of the matched low consumers agreed to participate in a double-blind placebo-controlled challenge study, in which they received 10 milligrams of caffeine or placebo each day for two weeks. On caffeine, the low-caffeine consumers were rated as more emotional, inattentive, and restless by their parents, while high-caffeine consumers were not rated as significantly changed.

The differences between low and high consumers could not be attributed to tolerance, withdrawal, or subject selection and thus suggest a possible physiological basis in children for dietary caffeine preference. Moreover, the study points out the importance of challenge studies. The initial data would have indicated that the caffeine caused the hyperactivity. Instead, the challenge data indicated that hyperactive children might selectively ingest caffeine, quite the contrary finding. Caffeine may serve to calm the hyperactive, a paradoxical phenomenon also found when stimulant drugs are given to hyperactive children to sedate them.

Those who experiment with alcohol and tobacco in early teenage years are more likely than their peers to consume illicit drugs a decade later. This has led some to believe that caffeine is a gateway drug. Most studies published since 1983 do not seem to support this premise in normal children at caffeine levels they consume.[42]

## Diet and School Performance

Can you give children a healthy, well-balanced diet that is low in food additives and sugar and see a difference in their intellectual performance?

First of all, you can be sure that your child has a good breakfast. A series of studies from Massachusetts General Hospital and the Harvard Medical School have shown that the National School

Breakfast Program improved academic performance and psychosocial behavior.[43]

"Our first two studies showed a relationship between hunger and behavior problems and obstacles to learning," said Dr. Ronald Kleinman, a Harvard Medical School research and past chair of the Committee on Nutrition of the American Academy of Pediatrics. "Our study of elementary school children in the Pittsburgh area links hunger to having a large number of behavior problems, especially fighting, stealing, having difficulties with teachers, not acknowledging rules, and clinging to parents," said Kleinman.

Between 1978 and 1983, a diet policy in 803 New York City schools was changed over a period of four years. The amount of sugary foods and synthetically colored and flavored foods as well as foods preserved with BHA and BHT was lowered over that four-year period.

The impact of a low-additive and sugar-reduced diet on academic performance in these schools was studied by Stephen J. Schoenthaler, Ph.D., Walter Doraz, Ph.D., and James Wakefield, Jr., Ph.D. They reported that the change in food policy was followed by a 15.7 percent increase in mean academic percentile, ranking above the rest of the nation's schools that used the same standardized tests. Prior to the 15.7-percent gain, the standard deviation of the annual change in national percentile ratings had been less than 1 percent. Each school's academic performance ranking was negatively correlated with the percent of children who ate school food before the diet policy changes. However, after the menu changes, the percent of students who ate school lunches and breakfasts within each school became positively correlated with that school's rate of gain. Before the diet change, very little change had occurred in mean academic percentile rank for the 803 schools.[44]

Dr. Schoenthaler and his colleagues say one question remains unanswered: Was the change in performance due to the combination of restriction of food additives, sucrose, and fat or to an unidentified factor which is correlated with all three, such as malnutrition?

The researchers said that lay people might be tempted to conclude that sugar and food additives directly caused the poor grades, with the fat being the least important factor. Most nutritionists, on the other hand, would assume that a reduction in malnutrition—rather than a reduction in sugar, fats, and food additives—is probably the primary cause of the improved academic performance, for three reasons:

1. A common factor exists in foods that contain high levels of fats, sucrose, and food additives. They tend to be low in the ratio of essential nutrients to calories. Foods that are laden with synthetic food colors and flavors tend to be the more processed foods that, in turn, have lost a substantial portion of their nutritional value in processing. Pure sucrose, by definition, contains no nutrient other than 4 calories per gram. Fat contains a few nutrients but has even more calories per gram—9 grams. When the consumption of empty calories (sucrose, fats, and processed foods) decreases, children normally eat other foods that contain a higher ratio of nutrients to calories. The uptake in foods that are more nutritious should lower any malnutrition that existed.
2. A substantial body of research supports the link between malnutrition and academic behavior in controlled laboratory studies.
3. The available data published in major journals that directly implicate food additives and sucrose consistently point to negative findings in general or else positive findings in a very select population.

Dr. Schoenthaler and his colleagues conclude:

> *Improvements in academic performance by comparison with other U.S. schools during the same time period appear to be due to the diet policies, which restricted fats, sucrose, and food additives. The cause will remain unverified without further research, but malnutrition may be the predominant cause since all students have the potential of being malnourished. Although malnutrition appears to be the most likely theoretical explanation for most of the improvements, selected children have improved due to restrictions of food additives and sucrose which cause "allergy" symptoms.*

The Centers for Disease Control and Prevention (CDC) offers the following guidelines for Vending Machine Foods Low in Saturated Fat that could be made available to youngsters at school:

Canned fruit

Fresh fruit (e.g., apples and oranges)*

Fresh vegetables (e.g., carrots)

Fruit juice and vegetable juice

Low-fat crackers and cookies (such as fig bars and gin-
gersnaps)

Pretzels

Bread products (e.g., bread sticks, rolls, bagels, and pita
bread)

Ready-to-eat low-sugar cereals

Granola bars made with unsaturated fat

Low-fat (1%) skim milk*

Low-fat or nonfat yogurt*

Snack mixes of cereal and dried fruit with a small
amount of nuts and seeds**

Raisins and other dried fruit**

Peanut butter and low-fat crackers†

*These foods are appropriate if the vending machine is refrigerated.
**Some schools might not want to offer these items because these foods can contribute to dental caries.
†Some schools might not want to offer peanut butter; it is low in saturated fatty acids, but high in total fat.

# The Feingold Diet and Food Additives

How many so-called selected children react to food additives and certain other ingredients in foods?

The Feingold Association believes there are thousands, many of them undiagnosed. The organization and the diet are based on the work of the late Dr. Benjamin Feingold, who was chief of allergy at Kaiser Permanente Medical Center in San Francisco. In 1973, Dr. Feingold presented a paper at a meeting of the American Medical Association purporting that adverse reactions to artificial food additives and natural salicylates were manifested as hyperactivity in some children. He said the adverse reactions did not involve the immune system but instead were due to druglike sensitivities. The following is an example of Feingold's premise:

*Harry, an engineer in his early thirties, had very severe headaches that would last up to three days. As time passed, they became increasingly frequent and severe, and he seemed to be constantly irritable. Harry went to a kaleidoscope of doctors and each time received a prescription for another painkiller. Because his stomach bothered him, he kept taking mints and antacids.*

*In the meantime, his small daughter, Laura, also had a very low tolerance for frustration. She was easily distracted, although she was not physically hyperactive.*

*Jane, the wife and mother in this family, taught art at a local grammar and junior high school. She felt she could not return to her job after Laura was born because she found it difficult to cope with the child's behavior. Jane talked to other mothers about her problem, and one of them suggested she buy a book that described a diet free of artificial colorings and flavorings and natural salicylates. Jane bought the book and started purchasing food and cooking meals according to the instructions.*

*Not only did Laura's behavior problems disappear, but so did Harry's headaches subside. Today, Laura is a seventeen-year-old honor student in high school. Harry is headache-free.*[45]

Today, Jane Hersey is executive director of the Feingold Association of the United States. The book she had read during her family's problems was a best seller, by Dr. Feingold, *Why Your Child Is Hyperactive* (Random House, 1975). Jane Hersey says there are 10,000 members of the Feingold organization and an estimated 200,000 families who follow the regimen. Many scientists, however, believe artificial food additives and natural salicylates are harmless, and argue that the diet and behavioral changes in families like the Herseys are merely coincidental. Despite the naysayers, the association is alive and thriving. You can check for yourself on the Internet at *www.Feingold.org* or write to them at 127 East Main St., Suite 106,

Riverhead, NY 11901 (telephone: 516-369-9340 or FAX: 516-369-2988). The Feingold Association lists the following symptoms as being possibly related to sensitivity to synthetic additives or salicylates:

**Symptoms**
Marked hyperactivity and fidgeting
Excitability, impulsivity
Poor sleep habits
Short attention span
Clumsiness
Poor hand-eye coordination
Difficulty with buttoning, writing, drawing, and speech
Trouble with comprehension and memory

## Substances on Feingold "Don't Eat" List

Synthetic (artificial) colors
Synthetic (artificial) flavors
Preservatives: BHA (butylated hydroxyanisole)

Dr. Bernard Weiss of the radiation biology and biophysics department at the University of Rochester School of Medicine and colleagues from the Kaiser Foundation Research Institute and the University of California did one of the first tightly controlled tests of the Feingold Diet and its effects on hyperactivity in children.[46] Twenty-two youngsters were maintained on a diet that excluded artificial flavorings and colorings and then were intermittently given a blend of seven artificial colors in a double-blind trial. That is, the investigators, the children, and the children's parents and teachers did not know when the artificial colors were given. The colors were in soft drinks identical to soft drinks that had inert substances.

Of the 22 youngsters, one responded mildly to the challenge and another responded dramatically. The latter, a 34-month-old girl, showed a significant increase in agitation. Dr. Weiss and his colleagues concluded that certain youngsters *are* sensitive to artificial additives and that the reason other studies had been negative was because insufficient amounts of the chemicals were used and there were deficiencies in analyses of the experimental data.

The National Institutes of Health held a consensus development conference on "Defined Diets and Hyperactivity" in January 1982.

A vocal contingent of physicians and families of hyperactive children contended that "defined diets" that are free of artificial colors, flavors, and preservatives are an effective treatment for childhood hyperactivity. An equally vocal contingent of medical researchers asserted that the diets' effects, if any, should be ascribed to faith healing.

Walking a tightrope between seeming to endorse the defined diets and condemning them outright as unproved in controlled studies, the consensus panel concluded that parents and physicians who believe in the diets may want to give them a try. But the panel made it clear that there is no firm evidence.

In 1985, an article was published in the British medical journal *Lancet* about the results of a well-controlled study. Seventy-six hyperactive children were given a diet consisting typically of two meats (such as lamb and chicken), two carbohydrates (such as potatoes and rice), two fruits, vegetables, water, calcium, and vitamins for the first four weeks. Those whose behavior was improved on the simple diet were then given fruit juices with artificial colorings and the preservative benzoic acid. If the symptoms returned, they were asked to participate in a double-blind study in which neither researchers nor subjects knew when the suspect chemicals were administered. The results were that, on the restricted diet, 62 children improved and a normal range of behavior was achieved in 21 of the children. Other symptoms such as headaches, abdominal pains, and tantrums also were relieved. Twenty-eight of the children who improved in the first weeks of the diet had their symptoms return or made worse when they were again given the additives, but not when they were given a placebo. In addition, one food dye, Yellow no. 5, and a preservative, sodium benzoate, produced the greatest adverse reactions in the children.

In another study published in 1993, researchers at the Institute of Child Health, London, worked with 78 children referred to a diet clinic because of hyperactive behavior.[47] The children were placed on a "few foods" elimination diet. Fifty-nine improved in behavior during the open trial. For 19 of these children, it was possible to disguise foods or additives, or both, that reliably provoked behavior problems by mixing them with other tolerated foods and to test their effect in a placebo-controlled double-blind challenge protocol. The results of the cross-over trial on these 19 children showed a significant effect for the provoking foods to worsen ratings of behavior and to impair psychological test performance. This study, the researchers concluded, shows that observations of change in behavior associated with diet made by parents and other people with a role in the child's care can be reproduced using double-blind methodology and objective assessments. "Clinicians should give weight to the accounts of parents and consider this treatment in selected children with a suggestive medical history," they advised. The University of Rochester's Dr. Weiss points out that Yellow no. 5 is banned in a number of European countries because it causes reactions in people who are sensitive to aspirin. He said there are a lot of questions about Yellow no. 6 and Red no. 40 because there are relatively high levels of these additives in food.

Jane Hersey of the Feingold Association says that the argument today is not over whether the Feingold Diet (which excludes artificial colorings and flavorings) works, but rather why it works and how many children can benefit.

## General Rules of a Healthy Diet for Children Today

Balance and moderation are the best rules to follow when it comes to diets for adults or for children. The following are the general regimens for a healthy diet for children, based on a compilation of sources from government and health organizations.[48]

From birth to 2 years, a period characterized by rapid growth, gains in weight and height are the primary indices of nutritional status. Breast-feeding is encouraged for at least the first 4 to 6 months of life for nutritional as well as immunological benefits to the infant.

Among the most common nutritional disorders during infancy is iron-deficiency anemia, which is routinely screened through blood tests of hemoglobin or hematocrit. "Solid" foods are usually introduced at about 4 to 6 months of age, particularly iron-fortified cereals, to help prevent this problem. Other foods such as strained fruits and vegetables and fruit juice are gradually introduced, until by about 12 months of age, when most babies are eating small, tender table foods.

In children under 2 years of age, dietary fat plays a key role in the formation of vital nerve and brain tissues. Health professionals do not recommend feeding fat-reduced foods to children of this age, as pointed out. For example, use of whole milk rather than low-fat or skim milk is advised.

Nutrition recommendations for teens and children over the age of 2 differ little from those for adults. The recommendations are designed, however, to promote optimal growth and development and, therefore, may not be as restrictive as those for adults. A wide variety of foods, rich in essential nutrients necessary for growing bodies, form the basis of recommendations.

Most children will grow about two inches per year and gain about four to seven pounds per year. Between the ages of 6 to 12, youngsters will grow an average of one to two feet and almost double in weight. Diminished weight-for-height may be indicative of acute undernutrition; a decreased height-for-age may suggest chronic undernutrition. Such growth failure may be due to malnutrition, psychosocial deprivation, eating disorders, underlying chronic disease, infection, or other factors.

While children often have definite food likes and dislikes, nutritionists recommend parents make available a wide variety of foods and encourage tasting new foods in small quantities without forcing the issue. In this manner, children will often come to accept and like new foods.

Adolescents need extra nutrients to support the adolescent growth spurt, which begins in girls at ages 10 or 11, reaches its peak at age 12, and is completed at about 15. In boys, it begins at 12 or 13 years of age, peaks at 14, and ends at about 19.

In addition to other nutrients, adequate amounts of iron and calcium are particularly important as the body undergoes this intensive growth period. From ages 11 to 24 years, both males and females are encouraged to consume a calcium-rich diet (1,200 milligrams daily) in order to help ensure adequate calcium deposition in the bones during the age at which peak bone mass is attained. This may help reduce the incidence of osteoporosis in later years. By eating at least three servings daily from the milk, yogurt and cheese group, the recommended calcium intake easily can be achieved.

Teens' caloric needs vary depending on their growth rate, degree of physical maturation, body composition, and activity level. Being overweight is one of the most serious nutrition problems of adolescents, and eating disorders are common among teens, whose food choices are often influenced by social pressure to achieve cultural ideals of thinness, gain peer acceptance, or assert independence from parental authority. According to the National Center for Health Statistics, one in 100 females between the ages of 12 and 18 has anorexia nervosa, a disorder causing people to severely limit their food intake. Both anorexia and bulimia, a disorder in which people binge and purge by vomiting or using laxatives, can lead to convulsions, kidney failure, irregular heartbeats, osteoporosis, and dental erosion. One in five children, according to the National Institutes of Health, is overweight.[49]

In general, the following is a consensus from private and government nutritionists about the general nutritional needs of teens and younger children.

## Meal Patterns

To meet energy needs throughout the day, children and teens should eat at least three meals a day, beginning with breakfast. Studies show eating breakfast affects both cognitive and physical performance; that is, if a child eats breakfast, he or she may be more alert in school and better able to learn and perform sports or other physical activities.

Snacks also form an integral part of meal patterns for children and teens. Young children one to ten years generally cannot eat large quantities at one sitting and get hungry long before the next regular mealtime. Midmorning and midafternoon snacks are generally advised.

Fast-growing, active teens may have tremendous energy needs. Even though their regular meals can be substantial, they still may need snacks to supply energy between meals and to meet their daily nutrient needs.

The following composition of diet is recommended by the experts for healthy children:

1. **Total fat** intake should be approximately 30 percent of calories, with 10 percent or less from saturated fat, about 10 percent from monounsaturated fat, and less than 10 percent from polyunsaturated fat. The emphasis should be on reduction of total fat and, especially, saturated fat rather than an increase in polyunsaturated fat.

2. **Daily cholesterol** intake should be approximately 100 milligrams of cholesterol per 1,000 calories, not to exceed 300 milligrams. This allows for differences in caloric intake in various age groups.

3. **Protein** should be about 15 percent of calories, derived from various sources.

4. **Carbohydrate** calories should be derived primarily from complex carbohydrate sources to provide necessary vitamins and minerals. Thus, the total calories from carbohydrates would be about 55 percent.

5. **Salt** intake should be reduced. On the whole, the American diet contains too much salt, so keep the salt shaker out of reach. High blood pressure in children does occur, and it is believed that the child who is in the ninetieth percentile for blood pressure will go on to develop high blood pressure by the age of 35 or 40 years.

Menu choices for children that fit the aforementioned criteria:

| Meal | Food | Serving Size |
|------|------|--------------|
| Breakfast | Protein | |
| | egg or | 1 |
| | peanut butter or | 1 ounce |
| | cheese | 1 ounce |
| | Fat | |
| | margarine or | |
| | butter | 1 pat |
| | Carbohydrate | |
| | bread or | 1 to 2 slices |
| | cereal | ½ to 1 cup |
| | Calcium | |
| | milk or | 1 cup |
| | yogurt | 1 cup |
| | Fruit | |
| | orange or | 1 |
| | fruit juice or | 1 cup |
| | apple | 1 |

| Meal | Food | Serving Size *(cont.)* |
|---|---|---|
| Lunch | Protein | |
| | chicken or | 3 ounces |
| | tuna or | 3 ounces |
| | cheese | 3 ounces |
| | Carbohydrate | |
| | bread or | 1 slice |
| | pasta | 1 cup |
| | Fat | |
| | butter or | 1 pat |
| | mayonnaise | 1 tablespoon |
| | Vegetable | |
| | lettuce and/or | several leaves |
| | carrot sticks or | 4 |
| | celery sticks | 2 |
| | Fruit | |
| | apple or | 1 |
| | orange or | 1 |
| | dried apricots | ½ cup |
| | Calcium | |
| | milk or | 1 cup |
| | yogurt | 1 cup |
| Dinner | Protein | |
| | broiled or baked | 4 to 6 ounces |
| | fish, poultry, or | |
| | beef or | |
| | legumes | 1 cup cooked |
| | Carbohydrate | |
| | pasta or | ¾ cup cooked |
| | bread or | 1 to 2 slices |
| | rice | ¾ cup cooked |
| | Vegetables | |
| | green salad or | small plate |
| | carrots or peas or | |
| | broccoli or spinach | ¾ cup cooked |
| | Fat | |
| | butter or | 1 pat |

| Meal | Food | Serving Size *(cont.)* |
|---|---|---|
| | margarine or | 1 pat |
| | mayonnaise or | 2 tablespoons |
| | salad dressing | 2 tablespoons |
| | Calcium | |
| | milk or | 1 glass |
| | ice cream or | 1 scoop |
| | frozen yogurt | 1 scoop |
| | Fruit | |
| | apple or orange or | 1 |
| | grapes or | 1 bunch |
| | fruit cup or | 1 cup |
| | fruit juice | 6 ounces |
| | Snacks | |
| | Any fruit or juice or | 1 piece or 1 cup |
| | nuts or | ⅓ cup |
| | popcorn or | 2 cups popped |
| | whole-wheat | |
| | crackers or | 4 |
| | fruit pops | 1 |

Doris L. Pertz, a learning disabilities teacher and consultant in the Caldwell–West Caldwell (New Jersey) public schools, and Lillian Putnam, director of the reading clinic at the Caldwell public schools and a professor at Kean College of New Jersey in Union, pointed out that eating a nutritious breakfast results in improved student attention in late-morning task performance.[50]

In early life, caloric deficits lead to reduction of activity—less play with peers, less verbalizing, and less sensory stimulation. Because of this, these children enter school with minimal readiness for learning. A low level of sensory stimulation in preschool years and poor attention in the school-age child are associated with later manifestations of intellectual deficit.

Poor nutrition also increases absenteeism because it reduces the body's capacity to resist disease and infections.

Anemia caused by an iron-deficient diet also affects learning. A child's brain uses about half of the oxygen supply carried in the blood. Iron-deficient blood does not carry a normal oxygen load.

There is some thought that a low blood-oxygen level due to iron deficiency may contribute to reading disability.[51]

In addition, as pointed out in the toxicology and allergy chapters, a child who is suffering an adverse reaction to foods can have reduced attention to the learning task. Pertz and Putnam suggest:

• Teachers should work with parents and school authorities to remove candy, soft drinks, and caffeine beverages from vending machines and school cafeterias. These should be replaced with fruits, nuts, milk, and fruit drinks.

• Teachers should discourage fund-raising projects that rely on the sale of candy. Sales can emphasize nuts, dried fruits, and nonedible items.

For more information concerning children and nutrition, contact:

**Weight-Control Information Network** (A service of the National Institutes of Diabetes, Digestive and Kidney Diseases)
1 Win Way
Bethesda, MD 20892-3665
Phone: (301) 984-7378 or (800) WIN-8098
e-mail: win@info.niddk.nih.gov

**The National Center for Nutrition and Dietetics**
The American Dietetic Association
216 West Jackson Boulevard
Chicago, IL 60606-6995
Consumer Nutrition Hotline: (800) 366-1655

**President's Council on Physical Fitness and Sports**
701 Pennsylvania Avenue NW, Suite 250
Washington, DC 20004
Phone: (202) 272-3421

As a parent, you should:

***Try not to use food to punish or reward your child.*** Withholding food as a punishment may lead children to worry that they will not get enough food. For example, sending children to bed without any dinner may cause them to worry that they will go hungry. As a result, children may try to eat whenever they get a chance. Similarly, when foods such as sweets are used as a reward, children may assume that these foods are better or more valuable than other foods. For example, telling children that they will get dessert if they eat all of their vegetables sends the wrong message about vegetables.

***Set a good example.*** Children are good learners, and they learn best by example. Setting a good example for your kids by eating a variety of foods and being physically active will teach your children healthy lifestyle habits that they can follow for the rest of their lives.

As a parent, one of the most important gifts you can give your children is a wise way of eating. It will help their brains and bodies develop to their full potential and will probably make your youngsters easier to live with.

# 8

# Vitamins, Minerals, and Your Mind

*Laura, a pretty, shy, twenty-four-year-old bank teller, developed Tourette's syndrome, a little-understood condition whose symptoms are twitching and uncontrollable utterances. Her head would jerk and she would start swearing, which frightened her coworkers and customers. She was given* haloperidol, *a drug that dampens the production of dopamine, a brain neurotransmitter involved with movement and stress. The drug stopped the symptoms, but it affected Laura's ability to think to the point where she could no longer cash checks correctly. The situation was even more frustrating because she had been in line to be promoted; instead, she was fired.*

*Many physicians tried, but none could help her. Finally, a young doctor suggested she take large doses of* nicotinic acid, or vitamin B₃. *The B vitamins are known to affect the central nervous system. A severe B₃ deficiency called* pellagra *causes mental aberrations including excitement, disorientation, memory impairment, confusion, and delirium.[1] Laura's symptoms cleared up within a month, and within two months she was rehired at her old job.*

*Unfortunately, after five months on B₃, Laura developed symptoms of nausea, fatigue, and yellowed skin. She had developed a chemical hepatitis, a liver problem caused by the massive doses of B₃. She was hospitalized, taken off the vitamin, detoxified, and then returned home. Several days later, her Tourette's syndrome returned, and she was again dismissed from her job.*

*In desperation, Laura's mother telephoned Herman*

*Baker, Ph.D., director of the Division of Nutrition and Metabolism at the Newark site of New Jersey Medical School and a professor of preventive medicine. Dr. Baker, a world-famous authority on vitamin research, suggested to Laura's physician that perhaps $B_3$, but in a smaller dose, should be tried. The Tourette's symptoms cleared, the liver problems did not return, and Laura is now employed at another bank.*[2]

*Dr. Baker explains that $B_3$ is not a conventional treatment for Tourette's syndrome; nor has it been tested as such, but it seemed to work for that young woman.*

*In another dramatic case involving a B vitamin, an eighty-one-year-old man, Mr. L., was admitted to a western hospital with a one-week history of irritable mood associated with hyperactivity, sleeplessness, grand delusions, sexual indiscretion, and reckless and agitated behavior. He felt his hometown was planning a day of celebration in his honor to which several Hollywood personalities were invited. He was so active, in fact, that six younger men were required to restrain him at the time of admission to the hospital. Mr. L. had no family history of mental illness. His test results were normal and he had not been taking medicines. The only test that came back abnormal was the test for vitamin $B_{12}$ levels in his blood.*

*Mr. L. received a daily dose of vitamin $B_{12}$ in his muscle while he was in the hospital, then monthly injections after discharge.*

*The supplemental $B_{12}$ returned Mr. L. to a normal mental state, and six months later he was still completely normal. This case supports other recent reports that psychiatric symptoms may antedate other major clinical manifestations of $B_{12}$ deficiency such as pernicious anemia.*[3]

There is much about vitamins that is yet unknown and untested. They are by no means always harmless, as demonstrated by Laura's experience. For nearly half a century, researchers have been trying to determine the complex ways in which vitamins and minerals interact with each other and with the other nutrients and elements.

There are more than forty chemical elements and compounds in your body that must follow a predetermined recipe to keep you "cooking" just right, physically and mentally. These substances are found in the vitamins, minerals, fats, proteins, and carbohydrates that are essential to your brain and body functions. Vitamins are the team players who work with the other substances to convert the food you eat into energy and tissue growth. They help repair damage, maintain immunity, and perform other important processes.

Minerals perform a variety of functions, including influencing the acid/base balance of your body fluids and the distribution of water throughout your body. They also play an essential role in the formation of bones and teeth and in the life processes of your cells. Vitamins and minerals are exquisitely measured; too much or too little of any one of them can throw your system off track.

What amounts of vitamins and minerals do you need?

The Food and Nutrition Board of the National Academy of Sciences periodically issues recommended dietary allowances (RDAs). The values given are estimates based on a review of the current nutrition literature and, hence, subject to controversy. In fact, when they met in 1985, there was so much debate among the members of the board that they could not agree, and consequently no new RDAs were issued until 1989.[4]

When the 1989 RDAs were released they had some significant changes. For the first time, they set RDAs for vitamin K and the mineral selenium. They also lowered the iron for women and teenage males and, as you will read later in this chapter, made a big mistake—they lowered the folic acid by 50 percent.

The RDAs are supposedly set at levels high enough to prevent classic deficiency symptoms such as the skin eruptions and mental disorders associated with pellagra. However, preventing classic deficiencies is now believed to be just one of the important functions of vitamins.

In 1997, the National Academy released the first in a series of new nutritional recommendations called Dietary Reference Intakes (DRIs). The nutrition experts agreed that while the RDAs were designed to meet the nutritional needs of almost all healthy people, times have changed.

"Our understanding of the relationship between nutrition and chronic disease has progressed to the point where we can now begin to recommend intakes that are thought to help people achieve measurable physical indicators of good health," says Vernon Young, Ph.D., chair of the committee overseeing the DRIs. A professor of nutritional biochemistry at Massachusetts Institute of Technology, Cambridge, he notes: "The new DRIs represent a major leap forward in nutrition science—from a primary concern for the prevention of deficiency to an emphasis on beneficial effects of healthy eating." Then the National Institute of Medicine of the National Academy went even further. They came up with some and are working on more estimated levels of vitamins and minerals. In addition to RDAs and DRIs, they are working on:

**Adequate intake (AI).** When sufficient scientific evidence is not available to estimate an average requirement. We, they say, should use the AI as a goal for intake where no RDAs exist. The AI is derived through experimental or observational data.

**Estimated average requirement.** The intake that meets the estimated nutrient need of half the individuals in a specific group. This figure is to be used as the basis for developing RDAs.

**Tolerable upper intake level.** The maximum intake by an individual that is unlikely to pose risks of adverse health effects in almost all healthy individuals in a specified group. This is bound to be the most controversial specification of all.

As you can tell by now, government and scientific agencies are trying to make regulations somewhere between new scientific research concerning vitamins and minerals and our desire to self-dose with high levels of nutrients about which we may have heard—often through the media or health store personnel—that are of benefit.

While a description of the research on vitamins alone could fill many volumes, in this book we are primarily concerned with the known and suspected effects of these nutrients on brain function.

## The Mystery of the Biotin Baby

The effects of a vitamin or mineral deficiency can be unrecognized, and when the missing nutrient is added, its benefits can be dramatic. Dr. Baker, for example, diagnosed a genetic condition when he was sent blood samples from a newborn who was having almost continuous convulsions. He found a deficiency of the B vitamin *biotin* and suggested that the pediatrician give the baby 75 micrograms of the nutrient. The baby's seizures continued. Dr. Baker then suggested increasing the dosage to 10 milligrams, which is a massive dose. After the new dosage was administered, the seizures stopped. The baby thrived because the high dose of biotin overcame a missing element in his body. When the child was three years old, the pediatrician decided that perhaps the seizure cessation was just coincidental to the biotin supplement, and he told the mother to stop giving it. Within a short time, the toddler again began to have convulsions.[5]

Dr. Baker believes that many current testing methods do not accurately identify vitamin levels and that there are other undetected vitamin deficiencies that contribute to subtle behavior effects that are escaping diagnosis by the usual methods of physical examination. "Classical deficiency diseases have all but disappeared in the United States because of improved nutritional knowledge and the enrichment of certain foods," he maintains, "but marginal or subclinical stages of vitamin deficiency certainly do exist."[6]

In a 1967–68 study of 674 New York City schoolchildren between the ages of ten and thirteen years, for example, 25 percent were found to have undetected marginal deficiencies that may have affected their intellectual performance.[7]

## Marginal Deficiency

Marginal deficiency, by definition, is a state of gradual vitamin depletion in which there is evidence of personal lack of well being associated with impairment of certain chemical reactions in the body.[8] The reactions impaired are those that depend on sufficient amounts of vitamins.

Vitamin deficiency is not something that occurs abruptly or acutely. There are four basic stages:

1. **The preliminary stage.** Body stores of a micronutrient are gradually depleted. When there is not enough of a particular vitamin to work for the body, the body's chemistry is impaired. In this preliminary stage, there is *no indication* of depletion in clinical terms of growth or appearance.

2. **The physiological stage.** These changes are ones that you might not associate with nutrient deficiencies—for example, loss of appetite, depression, irritability, anxiety, insomnia, or sleepiness. The person is not sufficiently ill to seek medical care or go to the hospital, yet his or her general health is less than optimal. If the deficiency continues symptoms of classic deficiency disease will appear.

3. **The clinical stage.** Something is obviously seriously wrong and if left untreated the person progresses to the next stage.

4. **The anatomical stage,** in which death will occur without nutritional intervention.[9]

Marginal deficiencies, since they are so subtle, are difficult to identify. Only in recent years has sufficient evidence accumulated to call attention to this gray area of nutrition. To demonstrate just how the stages of a vitamin deficiency occur, a former research assistant of Dr. Baker's placed himself on a diet deficient in folic acid (vitamin B complex).[10] That meant no green vegetables, beans, walnuts, or chicken liver, all good sources of the vitamin necessary for the manufacture of genetic material (DNA) and healthy red blood cells. What occurred?

- *Two and a half weeks* after he began the diet, he noticed a low level of folic acid in his blood.
- *Ten to twelve weeks,* he began to detect a biochemical sign—an abnormal waste product of metabolism in his urine.
- *Sixteen weeks* into the diet, a bone marrow examination was performed to see whether he had any signs

of anemia and cell changes. He began to see evidence of folic acid deficiency in his red blood cells.

- *Seventeen weeks* later, his body's new red blood cells were being formed with low folic acid.
- *Twenty-five weeks* after beginning the diet he saw the full-blown anemia due to folic acid deficiency.

Dr. Baker maintains that a clinician who looks at a blood picture and sees a patient suffering from an early, marginal deficiency, as in the case above when the research assistant first had low levels of folic acid, should treat that patient then, rather than wait for the clinical signs. In the case of folic acid deficiency, it took twenty-five to thirty weeks to show a full-blown anemia. Many clinicians, however, would just ignore these early signs. They would say vitamins are ubiquitous and there is no need for supplementation. However, if there were a similar picture as the research assistant's but instead of folic acid deficiency there was too much sugar in the blood, what would a physician do? He'd say, "Hey, I'm not going to wait around till this fellow goes blind and his kidneys fail," as can happen with advanced diabetes. He would begin to treat him with insulin. He wouldn't wait.[11]

Only a blood analysis of vitamins can help detect subclinical deficits and can avoid physiologic and eventually full-blown vitamin deficits, the same as one would do to check cholesterol levels to avoid eventual heart disease. According to Dr. Baker, many older persons suffer from undiagnosed marginal deficiencies that cause mental and physical problems. They have these nutrient deficiencies, even though they may be eating nutritious meals and taking supplemental vitamins orally, because they can no longer absorb sufficient nutrients. He and his colleagues proved this by testing the elderly residents.

"We found that the residents' livers were not able to bind enough vitamins as younger people can and that the residents were also taking drugs that deplete nutrients. Since they could not absorb sufficient vitamins from food or supplementation by mouth to saturate the liver, we gave them an injection of a bolus of vitamins, more than the conventional RDAs. We continued to monitor them and found their vitamin levels were normal for three months; then began to decline after that until they were back to deficient after a year. Therefore, we felt they needed vitamin injections every three months.

"The nurses told us the patients improved following the injection. Some who were bedridden were able to get out of bed. Others were able to return to a sheltered workshop. All seemed to function better mentally. In fact, the nurses asked us if we wouldn't give them vitamin injections, too."[12]

Among common nutritional deficiencies with potential relevance to mental problems, folate deficiency appears to be the most closely linked to depression.[13] Borderline low or deficient blood folate levels have been detected in 15 to 38 percent of adults diagnosed with depressive disorders, according to Harvard Medical School researchers Dr. Jonathan Alpert and Dr. Maurizio Fava. They also note low folate levels have been linked to poorer response to antidepressants that affect serotonin levels. In a retrospective survey, psychiatric patients treated with folic acid spent less time in the hospital and exhibited mood improvement and better social functioning than those with low folate levels who did not receive supplemental folate.

New Jersey Medical School's Dr. Baker feels that many clinicians are unaware that widespread subclinical or marginal vitamin deficiencies exist and do not know how to test for these deficiencies.[14]

## How Do You Know If You Have a Marginal Deficiency?

Dr. Baker says:

- You'll always feel tired.
- You may have insomnia.
- You may have a loss of appetite.
- You may have a decreased ability to concentrate.
- Your brain does not function well.
- You complain to your physician, "I feel under the weather. I don't know what is bothering me but I keep getting colds."

"The doctor examines you and tells you he can find nothing wrong. So he says, 'Take some vitamins!' If you have an absorption problem or the liver cannot bind or store vitamins, you can take a ton of vitamins but you will just enrich the sewage system. You can take one-tenth or three-tenths of a milligram of vitamin $B_{12}$, and you won't absorb any more than one-tenth milligram since that is all your body can absorb at one time. The rest is wasted. But if you break the dose into three times a day, you can absorb a total of three-tenths of a milligram of thiamine a day."[15]

According to Dr. Baker, taking vitamins with food will aid absorption, while mineral supplements are best absorbed when taken between meals. "Not only lay persons but physicians are often unaware of these simple facts," he maintains.[16]

The following provides descriptions of functions of vitamins and minerals. Some of it is on the cutting edge of research.

## Bs Are for the Brain

A trio of B vitamins given to a group of people who had suffered a stroke reduced two biochemical markers that could damage their arteries and lead to another stroke. The two were:

- *Homocysteine,* a natural byproduct of the body's metabolism of protein and other nutrients that in high levels in laboratory studies have been shown to damage blood vessels.
- *Thrombomodulin,* produced by injured cells lining blood vessels and involved in blood clotting.[17]

Scientists reported significant reduction in these two biochemical markers in 27 patients who received a vitamin supplement with folic acid, $B_6$, and $B_{12}$ added to it, compared to 23 patients who got the vitamin preparation without the B vitamins.

The study was not designed to determine whether giving the B vitamins would reduce the risk of a second stroke, but the results show the ability to manipulate these markers and indicate the need for further work on the potential protective benefits of the B vitamins, says Richard F. Macko, M.D., of the Baltimore Veterans Administration Medical Center and assistant professor of neurology and geriatrics at the University of Maryland. "It now appears, based on numerous epidemiological studies, that homocysteine increases the risk of stroke and heart attack even when elevated to mild amounts in the bloodstream."

"It is remarkable that only three months of vitamin therapy can produce these kinds of changes," Dr. Macko says.

## New B Vitamin?

In another development, a new B vitamin, NADH, the abbreviation for *nicotinamide adenine dinucleotide,* is expected to be named. At this writing, it is called coenzyme #1. A coenzyme is any of a group of relatively small organic molecules that make up the nonprotein portion of an enzyme, the workhorse of the cell that processes a substance. The enzyme is inactive without the coenzyme. Vitamins can act as coenzymes. NADH stimulates the neurotransmitter production of dopamine, which enhances the body's ability to repair or replace damaged and wounded cells. It also is the neurotransmitter involved in Parkinson's disease. Patients given NADH showed elevated levels of L-dopa and dopamine in the blood. The FDA is expected to name it a "B" vitamin after it completes evaluating testing efforts in the medical treatment of degenerative and chronic diseases.[18]

The water-soluble B-complex vitamins are usually found in the same foods but here are some of the symptoms of deficiency and benefits of supplementation for individual Bs.

*Vitamin B₁ (thiamine).* The link between vitamin B₁ and brain function is direct and strong. Our bodies cannot manufacture vitamin B₁ yet it is needed to process the only fuel the brain can use: glucose. Because of this vital need in thiamine-dependent carbohydrate (sugar and starch) metabolism, the nervous system is particularly susceptible to thiamine deficiency.[19] Vitamin B₁ is necessary not only for the health of your nerve tissue, for your intestinal and cardiovascular functions, your appetite and your growth.

Deficiency in its early stages produces:

- Fatigue
- Irritation
- Poor memory
- Sleep disturbance
- Chest pain
- Loss of appetite
- Abdominal discomfort

- Constipation
- Later symptoms are numbness, a burning sensation in the feet, calf muscle cramps, and leg pains.

A combination of decreased intake, impaired absorption, inadequate utilization, and increased requirements occur in alcoholism. Even a glass of wine or a cocktail reduces absorption of thiamine by your gut. Incidentally, marinating meat in wine, soy sauce, or vinegar depletes between 50 and 75 percent of its thiamine content.

Thiamine treatment—as much as 300 milligrams per day—is used in cases of Wernicke's encephalopathy, an acute brain disorder sometimes called "cerebral beriberi" in which, in the early stages, there is mental confusion, inability to think of a word, and making up of "facts." As it progresses, there are delusions, loss of memory, loss of balance, and eye problems. This syndrome is associated with thiamine deficiency. In industrialized countries, the disorder occurs most frequently in alcoholics. In fact, the brain damage caused by alcohol in this syndrome has only recently been directly attributed to a lack of thiamine. Australian psychiatrists, as a result, want to add thiamine to alcoholic beverages—beer, in particular—to prevent brain damage. They calculated that the annual cost of adding thiamine to the entire supply of Australian beer would be no higher than the cost of supporting eight alcoholics with Wernicke's psychosis for one year.[20] Many other Australian researchers believe that treatment with thiamine and abstinence from alcohol can reverse brain damage, including the shrinkage, caused by alcohol.[21] Cerebral beriberi has also been associated with intravenous feedings, starvation, neurological disease, chronic infection, kidney dialysis, cancer, anemia, and scurvy.[22]

## What About Marginal Deficiency?

As early as 1946, one scientist noted a liberal thiamine intake improved a number of mental and physical skills of children in orphanages.[23]

In a study concerning human starvation, another investigator observed thiamine deficiency in close detail and found that lack of well-being, anxiety, hysteria, nausea, depression, and loss of appetite preceded any aspect of the clinical state of beriberi. These

## VITAMIN B₁ Sources

| Very Good | Good |
|---|---|
| Wheat germ | Collard greens |
| Lobster | Enriched or whole-wheat spaghetti |
| Pinto beans | Enriched or brown rice |
| Roast pork | Fortified milk |
| Kasha | Asparagus |
| Oat flakes | Lima beans |
| Sunflower seeds | Cauliflower |
| Brewer's yeast | Pecans |
| Soybeans | Shredded wheat |
| Black-eyed peas | Broccoli |
| Green peas | |
| Whole-wheat bread | |

personality changes were all typical of pure thiamine deficiency and were normalized within a short period following the addition of thiamine to the diet.[24]

Other studies, using a behavior test called the Minnesota Multiphasic Personality Index (MMPI), have demonstrated that adverse behavioral changes precede physical findings in thiamine deficiency, as shown in Mr. L.'s case at the beginning of this chapter, as well as in deficiencies of vitamin C and riboflavin. The deficiencies of these nutrients were induced in human subjects under carefully controlled laboratory conditions; then subjects were given the MMPI test. Hypochondria, depression, hysteria, and, in some cases, manic and crazy behavior were described by the investigators as occurring before any specific physical signs of vitamin deficiency were observed.[25]

Extensive studies on the effects of thiamine depletion on human red blood cells have definitely been correlated with changes in behavior.[26] Depleted subjects most commonly complained of lethargy, loss of appetite, and fatigue. Since no obvious physical signs of thiamine deficiency were noted, such symptoms were believed to be caused by a marginal deficiency. This belief was proven true when the behavior of subjects reverted to normal within two to three days after thiamine was again present in their diets.[27]

A group of enzymes called *thiaminases,* which destroy thiamine, have been found in raw fish (as in an increasingly popular Japanese dish, sushi), shellfish, some berries, Brussels sprouts, and red cabbage. However, these enzymes are inactivated by cooking. The Reference Daily Intake for thiamine is 1.5 milligrams for adults and 0.3 to 1.1 milligrams for infants and children.

***Vitamin $B_2$ (riboflavin).*** Vitamin $B_2$ is also called *lactoflavin* or *hepatoflavin* because milk and liver are its main natural sources. Deficiency is associated with:

- Lip and mouth lesions
- Flaky skin around the nose, eyebrows, and hairline
- Teary, bloodshot eyes
- Indigestion, since $B_2$ aids in the digestion of fats
- Easy fatigability
- Irritability

This vitamin is believed to fight stress. Riboflavin has a high affinity for your brain and helps to explain the long-standing observation that even in severe riboflavin deficiency its concentration in the brain does not decline appreciably. Ironically, while riboflavin reportedly fights stress and is similar in chemical structure to the tranquilizer chlorpromazine (Thorazine), the medication depletes riboflavin. Inhibition of riboflavin metabolism is also observed with the tricyclic antidepressant drugs imipramine and amitriptyline.[28]

The Reference Daily Intake for vitamin $B_2$ is 1.7 milligrams for men, 1.2 to 1.3 milligrams for women, and 0.4 to 1.6 milligrams for infants and children.

## VITAMIN B$_2$ Sources

| Very Good | Good |
|---|---|
| Beef and beef liver | Noodles |
| Milk | Peas |
| Brewer's yeast | Spinach |
| Ham | Puffed and flaked wheat |
| Sunflower seeds | Chocolate chip cookies |
| Broccoli | Oatmeal with raisins |
| Butternut squash | Custard |
| Wild rice | Asparagus |
| Almonds | |
| Cottage cheese | |

*Niacin (B$_3$ or niacinamide, or nicotinic acid).* At least forty biochemical reactions depend on this B vitamin, niacin. Perhaps the most important involves red blood cells, which carry oxygen to all parts of your body, including your brain. Niacin, when taken in large doses, causes flushing, itching, dilation of the blood vessels, increased blood flow in the brain, and decreased blood pressure. It can lower blood cholesterol and is being used for that purpose. Niacin also has been found to counteract some of the effects of caffeine. Pellagra is a disease caused by the lack of the vitamin niacin or of the amino acid tryptophan (which is converted in the body to nicotinic acid). It afflicts people whose dietary protein comes mainly from corn. It also occurs in vegetarians and in some alcoholics or in people with disorders of absorption. The clinical signs of pellagra are the three Ds—dermatitis, diarrhea, and dementia.

Niacin is made in your gut from the amino acid tryptophan, which derives from protein. Tryptophan also serves as the raw material for the manufacture of the calming neurotransmitter serotonin. Therefore, it is not surprising that striking and profound mental disturbance may frequently occur as part of this B-vitamin deficiency. The brain and nerve symptoms caused by B deficiency are not completely understood, but problems with brain nerve messenger (neurotransmitter) serotonin have been suggested as the basis.[29]

Large doses of niacin have been used to treat schizophrenia. Drs. Abram Hoffer and Humphry Osmond, who consider the disease to be caused by a biochemical abnormality, reported outstanding improvement in many of the thousands of patients treated. But other investigators reported that they could not duplicate those results. There is a theory that schizophrenia is actually many diseases, some of which are responsive to niacin. This seems to be backed by a study made by Dr. J. Richard Wittenborn of Rutgers University. Dr. Wittenborn studied schizophrenics for two years at a New Jersey state hospital. At first he found that patients receiving the vitamin showed no impressive gains as compared to patients not receiving it. But when Dr. Wittenborn went back over the original study, he decided that some patients treated with the vitamin had responded more than others and that the response was significant.[30]

Usually, not enough niacin is manufactured from tryptophan by bacteria in your gut to keep you in good health. You need to obtain more of it from your diet. The Reference Daily Intake for adults is 20 milligrams and for infants and children, 6 to 16 milligrams.

## VITAMIN $B_3$ Sources

| Very Good | Good |
|---|---|
| Turkey | Muffins made with enriched flour |
| Tofu | Peanuts |
| Calf's liver | Enriched or whole-wheat noodles |
| Bulgur wheat | Oats |
| Puffed wheat | Corn flakes |
| Halibut | Barley |
| Peanuts | Bagels |
| Hamburger | Kale |
| Tuna | Broccoli |
| Coffee | Enriched French bread |
| Cottage Cheese | Corn tortilla |
| Peas | Enriched spaghetti |
| Beans | Brown rice |
| Milk | Mangos |

*Vitamin $B_6$ (pyridoxine).* Vitamin $B_6$ is believed to act as a partner for more than one hundred different enzymes. A number of the

## VITAMIN B$_6$ Sources

| Very Good | Good |
|-----------|------|
| Wheat germ | Brown rice |
| Brewer's yeast | Ham |
| Bananas | Spinach |
| Fish | Peanuts |
| Soybeans | Cantaloupe |
| Tomatoes | Milk |
| Salmon | Cabbage |
| Kale | Raisins |
| Spinach | Broccoli |
| Beans | Asparagus |
| Sunflower seeds | Cauliflower |

brain's neurotransmitters depend on B$_6$ for formation. A deficiency in this vitamin is known to cause depression and mental confusion. The occurrence of seizures in experimental animals in response to vitamin B$_6$ antagonists have been observed by many. Similar seizures were observed in human infants made vitamin B$_6$ deficient intentionally or inadvertently when they were fed a commercial infant formula in which the vitamin had not been properly preserved. Certain substances that deplete B$_6$ also produce deficiency seizures.[31]

Vitamin B$_6$ also reportedly helps rid the body tissues of the excess fluid that causes some of the symptoms of premenstrual tension.

Two possible causes have been suggested for the frequent deficiency of vitamin B$_6$ in alcoholics. Alcohol may inhibit the body's absorption of the vitamin from the intestine and it may cause B$_6$ to break down prematurely in the blood. Reduced levels of vitamin B$_6$ have also been found in smokers, but this may be due to their higher alcohol use.

Estrogen and cortisone deplete B$_6$. Storage over a long period of time diminishes the vitamin. Freezing vegetables results in 57 to 77 percent reduction of their B$_6$ content.

Overdosing on B$_6$, on the other hand, is very unwise. A study in the *New England Journal of Medicine* in 1983 reported the loss of balance and numbness suffered by seven young adults who took from 2 to 6 grams of pyridoxine daily for several months to a year.[32] Discontinuation of the supplements resulted in improvement in all subjects, although a few continued to have residual abnormalities in nerve conduction as late as six months afterward.

The Reference Daily Intakes for vitamin $B_6$ are 2.2 milligrams for adults and 0.3 to 1.6 milligrams for infants and children.

***Vitamin $B_{12}$*** is one vitamin that is believed to be deficient and yet vitally needed for the aging brain. It is known to be necessary for normal growth, a healthy nervous system, and normal red blood cell formation. It can be found only in animal and dairy products. A $B_{12}$ deficiency produces pernicious anemia, a severe anemia similar to that caused by a $B_6$ deficiency. Vitamin $B_{12}$ anemia is rarely the result of dietary deficiency, except in vegans (vegetarians who consume no animal food or dairy products), since the liver stores sufficient quantities to sustain the body's needs for three to five years. Vegetarians may obtain vitamin $B_{12}$ by eating fermented foods such as tamari or tofu or by eating large amounts of raw fruits and vegetables. It is believed that they can then manufacture $B_{12}$ in their own systems with the aid of friendly bacteria in fermented or raw edibles. Like the other B vitamins, a deficiency in $B_{12}$ can lead to brain and nerve damage. In most patients, the symptoms develop insidiously and progressively as the large liver stores of $B_{12}$ are depleted. As has been noted, as we grow older, there is less stomach acid to process $B_{12}$ and taking the vitamin by mouth is often ineffective. It must be given by injection about once a month.

Symptoms of deficiency include:

- Loss of appetite
- Intermittent constipation and diarrhea
- Stomach pain
- Fatigue
- Patchy, diffuse, and progressive nerve degeneration; there may be a loss of balance, numbness, and weakness of the limbs
- Irritability
- Mild depression
- Paranoia, a condition known as megaloblastic madness[33]

Alcohol, estrogen, and sleeping pills can lower $B_{12}$ levels in the body. Vitamin C, however, does not destroy vitamin $B_{12}$, as some medical reports have proposed. Dr. Baker and associates tested Nobelist Linus Pauling, an advocate of massive doses of vitamin C, and Dr. Pauling's colleagues, all of whom had taken large amounts of vitamin C for years. Dr. Baker found that all of the vitamin C takers had normal levels of $B_{12}$.[34]

The Reference Daily Intake for $B_{12}$ is 6 micrograms for adults and 0.5 to 3 micrograms for infants and children.

## Vitamin $B_{12}$ Sources

| Very Good | Good |
| --- | --- |
| Beef liver | Swiss cheese |
| Roast beef | Whole or skim milk |
| Ham | Eggs |
| Filet of sole | Cottage cheese |
| Oysters | Yogurt |
| Sardines | |
| Crab | |
| Herring | |

***Fortifying with folic acid.*** This B complex vitamin, folic acid, is necessary for the division and replacement of red blood cells. It is needed for protein metabolism and the utilization of sugar. A deficiency anemia may occur, especially in menstruating women, but it is less common than other anemias caused by a B deficiency. Folic acid is needed in the manufacture of genetic material. Folic acid supplementation has been used in the treatment of alcohol withdrawal. A deficiency can also cause gastrointestinal upsets and emotional irritability.

Newer research shows that folic acid protects against blood vessel disease and also confers protection against serious birth defects. Women who take multivitamins with folic acid several months before and after they become pregnant can greatly reduce their risk of having a baby with a neural tube birth defect such as spina bifida. The U.S. Public Health Service has officially recommended that all

## FOLIC ACID SOURCES

| Very Good | Good |
|---|---|
| Deep-green leafy vegetables | Cantaloupe |
| Carrots | Dark rye flour |
| Apricots | Shredded wheat |
| Asparagus | Cottage cheese |
| Navy beans | Chuck pot roast |
| Chicken liver | Avocados |
| Wheat bran | Eggs |
| Walnuts | Sweet potatoes |
| Brewer's yeast | Grapefruit juice |
| Beans, especially soybeans | Potatoes |
| Orange juice | Bananas |

women of childbearing age should get 0.4 milligrams (400 micrograms) of folic acid daily, for the prevention of birth defects.

Every study that has been done to prove this effect has been done with multivitamin supplements containing folic acid or with folic acid alone. Yet public health officials in the U.S. have bent over backwards to think of ways to deliver the recommended amount of folic acid without endorsing the use of supplements. The Food and Drug Administration has mandated folic acid fortification of enriched breads and other grain products, at 140 micrograms per 100 grams of cereal grain. The Centers for Disease Control and Prevention advocates 300 micrograms per 100 grams. Other groups such as the AMA are against fortifying food with folic acid because they say it may harm some that do not need the supplementation.

Nevertheless, many believe the proposed fortification is not high enough. Dr. Godfrey Oakley of the Centers for Disease Control and Prevention believes that to obtain 800 micrograms per day of folic acid from foods would require consuming:[35]

- 6 cups orange juice;
- 11 cups romaine lettuce;
- 33 eggs; or
- 7 cups broccoli.

The trade organization for supplements is the Council for Responsible Nutrition (CRN). President and Chief Executive Officer John Cordaro added, "Federal policy makers should move quickly to inform consumers about these life-saving findings, and the rational use of supplements to achieve protective intakes of these and other essential nutrients."[36]

Alcohol and contraceptives reduce the body's absorption of this vitamin and thus increase the risk of deficiency. Sunlight and aspirin can deplete it. The sugar from fruit, vegetables, and grain enhances the absorption of folic acid.

The Reference Daily Intake for folic acid is 400 micrograms or 0.4 milligrams for adults and 30 to 300 micrograms for infants and children.

**Biotin.** Biotin is a B vitamin involved in many of your body's functions, including the metabolism of sugar and the formation of certain fatty acids. It was once thought that biotin deficiencies occur only in infants. However, in a 1942 study, seven adult volunteers were fed 200 grams of dehydrated egg whites per day, in addition to an otherwise balanced diet.[37] (A vitamin antagonist in raw eggs contains avidin, a substance that binds up biotin and makes it nonabsorbable; cooking destroys the avidin.) After five weeks, the subjects displayed symptoms of mild depression, lassitude, sleepiness, hallucinations, anxiety with muscle pain, and oversensitivity to pain stimuli. After eight weeks, loss of appetite, a grayish pallor, and a skin rash occurred. The experiment was terminated because of the falling food intake. The symptoms disappeared within five days of treatment with 75 to 300 milligrams per day of intravenous biotin.

A biotin deficiency is rare, except in children born with an inborn error of metabolism. The Reference Daily Intake is 0.3 milligrams for both adults and children. The RDA is 100 to 200 mcg.

## BIOTIN SOURCES

| Very Good | Good |
| --- | --- |
| Peanuts | Chicken |
| Liver | Halibut |
| Mushrooms | Cauliflower |
| Yeast | Milk |
| Cauliflower | Lamb |
| Egg yolks | |

***Pantothenic Acid.*** Pantothenic acid is needed for the adrenal glands, which are located above the kidneys and which secrete adrenaline, and to convert fat and glucose into energy. In studies with both rats and humans, those with high levels of pantothenic acid had more endurance when swimming in cold water.[38] The rats with low levels of the vitamin were able to swim only sixteen minutes in the cold water, while those with high levels were able to swim sixty-two minutes. The humans with high levels of the vitamin showed less wear and tear on a biochemical level than did those with low levels during a ten-minute swim in forty-five-degree water.

Some researchers believe that when the adrenal glands contain high levels of pantothenic acid, the body is better able to deal with stress.[39] In fact, the discoverer of pantothenic acid, Dr. Roger Williams, named it the Latin word for "from all sides." Pantothenic acid deficiency is rare, because the vitamin is found in most foods. However, food processing such as canning or freezing destroys as much as 75 percent of a food's pantothenic acid content. Sleeping pills, alcohol, caffeine, and estrogen also destroy it. A deficiency may result in such symptoms as malaise, abdominal distress, and a burning sensation in the feet associated with numbness.[40]

The Reference Daily Intake is 10 milligrams daily for adults, 35 to 40 nanograms for infants, and 65 to 120 nanograms for children and adolescents.

| PANTOTHENIC ACID SOURCES | |
|---|---|
| **Very Good** | **Good** |
| Brewer's yeast | Eggs |
| Beef liver | Milk |
| Bran | Fresh vegetables |
| Cereal | |

***Vitamin C (ascorbic acid).*** The level of vitamin C in the brain is second only to that found in the adrenal glands. This has led researchers to believe that vitamin C plays an important role in fighting stress. Since vitamin C is so abundant in the brain, it is assumed to be needed there, but its full role has yet to be identified. Numerous studies have noted a relationship between vitamin C and brain function, and behavior. The interplay between vitamin C and the amino acids suggests it may play a vital role in the regulation of the brain nerve cells' messengers, the neurotransmitters. Vitamin C, for example, has been found to be needed as a helper in the manufacture of norepinephrine, a major brain neurotransmitter that acts as a stimulant.[41]

The blood-brain barrier has long been regarded as the body's most formidable gatekeeper. It seems to prevent much vitamin C from entering the brain, but the brain has more vitamin C concentration than any other organ of the body. Vitamin C is an antioxidant that is essential to keep the central nervous system functioning properly.[42] Now, researchers at the Memorial Sloan-Kettering Cancer Center in New York City have discovered how to get large amounts of vitamin C past the blood-brain barrier. This finding may prove useful in efforts to slow the progression of certain neurodegenerative diseases, such as Alzheimer's. Oncologist Dr. David Agus and his colleagues had established that specific "sugar train" (glucose transporter) molecules were responsible for railroading vitamin C into cells. This process occurs when vitamin C, which is used by cells in the form of ascorbic acid, is converted into dehydroascorbic acid and transported by the "sugar train" into the cell. Once inside, the vitamin is converted back to ascorbic acid.

Although scientists do not know the exact role that vitamin C plays in the brain, recent studies have shown that various vitamin compounds with antioxidant-like properties can slow the progres-

## VITAMIN C SOURCES

| Very Good | Good |
|---|---|
| Brussels sprouts | Enriched flour |
| Cauliflower | Tomatoes |
| Freshly squeezed orange juice | Puffed wheat |
| Sweet potatoes | Waffles |
| Broccoli | Potatoes |
| Papaya | Collard greens |
| Cabbage | Spinach |
| Watermelon | Apricots |
| Grapefruit | Avocados |
| Green and red peppers | Pineapple |
| Honeydew melon | Corn flakes |
| Strawberries | |
| Kale | |

sion of moderately severe Alzheimer's disease. In addition, vitamin C is also known to act as a scavenger of free radicals—substances that play a role in causing diseases. The Sloan-Kettering scientists believe brain vitamin C can be increased by increasing dehydroascorbic acid in the blood but they say it can not be done by just taking an oral supplement because most of it would be excreted in the urine.[43]

If you smoke and drink alcohol, you may want to take vitamin C to make these bad habits less harmful. This is because vitamin C helps prevent damage from free radicals, the extremely reactive unstable molecules that are produced in the body through normal biologic processes as well as in the environment through radiation, sunlight, air pollution, cigarette smoke, and other chemical processes. Free radicals have been linked to aging, cancer, arthritis, lung inflammation, and senility. (*See* pages 199 and Glossary.) This may explain why, on average, heavy smokers are known to have lower levels of vitamin C in their blood than do nonsmokers.

Vitamin C is also needed for teeth and bone formation, bone fracture healing, wound and burn healing, and resistance to infections and other diseases. A deficiency can produce weakness, swollen and tender joints, loose teeth, delayed wound healing, easy bruising, and loss of appetite.

The Reference Daily Intake for vitamin C is 60 milligrams for adults and 35 to 45 milligrams for children. Vitamin C is reduced by aspirin. Cooking can destroy a food's vitamin C content.

**Vitamin D (calciferol).** Vitamin D is needed to absorb calcium, the building block of bone, so a deficiency of this vitamin will cause rickets and other bone diseases. Alcohol may impair the body's processing of vitamin D, causing it to build up to dangerous levels. Too much vitamin D can cause:

- Loss of appetite
- Elevated cholesterol
- Drowsiness, headache
- Kidney failure
- Calcium deposits in organs[44]

Most of the natural foodstuffs we consume contain only trivial quantities of vitamin D. Because these small amounts appear to have little effect on the status of vitamin D in our bodies, researchers believe that there are several means by which the body obtains it, one of which is through the action of sunshine on the skin. Conversion of vitamin D to its active forms involves the liver and kidneys, both of which may become less efficient with aging.

The Reference Daily Intake for vitamin D is 400 international units for adults and children.

### VITAMIN D SOURCES

| Very Good | Good |
|---|---|
| Cod liver oil | Fortified milk |
| Sardines | Fortified soybean milk |
| Salmon | Cheese |
| Egg yolk | |
| Tuna | |

**Vitamin A.** The nutritional requirement for the fat-soluble vitamin A for you, as an individual, will depend on a number of related factors, including age, growth rate, sex, your body's efficiency in absorbing and storing the vitamin, and the efficiency of transporting

## VITAMIN A SOURCES

| Very Good | Good |
| --- | --- |
| Beef liver | Milk |
| Bok choy | Prunes |
| Spinach | Asparagus |
| Cantaloupe | Green beans |
| Kale | Brussels sprouts |
| Carrots | Corn |
| Broccoli | Eggs |
| Apricots | Orange, tomato, or |
| Red peppers | Grapefruit juice |
| Fish oil | Margarine |
| Sweet potatoes | Peas |
| Butternut squash | Yogurt |
| Papaya | Peaches |

it in your blood and utilizing it by your cells. Intestinal, kidney, and liver disease tend to increase the need for vitamin A. Other vitamin A depleters include alcohol, cortisone (often used to treat inflammation), and mineral oil (taken frequently, especially by older people, in laxatives). Vitamin A is needed for the health of the skin and the inner lining of the body—the mucous membranes that protect the throat, nasal passages, bronchial tubes, digestive system, and genitourinary tract. It helps to maintain the structure of cell membranes and is necessary for the healthy functioning of your immune system.

Primary deficiency of vitamin A, of course, occurs from inadequate intake. Secondary deficiency arises from an increased requirement due to an overactive thyroid gland, pregnancy, breastfeeding, or fever. It also results from impaired absorption, as in chronic diarrhea, and from inadequate utilization, as in severe liver disease. A government survey showed that half of the people aged eighteen to forty-four years in the United States take in less than the RDA of vitamin A.[45] The Reference Daily Intake is 5,000 international units for men, 4,000 international units for women, and 1,400 to 3,000 international units for infants and children.

One major problem, as far as the brain is concerned, is vitamin A overdosing. It can cause:

- Drowsiness
- Irritability
- Headache
- Vomiting
- Pressure on the brain that produces tumorlike symptoms

Overdosing on beta-carotene, the vegetable form of vitamin A, does not produce the serious side effects of a vitamin A overdose but may cause your skin to turn yellow.[46]

***Vitamin E (tocopherol).*** New research has shown vitamins E and C collaborate in protecting the blood vessels and other tissues against damage by oxidation. They slow down the process of deterioration of the brain and body and help prevent strokes.

A stroke is a form of cardiovascular disease, so it is vital to keep blood vessels feeding the heart and brain healthy. Stroke—the third leading cause of death in the United States—occurs when part of the brain is damaged by not receiving a sufficient blood supply. There are several types of stroke:

> *Cerebral thrombosis,* the most common, occurs when a blood clot forms and blocks blood flow in an artery bringing blood to the brain. It usually develops in arteries damaged by atherosclerosis.
> *Cerebral embolus,* which also involves a block, but is usually caused by a wandering blood clot.
> *Subarachnoid hemorrhage* occurs when a blood vessel on the surface of the brain ruptures and bleeds into the space between the brain and the skull, causing pressure on the brain.
> *Cerebral hemorrhage* is caused by a defective artery in the brain that bursts.

A very common cause of stroke is a blockage in a carotid artery. One of these two major conveyors of blood to your brain lies on each side of your neck.

The National Institute of Neurological Disorders and Stroke of the National Institutes of Health (NINDS) is sponsoring the Asymptomatic Carotid Atherosclerosis Study (ACAS), a major multicenter prevention trial. The carotids on either side of the neck are the major arteries feeding blood to the brain. One result reported thus far is that an operation to clean out the carotid artery in the neck is significantly better than the best medical treatment in preventing strokes.

At this writing, the NINDS is sponsoring a major multicenter trial to determine if a healthy diet and common nutrients can prevent strokes from recurring. The study involving 3,600 patients at about 36 medical centers. Dr. James F. Toole of Bowman Gray School of Medicine—the coordinating center—says that the trial is measuring whether the nutrients prevent second strokes or heart attacks in patients who already have had one mild, nondisabling stroke. The incidence of second stroke in patients who have had first strokes is between 7 and 10 percent per year. In addition, many first stroke patients soon have a heart attack. Can both conditions be headed off by the nutrients?[47]

Stephen Kritchevsky, Ph.D., of the division of Biostatistics and Epidemiology, Department of Preventive Medicine, University of Tennessee, and his colleagues have already studied the average carotid artery wall thickness in 6,318 female and 4,989 male participants 45 to 64 years old in the Atherosclerosis Risk Communities Study. They used a food-frequency questionnaire and correlated the answers with the thickness of the study participant's carotid arteries. They found that among men and women older than 55 years old there was an inverse relationship between vitamin C intake and average artery wall thickness. An inverse relationship was also seen between wall thickness and vitamin E intake but was significant only in women.[48]

Vitamin E may also protect against or slow down Alzheimer's disease, that memory-robbing, degenerative brain disease. A two-year clinical trial funded by the NIH, determined that 2,000 international units of alpha-tocopherol (vitamin E) daily, 10 milligrams of the medication selegiline daily, or a combination of the two slowed the functional deterioration seen in moderately severe Alzheimer's patients.[49] There are characteristic nerve tangles and amyloid deposits in victims' brains. Amyloid is a protein substance in tissues and organs that are undergoing degeneration. When excessive amyloid builds up on the brain, it interferes with the brain's nerve network, disrupting normal function. Some researchers believe it is oxidation of free radicals (see Glossary) that causes the build up of amyloid that eventually leads to Alzheimer's.[50] Vitamin E, of course, is an antioxidant.

## VITAMIN E AND PARKINSON'S DISEASE

Parkinson's, a chronic neurologic disease of unknown cause, is characterized by tremors, rigidity, and abnormal gait. Does oxygen damage to cells caused by environmental factors contribute to the development of Parkinsonism? If so, then antioxidants such as vitamin E may be effective in early treatment of the disease.[51]

A preliminary trial with vitamin E in Parkinson's patients was encouraging, and some Parkinson's patients, who were self-supplementing with vitamin E, reportedly had significantly less severe disease symptoms than those matched controls.[52]

In addition, patients with tardive dyskinesia showed some improvement on vitamin E. This is a disorder caused by long-term use of certain tranquilizers and other drugs that affect the brain. One of the theories is that the uncontrolled movements associated with the disorder may be the result of oxidation damage to nerve endings. A controlled study of 15 patients with tardive dyskinesia was conducted with 1200 international units of a tocopherol for two-week periods. The supplemented group exhibited a 43 percent reduction in scores of abnormal involuntary movement test. The scores of patients not on vitamin E were not changed significantly.[53]

Therefore, in 1987, there was heightened enthusiasm when a multicenter controlled clinical trial of deprenyl, which inhibits a brain chemical involved in depression (monoamine oxidase), and vitamin E in the treatment of early Parkinson's disease got underway with 800 patients.[54] The beneficial effects of deprenyl, which occurred largely during the first twelve months of treatment, remained strong and significantly delayed the onset of disability for about an average of nine months. The high dose of vitamin E (2,000 internal units per day) was not deemed affective.[55]

Still, nerve and muscle abnormalities are associated with vitamin E deficiencies. The mechanism of action on vitamin E is assumed to be through antioxidant protection of membranes and/or membrane's stabilization. It has been suggested that the large surface area of certain nerves is particularly susceptible to oxidative damage.[56] And perhaps new studies at a different dosage or in combination with something else will demonstrate that vitamin E can be beneficial in the treatment of Parkinson's.

The US Recommended Daily Allowance (RDA) in 1973 was then set at 30 international units daily for adults. This was intended to be an amount that would allow for increased consumption of polyunsaturated fatty acids. Polyunsaturates are those fats from vegetable sources that are liquid at room temperature as opposed to saturated fats from animals that are usually solid at room temperature. The recognition that saturated fats contributes to the buildup of plaques in the arteries caused government and health organizations to encourage the public to replace saturated fats with unsaturated ones. Unsaturated fats, however, deplete vitamin E. Low-cholesterol or fat-modified diets rich in polyunsaturated fats raise the body's need for vitamin E.

The intake of vitamin E in our diets, according to government surveys, was 10.4 to 13.4 international units per day in 1989.[57] The Reference Daily Intake is 9 milligrams or 30 IU.

Be aware that heat and freezing destroy vitamin E!

| VITAMIN E SOURCES | |
|---|---|
| **Very Good** | **Good** |
| Walnuts | Coconut |
| Almonds | Olive oil |
| Sunflower seeds | Pears |
| Wheat germ | Peanuts |
| Whole wheat | Filberts |
| Oils: corn, peanut, | Broccoli |
| safflower, sesame, | Brussels sprouts |
| soybean, sunflower, | Blackberries |
| walnut, cod liver, | Apples |
| wheat germ | |
| Sweet potatoes | |
| Leeks | |
| Spinach | |
| Asparagus | |
| Beet greens | |
| Margarine | |

## Minerals for the Mind

Vitamins are organic and minerals are inorganic. Minerals, however, are generally dependent on organic molecules for transport, storage, and actual function. This characteristic binding pattern can lead to problems if high amounts of some nonessential and essential elements are present in the diet. Like vitamins, much remains unknown about how the minerals in your food and water affect your brain. The following are minerals that are known to play an important role in your brain function and general health. Sodium, chloride, and aluminum are not listed, as they will be discussed in detail in later chapters.

Minerals perform a variety of functions in your body. There are two classes of minerals: *macronutrients* and *micronutrients*. Your body contains more of the macronutrients—magnesium, sodium, potassium, and chloride—and you require more of them in your diet. The amounts range from hundreds of milligrams to grams. The micronutrients include iron, manganese, copper, iodine, zinc, fluoride, selenium, molybdenum, chromium, aluminum, boron, nickel, silicon, and vanadium. Micronutrients, also called trace elements, are found in tiny amounts—so small they are often measured in micrograms. Your body contains some trace elements even though there is no known need for them. These include aluminum, antimony, barium, boron, bromine, gallium, germanium, gold, lithium, mercury, silver, strontium, and titanium.

Lithium, a light metal that exists in the earth's crust, has been used as a medicine since ancient Greece, when it was prescribed for gout, rheumatism, and kidney stones. Small amounts of the salts of lithium are being used to treat manic-depressive disorder (bipolar disorder), which is characterized by wide swings between deep depression and overexcitement. Lithium has also been reported to cause alcoholics to lose their taste for liquor. Exactly why it works in either case is unknown.

In 1997, Japanese scientists studied the incidence in the western Pacific, including Japan, to determine if environmental factors that may contribute to the nerve-destroying disease amyotrophic lateral sclerosis (ALS) and Parkinsonism dementia. They found the condition of unbalanced minerals—a low content of calcium and magnesium, and a high content of aluminum in the soil and drinking water. They were able to reproduce ALS in rats by mimicking the mineral situation they found in their epidemiological studies.[58]

The Japanese scientists concluded that insufficient dietary intake of calcium and magnesium over a prolonged period of time may cause deterioration in the physical condition, and may lead to an abnormal accumulation of other toxic metals such as aluminum and manganese. Lack of calcium and magnesium may also cause a reduction of essential elements such as zinc.

So, just as there is a lot to learn about vitamins, there is even more to learn about minerals and their effects on the body and mind. The following are descriptions of some of the known and potential effects of minerals.

**Calcium.** Calcium is the most abundant mineral in your body. You need it for blood clotting, the development of normal nerve tissue, regular heartbeat, iron metabolism, and healthy teeth and bones.

Could calcium turn a message sent between nerve cells into a memory? Scientists know that the synapses—the minute spaces between two neurons or between a neuron and an organ across which nerve impulses are chemically transmitted—are stronger during and just after periods of high-frequency signaling. This short-term enhancement contributes to short-term memory, the kind you use when you remember a new phone number long enough to make a call.[59] Dr. Walter Regher of the Department of Neurobiology at Harvard Medical School, Boston, and his colleagues are looking at calcium ions. Calcium actually triggers the cell to release its chemical messengers, but Regehr's work, and the work of others, is showing that calcium is also involved in controlling synaptic strength. By measuring calcium at the site of release in the sending nerve cell, they have found that calcium persists for tens of seconds after triggering the messengers and that these elevations in calcium can enhance subsequent responses between nerve cells. The researchers are now trying to learn how synaptic calcium dynamics help to define the time, course and magnitude of short-term enhancement.[60]

There is a long way to go before some form of calcium can enhance short-term memory. The level of calcium in blood plasma is remarkably constant at concentrations of about 10 milligrams per deciliter. Calcium within the cells is also tightly controlled. Calcium is absorbed from the intestine by a process requiring vitamin D. Milk sugar (lactose) and vitamin D can both increase calcium absorption, which is why milk and milk-based products like yogurt are excellent sources of calcium. Calcium absorption is also aided by acidity in the digestive tract. Too much fat, oxalic acid (found in spinach, rhubarb, and chocolate), and phytic acid (found in grains) in the diet can result in calcium not being absorbed. The recommended calcium-phosphorus ratio is one-to-one, but this is almost impossible to achieve, especially in diets as high in protein as that of the average American. In general, meats, poultry, and fish supply fifteen to twenty times more phosphorus than calcium, whereas eggs, grains, nuts, dried beans, and lentils provide about twice as much phosphorus. Data from studies suggest that high phosphorus intakes or low calcium-to-phosphorus ratios cause bone demineralization and soft tissue calcification. Evidence indicates that both protein and phosphorus affect the calcium requirements in humans. Calcium retention is believed to be reduced by increases in protein, which intensifies the loss of calcium in urine.[61]

Calcium ingestion may have an effect on mood. Kaymar Arasteh, Ph.D., of Texas A&M University reported that depressed patients given 1,000 milligrams of calcium gluconate plus 600 international units of vitamin D twice a day for four weeks showed a significant elevation in mood compared to a control group of depressed patients who received placebos. Dr. Arasteh noted that calcium's effect on nerves in the brain and on mood is biphasic—that is, a little stimulates the nerves and elevates mood, but a lot can depress nerve activity and moods.[62]

The Reference Daily Intake for calcium is 800 to 1,200 milligrams for adults and 360 to 1,200 milligrams for infants and children, but because of the interrelationships among calcium, protein, and phosphorus, many researchers believe it is almost impossible to select a single requirement for any age group.[63] Surveys have shown that American women consume approximately 450 to 550 milligrams of calcium a day, only about half of the amount believed to be needed to help slow age-related bone loss. On the other hand, too much calcium can cause kidney failure, intestinal sluggishness, and psychosis.[64]

## CALCIUM SOURCES

| Very Good | Good |
|---|---|
| Milk, especially skim and low-fat yogurt | Potatoes |
| Cheese | Oranges |
| Sardines | Figs |
| Kidney beans | Oysters |
| Almonds | Sunflower seeds |
| Beet greens | Kelp |
| Broccoli | Soybeans |
| Salmon | Tofu |
| Kale | |
| Watercress | |
| Bok choy | |

***Chromium.*** Chromium allows insulin to regulate blood sugar, which is of vital importance to your brain (*see* Chapter 4). It is believed that a marginal chromium deficiency exists in a large percentage of the population. However, knowledge of chromium absorption and availability is incomplete. Three scientifically sound studies have reported that the elderly and even younger adults may have low levels of chromium and that supplemental chromium seems to have a beneficial effect on carbohydrate tolerance and cholesterol levels. Therefore, some researchers believe that chromium deficiency may play a part in diabetes and arterial disease. Since chromium and insulin work hand in hand, this is not improbable; however, not enough is known about the mineral to set a RDA.[65]

## CHROMIUM SOURCES

| Very Good | Good |
|---|---|
| Black pepper | Corn oil |
| Brewer's yeast | Shellfish |
| Mushrooms | Chicken |
| Meat products | |
| Whole grains | |

The estimated SDIs for chromium are 0.05 to 0.2 milligrams for adults and 0.1 to 0.08 milligrams for infants and children.

***Cobalt.*** Cobalt, an essential constituent of vitamin $B_{12}$, was first shown to cause a debilitating, wasting disease in sheep when the amount in the diet was insufficient. Data on the human need for cobalt is sparse and controversial. In research reported by the Russians, cobalt deficiency has been associated with disturbances in thyroid function—and, of course, thyroid hormone is needed for proper brain function.[66] Too much thyroid causes agitation. Too little produces lethargy in adults.[67] Cobalt is most useful when absorbed as part of $B_{12}$.[68] Vitamin $B_{12}$ is a cobalt-containing compound. Cobalt is also found in green leafy vegetables.

***Copper.*** Copper is a component of several enzymes, including the enzyme needed to make skin, hair, and other pigments. It stimulates iron absorption and is needed to make red blood cells, connective tissue, and nerve fibers. It helps the amino acid tyrosine do its work (tyrosine serves as a raw material for certain brain neurotransmitters). Copper deficiency is rare. A deficiency in copper, as you can read under magnesium, can cause rats to be hyperactive and develop learning or memory deficits. Women who use birth control pills have an elevated level of copper in their blood, but the significance of this is unclear.

In Wilson's disease, copper accumulates to toxic levels in several organs, especially the liver and the brain. In the brain, the copper deposits cause profound psychiatric and neurological symptoms. WD is fatal unless treated with agents to remove copper. Researchers at Massachusetts General Hospital have isolated a gene that causes Wilson's disease and that is responsible for copper transport in cells throughout the body. The WD gene also shows a striking similarity to a protein involved in Menkes's disease, another metabolic disorder involving a shortage of copper in cells that need it. The findings may both improve diagnosis of the two diseases and open the door to developing better treatments.[69]

The estimated Reference Daily Intakes for copper are 2 milligrams for adults and 0.5 to 1.5 milligrams for infants and children.

## COPPER SOURCES

| Very Good | Good |
|-----------|------|
| Almonds | Beans |
| Avocados | Dried prunes |
| Oysters | Walnuts |
| Margarine | Shrimp |
| Mushrooms | Bananas |
| Cocoa | |
| Seeds | |

*Iodine.* Two-thirds of your body's iodine is in your thyroid gland, located in your neck. Since the thyroid controls metabolism, and iodine influences the thyroid, an iodine deficiency can result in:

- Cloudy thinking
- Depressed mood
- Weight gain
- Lack of energy in adults
- In newborns, cretinism (stunted growth, swollen features, and mental deficiency) occurs with iodine deficiency
- A long-term iodine deficiency in adults can result in goiter, the extreme enlargement of the thyroid gland

Foods with *goitrogens* that can block the thyroid's uptake of iodine include cabbage, broccoli, Brussels sprouts, kale, turnips, rutabagas, cauliflower, mustard seed, and horseradish. Fortunately, because of iodized salt, goiter is rare today.

The Reference Daily Intake for iodine is 150 micrograms for adults and 40 to 120 micrograms for infants and children.

## IODINE SOURCES

| Very Good | Good |
|-----------|------|
| Kelp and other seaweed | Onions |
| Seafood | Vegetables grown in iodine-rich soil |

*Iron.* Iron deficiency is the most common single-nutrient deficiency disease in the world.[70] Many studies have consistently shown that iron-deficient children have alterations in attention span, lower intelligence scores, and some degree of perceptual disturbance.[71] Iron is essential for making hemoglobin, the red substance in blood that carries oxygen to your brain cells, and for making use of that oxygen when it arrives. Although some believe iron deficiency mainly affects the cognition of children, some studies have shown alterations in brain functions in adults.[72] An overload of iron is also being studied in the older adult population. Iron is widely distributed in the body, mostly in the blood, with relatively large amounts in the liver, spleen, and bone marrow. Your body loses iron mainly through blood loss. Iron-deficiency anemia occurs when there is an inadequate diet, impaired absorption of iron, blood loss, repeated pregnancy, chronic diarrhea, or a greater need for manufacturing blood. This is why women of childbearing age, pregnant women, and growing children are most likely to suffer from iron-deficiency anemia. Symptoms of deficiency include:

- Weakness
- Fatigue
- Pale skin
- Cold feet

When plant foods containing iron, such as asparagus and spinach, are eaten with citrus fruits, tomatoes and peppers, or other foods containing vitamin C, iron absorption is increased. Caffeine decreases the absorption of iron, so iron supplements should certainly not be taken with a cup of coffee or cola. Too much iron can also adversely affect the brain. Brain dysfunction in patients with Alzheimer's disease may relate to iron since the mineral is found in the senile plaques in the brain characteristic of the disease.[73] Iron has also been found to be at high levels in the brains of patients with Parkinson's disease.[74]

The Reference Daily Intake for iron is 18 milligrams for adults and 10 to 15 milligrams for infants and children. The average diet yields only 6 milligrams of iron.

## IRON SOURCES

| Very Good | Good |
|---|---|
| Blackstrap molasses | Green leafy vegetables |
| Clams | Nuts |
| Brewer's yeast | Asparagus |
| Eggs | Oatmeal |
| Organ meats | Dried peaches |
| Oysters | Dates, raisins, and prunes |
| Prune juice | Tofu |
| Most beans, | Tomato juice |
|   especially garbanzo and black | |
| Pumpkin seeds | |

*Magnesium.* Magnesium conducts nerve impulses and keeps the messages going in the brain. It maintains metabolism, aids normal muscle contraction, including that of the heart muscle, and is necessary for kidney, liver, and other organ functions. It is needed by cells for the creation of genetic material. It helps calcium, vitamin C, phosphorus, sodium, and potassium do their jobs in the body. Magnesium is important to the conversion of blood sugar into energy, and it has a reputation for being an antistress mineral because a magnesium deficiency can cause nervousness, irritability, and depression.

Rats deficient in magnesium or copper have been found to be hyperactive and had either memory or learning deficiencies. U.S. Department of Agriculture researchers tested the psychological impact of each mineral because previous experiments have shown that both have important roles in brain function. In one study, they fed rats diets containing either adequate copper or about one-tenth the adequate level for ten weeks. In a second study, they altered the magnesium content of the diets in the same manner.[75]

Deficiencies of both minerals prompted the rats to be more active in general. That's consistent with symptoms of magnesium deficiency in people who often experience tremors and disrupted sleep.

It is also reported to be vital to exercise endurance. A deficiency also causes muscle weakness, twitching, cramps, and irregular heartbeats. An overdose of magnesium can cause nervous system disorders and can be fatal to people with kidney disease. Ingesting diuretics and alcohol will deplete the level of magnesium in your body.

The Reference Daily Intakes for magnesium are 400 milligrams for adults and 50 to 250 milligrams for infants and children.

| MAGNESIUM SOURCES | |
|---|---|
| **Very Good** | **Good** |
| Bran buds | Green leafy vegetables |
| Tofu | Figs |
| Spinach | Lemons |
| Brown rice | Yellow corn |
| Oatmeal | Apples |
| Soybeans | Apricots |
| Avocados | Bananas |
| Beef | Cashews |
| Blackstrap molasses | Wheat flakes |

**Manganese.** Manganese is essential to enzymes that extract energy from food and convert proteins into amino acids and neurotransmitters. It is needed for normal tendon and bone structure and for some enzymes important to metabolism, particularly in processing glucose and fatty acids. A manganese deficiency in humans is unknown. Animal studies have shown that manganese turns off neuromuscular transmission of signals. It has been suggested that changes in the manganese concentration in human body fluids may be associated with some neurological disorders.[76] See the Japanese study on page 178.

The estimated DIs for manganese are 2.5 to 5 milligrams for adults and 0.5 to 3 milligrams for infants and children.

| MANGANESE SOURCES | |
|---|---|
| **Very Good** | **Good** |
| Nuts | Tea |
| Unrefined grains | Vegetables |
| Legumes | Fruits |
| Soybeans | Coffee |

***Phosphorus.*** Phosphorus is involved in nearly all metabolic reactions in the body. It is necessary for nerve and muscle function and for the transmission of messages in the brain. It works with calcium and vitamin D to build strong bones and teeth. Calcium and phosphorus should be consumed in a ratio of two calcium to one phosphorus, but rarely is in the Western diet. Antacids destroy phosphorous. A deficiency causes weakness and bone pain. An overdose hinders the body's absorption of calcium.

The Reference Daily Intakes for phosphorus is for children nine to eighteen years is 1000 milligrams.

| PHOSPHORUS SOURCES | |
| --- | --- |
| **Very Good** | **Good** |
| Meat | Peas |
| Nuts | Cereal |
| Seeds | Cheese |
| Fish | Apricots |
| Bran | Cocoa |
| Most beans | Tofu |
| especially pinto, black | Corn |
| Cottage cheese | Almonds |
| Milk | Broccoli |
| Yogurt | |

***Selenium.*** Selenium interacts with vitamin E to serve as part of the body's antioxidant defense system. Interest in selenium in human nutrition has grown and the element has been shown to be an essential nutrient.[77] Knowledge about selenium deficiencies and supplementation is sparse. Newer investigations have reported that certain enzymes important to brain function are dependent upon selenium. There is a decline in these enzymes with aging. A deficiency of selenium is believed to alter neurotransmitter metabolism in an as yet unknown way. The depletion of three important brain messengers—noradrenaline, serotonin, and dopamine—was found to occur in selenium-deficient adult rats. All three neurotransmitters are critical to processes of attention, arousal, and memory, in addition to their roles in motor activities. In another study, two children were shown to have low selenium status and intractable seizures.

The older child was given selenium to reduce the frequency of epileptic seizures, which suggests that selenium status may play a role in the neurobiology of epilepsy.[78] The range between benefit and toxicity is very narrow with this mineral.[79] Selenium in very small amounts is essential to life, but it is more toxic than arsenic and mercury and less abundant in the earth's crust than gold.

A provisional RDA of selenium is 50 to 200 micrograms for adults. The amount of selenium in the diet depends on the amount contained in the soil and water.

### SELENIUM SOURCES

| Very Good | Good |
| --- | --- |
| Wheat germ | Onions |
| Bran | Tomatoes |
| Tuna | Broccoli |
| Garlic | |
| Liver | |

**Zinc.** Zinc may help regulate chemical communication between brain cells and could be a clue to the chemical basis of learning. It may also help explain how the brain protects itself from certain forms of injury.[80] Zinc aids wound healing, affects reproduction, and counteracts the harmful effects of cadmium. Low zinc levels have been reported in the brains of epileptics and in men suffering from hardening of the arteries. A deficiency in zinc causes impaired cell growth and repair and a reduced sense of taste, and profoundly affects growth in fetuses and children.

Zinc is highly concentrated in the hippocampus, the area deep within the brain involved with memory function. Zinc also has been found to calm nerve cells in the brain when they become overexcited and begin firing too rapidly.[81]

A zinc deficiency is also suspected of playing a part in anorexia (self-starvation) and bulimia (characterized by gorging and purging). Alexander G. Schauss, Ph.D., director of the American Institute of Biosocial Research in Tacoma, Washington, says that the initial reduction of food intake in anorexics probably results from social influences, but that during adolescence, there are increased demands for most nutrients and for zinc in particular.[82] According to

## ZINC SOURCES

| Very Good | Good |
|---|---|
| Oysters | Clams |
| Whole-wheat bread | Cranberry juice |
| Wheat bran and wheat germ | Tuna |
| Beef | Applesauce |
| Lamb | Cocoa powder |
| Liver | Peanut butter |
| Herring | Rice cereal |
| Most beans, | Eggs |
|    especially black-eyed peas, | Cooked spinach |
|    garbanzos, lentils, | |
|    and green peas | |
| Brown rice | |
| Oatmeal | |
| Soy products | |

Dr. Schauss, the further zinc levels decline, the more the zinc-dependent senses of taste and smell reduce the desire for food.

When Dr. Schauss and his colleague, Dr. Derek Bryce-Smith, tested the anorexics, they found a zinc deficiency. They described one thirteen-year-old anorexic girl who weighed only 69.5 pounds. She was given 15 milligrams of zinc three times a day. After two weeks, her mood and appetite improved and she smiled; her weight had increased by 3.3 pounds. After several weeks on zinc, her weight rose to 97 pounds and her mood and appetite were reported normal.

There is no doubt that zinc is an essential trace element in humans. When zinc is present in the diet in adequate amounts, the body makes better use of vitamin A. A lack of zinc can cause night blindness indirectly, by not helping vitamin A to be released from liver stores, even when the diet is sufficient in vitamin A.

Zinc, however, is increasingly suspect in the brain degenerative disease, Alzheimer's.[83] Large medical doses of zinc may cause nerve death. Increased levels of zinc have been shown to be present in cell cultures of dying immune cells. Australian researchers say that changes in zinc metabolism which occur during oxidative stress may be important in neurological diseases such as

Alzheimer's, Parkinson's disease, and amyotrophic lateral sclerosis (ALS). They maintain the role of zinc in nerve damage must be further studied.[84] Several studies show that zinc promotes aggregations of the main component of the senile-plaques frequently found in Alzheimer's disease brains. While controversial, some studies indicate that total tissue zinc is markedly reduced in several brain regions of Alzheimer's patients.[85]

The Reference Daily Intakes for zinc are 15 milligrams for adults and 3 to 10 milligrams for infants and children.

## Nutrient Depleters

There are dietary factors that can affect the absorption and utilization of both vitamins and minerals. It may surprise you to know that fiber—that much-touted anticancer ingredient—and other plant material may interfere. Fiber, phytates, oxalates, and tannins found in plants can attach themselves to certain nutrients and render them incapable of being absorbed through the intestinal wall. The nutrients most commonly affected are calcium, iron, zinc, copper, magnesium, protein, and vitamin $B_6$.

Fibers, such as bran, that provide bulk in the diet interfere with nutrient availability. Phytates—substances in whole grains, beans, and nuts that bind with zinc, calcium, magnesium, and iron to form a compound the body can't absorb—may lower the levels of these metals, so going overboard and loading yourself with fiber is not a good idea. Oxalates, which are abundant in spinach, rhubarb, beef, collard greens, soybean products, wheat germ, and Swiss chard, deplete foods of their calcium, even those that are naturally high in calcium, because they keep the calcium from being absorbed. Almonds, cashews, chocolate, and cocoa also contain oxalates. Tannin and other phenols found in tea and red wine can reduce the availability of iron, vitamin $B_{12}$, and protein by forming chemical complexes with the enzymes needed to metabolize these nutrients.

Aging, about which we can do little, of course, causes the reduced secretion of stomach acid, which can affect absorption of many important nutrients. Protein, iron, zinc, calcium, and vitamins A, E, folic acid, and $B_{12}$ are among the nutrients possibly affected.

Alcohol and tobacco, as mentioned earlier, generally deplete the body of vitamins. In fact, alcohol interferes with the absorption of all nutrients. You must age, but if you also smoke and drink, dietary supplementation is advisable as an antidote to the effects of abuse. Dietary supplementation may assist the body in other ways in its handling of abuse of these popular drugs and the malabsorption and poor utilization that may occur with aging. Younger people under the stress of striving for athletic or career achievements also may need supplementation. In fact, we may all need vitamin and mineral supplementation, but, as Dr. Baker cautions, "Too much of a good thing is always bad."[86]

## Using Your Brain About Vitamins and Minerals

Cognitive impairment—deficits in memory function, orientation or problem solving—may be delayed or alleviated by diet in some cases. There are sparse scientific studies on the relationship between nutrition and cognitive function in healthy adults. In two recent investigations, one in Spain and the other in the Netherlands, dietary antioxidants and cognitive function in a variety of adult groups were evaluated. In the Spanish study at Universidad Complutense, Madrid, 260 elderly individuals (65 to 90 years) who were free of significant cognitive impairment participated. Results showed that subjects who scored highest on cognitive function tests had greater dietary intakes of fruits and vegetables. Subjects with higher test scores had greater dietary intakes of beta-carotene, vitamin C, vitamin E, folate, zinc, iron, fiber, and carbohydrate, and lower intakes of saturated fatty acids and cholesterol compared with those people with lower test scores.[87]

In the Netherlands study, the researchers at Reassume University Medical School found no benefit for cognitive function and intake of vitamins C and E but they did conclude that beta-carotene–rich food may protect cognitive function in older people.[88] Beta-carotene is found in all plants and in many animal tissues. It is the chief yellow coloring matter of carrots. In this study, 5,182 community participants aged 55 to 95 years were tested over a period of three years.

As you can determine, there is a lot yet to be learned about nutrients and your brain. There is a great deal of exciting scientific work in progress. In the meantime, here are some hints about getting the most nutrients out of your food:

**Buy wisely.** Some foods have more nutrients than others. Wholegrain cereals and breads are better than refined ones because some of the nutrients are lost during milling and are not restored by "enrichment." Fresh or frozen fruits and vegetables are preferable to canned ones, which have been exposed to vitamin-destroying high temperatures. If you do find canned vegetables and fruits more convenient, don't throw out the liquid. Use it in casseroles or soups, because these liquids contain the water-soluble B and C vitamins.

**For keep sake.** Store frozen foods at zero degrees Fahrenheit or below, and try to use the products within two months. Keep canned foods at about sixty-five degrees and refrigerate greens promptly. Keep milk and bread in opaque containers, as strong light destroys riboflavin. Try to use freshly squeezed oranges or, if you buy cartons of juice, use it as soon as possible. Even overnight storage can deplete orange juice of some of its vitamin C.

**Cook right.** If you can find your grandmother's old iron cooking pots, you can add this mineral to your meals without cost. To retain water-soluble vitamins, avoid soaking fresh vegetables. Vitamin C can be preserved by preparing salads and vegetables just before serving and by boiling or baking potatoes in the skin. Boil or steam vegetables until just tender, using the least amount of water possible. Pressure-cooking preserves the most vitamins; steaming is second best. Broiling, frying, or roasting meats preserves more B vitamins than does braising or stewing, unless the broth is also consumed.

**One potato two.** The white potato, like the banana, is loaded with nutrition. In addition to fiber, it contains B vitamins, vitamin C, potassium, iron, copper, magnesium, phosphorus, iodine, and zinc. The sweet potato has all the above as well as a lot of vitamin A. Eat the peel as well as the inside, because the peel not only seals in the nutrients during cooking, it also contains most of the potato's vitamins and minerals.

**Have your vitamin levels checked.** If you recognize any of the symptoms of deficiency mentioned in this chapter, ask your physician to take a sample of your blood for testing at a laboratory approved for testing vitamin and mineral levels. You may need some supplementation.

**Avoid megadoses of vitamins and minerals.** In large doses, vitamins are pharmaceuticals. Without medical supervision, loading yourself with one or more of a vitamin or mineral is unwise.

**Eat a varied diet.** Avoid eating the same thing day after day, and forgo those fad diets that emphasize one food over all others. A well-balanced, varied diet is the best insurance for your brain and body.

# 9

# Your Hungry Brain:
# Why You Eat and Why You Stop

It's 10:00 P.M. and you have a craving for a ham sandwich. It's 10:00 A.M. and you are longing for a jelly doughnut and a cup of coffee.

Most of us frequently have a compelling urge to eat a particular item. Food cravings can crop up at any time for any number of reasons, including pregnancy, menstruation, and stress.

A craving could also be a signal that your body's store of a certain nutrient is running low, especially if it is for a food you normally don't select. This can happen when you are on a stringent diet and you suddenly crave a high-fat food such as a cheeseburger. There is evidence that when you lose a lot of weight, your fat cells shrink and they try to plump up again by signaling your brain to get the cheeseburger.

A late-afternoon craving can be a signal to your body that your blood sugar is low and that it's time to eat again. Hence the British tea and the American afternoon snack habits. Cravings can also be switched on by emotions. Early associations with sweets and comfort or rewards often stick with us when we grow up.

Salt appetite is one of a group of so-called specific hungers that are known to develop in states of need.

A craving can cause you to overcome obstacles to obtain your desired food, even though it may not be healthy for you. The cause of the craving could be psychological rather than physiological or it could be a combination of both. It is just one reason, however, for ingesting food.

Why do you eat?

Have you eaten when you had no appetite, just to be sociable or because it's time for a meal?

Do you continue to eat when you're no longer hungry?

What's the difference between hunger and appetite?

Is your hunger in your brain or in your heart?

The answers to all of the above lie within your brain and the messages it sends and receives from other parts of your body. First of all, hunger is the *need* for food. Appetite is the *desire* for food. You can have an appetite without being hungry, and you can be hungry and not have an appetite, as in the case of anoretics who literally starve themselves. While your hunger may be based more on your physical needs and your appetite influenced more by culture and experience, your brain regulates both and both affect your brain function.

It was believed, at one time, that your stomach contractions and "growling" informed your brain when you were hungry. We now know that the message is much more complicated and involves a variety of chemical signals to and from your brain that turn on and off your hunger. Most of us have a greater problem not with starting to eat but with stopping.[1]

There are now believed to be two signal systems for hunger and satiety:

1. Signals are sent out when food passes through your gastrointestinal tract.
2. Signals are sent from your brain that integrate the information from your gut and send out further instructions.[2]

## Satiety Center

The search for the "stop-eating" control—the satiety center—in the brain began around 1940, when researchers inserted electrodes in the brains of rats and created various lesions. When a place in the center of an area of the brain, the *ventromedial hypothalamus (VMH)*, was destroyed, the rats ate excessively and became obese.[3] The VMH seemed to be the long-sought satiety center.

A similar condition of insatiable hunger occurs in human victims of Prader-Willis syndrome, a congenital defect of unknown origin in which a person is retarded and tremendously obese. These individuals are constantly preoccupied with food and will eat as long as food is available. They will steal food and gobble down garbage or pet food if meals are restricted. Researchers believe Prader-Willis victims never reach satiety.[4]

The hypothalamus, a tiny segment of nerve cells in the brain weighing less than four grams, acts like a central computer. It receives and integrates information about body weight, temperature, activity level, season, and reproductive cycle (in women) and estimates how much food is needed. Since the hypothalamus is the control center for so many functions, it is easy to see how one of its duties—control of eating behavior—can be influenced by its other jobs, such as control over sexual excitement, mood, or temperature. If you are in a very hot dining room without air conditioning, for example, your appetite will certainly be dampened. And a starving person is more interested in finding food than in finding someone with whom to have a sexual encounter.

The search for the chemical signals in the brain—the neurotransmitters that have to do with satiety—has heated up. Neuroscientists at the Yerkes Primate Research Center of Emory University have discovered in the brain a novel neurotransmitter that helps control food intake and seems to be partially responsible for the feeling of satiety. The finding may eventually be used to develop medications for obesity, a life-threatening yet common condition that often lies at the root of other serious illnesses, such as diabetes and cardiovascular diseases.

The neurotransmitter is called *CART,* for *Cocaine and Amphetamine Regulated Transcript,* and its role in feeding was found during studies on the effects of cocaine on the brain. Yerkes neuroscientist Pastor Couceyro was one of the first to notice in rodents that CART increased in a specific area of the brain when cocaine was administered.

"We tested CART to see if it could be an agent responsible for loss of appetite for two reasons," says Mike Kuhar, Ph.D., Chief of Neuroscience Division at Yerkes. "First, CART is associated with cocaine and cocaine reduces food intake. Also, CART peptides are found in regions of the brain that control food intake."

When the Yerkes research team injected CART into the brains of normal rats, their food intake was significantly inhibited by as much as 30 percent, according to Phil Lambert, Ph.D., who completed the behavioral aspect of the work. "In normal rats, CART was present in high levels in the hypothalamus, meaning that CART is apparently involved in a variety of physiologic processes, not just in cocaine addiction," says Dr. Lambert.

Next Lambert tried the flip side of the experiment in blocking the brain's naturally occurring CART by injecting antibodies (which bind to the CART and renders it nonfunctional). Without CART to put the brakes on appetite, the rats' feeding increased. "This antibody data is what makes us think CART is responsible, at least partially, for making you feel sated—whether it's after eating, or perhaps after cocaine use," explains Dr. Lambert. To further support the evidence that CART plays a major role in influencing appetite, Dr. Lambert found that CART interacts anatomically and functionally with a substance called *neuropeptide Y (NPY)*, a neurotransmitter known for years as a strong hunger stimulant. "We may be completing more of the food intake picture," says Dr. Kuhar. "Although NPY has been well characterized as a catalyst for hunger, agents that mediate satiety are not fully identified. This seems to be a part of the puzzle."

The next steps are to identify the precise structure of the CART and to further explore its role in managing an animal's body weight, especially long-term. This could prove especially important to the 59 percent of Americans who, according to the Institute of Medicine, are clinically obese. It could also help those suffering from bulimia and anorexia nervosa. The fact that CART appears to be a neurotransmitter is significant, because neurotransmitters are by definition related to the control of normal physiological processes and are easily modulated for treatment purposes.

Yerkes scientists caution that CART is only part of the feeding story. There are many chemicals in the brain regulating food intake and if one is knocked out of commission, the brain will eventually learn to compensate.

"Eating is too important an activity for survival to have just one pathway responsible," says Dr. Lambert. The Yerkes team is looking for a final common pathway traveled by all the feeding-related peptides and their receptors. "Using rodents for such studies is necessary for these early studies because humans don't necessarily eat just when they're hungry," says Dr. Lambert. "They are more dependent than most animals on social cues and timetables."

The CART studies show potential for more than just obesity studies. Dr. Kuhar and his colleagues believe the family of CART peptides can still reveal much about the mechanisms of addiction, and possibly even stress-related disorders because the CART peptides are also localized in areas of the brain involved in stress. The National Institute of Drug Abuse funded this study.

## Hunger Center

Scientists reasoned that if the ventromedial hypothalamus (VMH) contained the satiety center, then perhaps there was another area of the hypothalamus that contained the hunger center. In 1951, researchers reported that rats who had a specific area of the hypothalamus destroyed would never eat again and would eventually die of starvation.[5] Three years later, Elliot Stellar, Ph.D., of the University of Pennsylvania's Department of Psychology, formally proposed that the center of the hypothalamus, the VMH, is the brain's satiety center and the side of the hypothalamus, the *lateral hypothalamus (LH),* is its hunger center.

Although he acknowledged that there must be other factors involved, he maintained that these centers in the brain receive information through special sensory receptors in the hypothalamus that process the information and cause an action. The hypothalamus,

**HUNGER CONTROL AREAS**

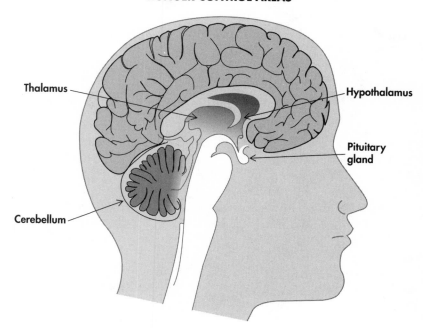

Thalamus

Hypothalamus

Pituitary gland

Cerebellum

like any executive, must receive feedback from the field. It is generally agreed that those signals must be carried in the blood.[6]

The glucostatic theory of hunger says that the signal to stop eating comes from the level of sugar in the blood. Dr. Jean Mayer, former president of Tufts University and an internationally known physiologist and nutritionist, concluded in 1952 that circulating sugar levels indicate the amount of immediately available or needed energy. Other substances such as fat or protein do not fit the picture because their concentration in the blood varies very little. Blood sugar, in contrast, increases quickly following eating and slowly decreases until the next meal.[7] Blood sugar is also known to be the primary energy source for the brain.

Sugar is part of the body's natural defense system. When in trouble, we instinctively seek more sugar to fuel our fight-or-flight response. (Now, you have a good excuse for eating sugary foods while under stress.)

When the blood-sugar sensory receptor cells are destroyed in the hypothalamus, the same obesity syndrome in the rats with VMH lesions and victims of Prader-Willis syndrome occurs.

Researchers have shown that when people feel hungry, their blood-sugar level is low, and when they are not hungry, their blood-sugar level is high. In normal people, the pancreas gland releases insulin, a hormone that enables the tissues of the body to use blood sugar. Without insulin, blood sugar is not taken into the cells but remains in the blood, building up to very high levels. In diabetes, the pancreas falls down on the job of producing enough usable insulin, resulting in high blood-sugar levels and tissue starvation. (A sudden drop in weight is often the first symptom of diabetes.) If you were not hungry and you were given a dose of insulin, thus lowering your blood-sugar levels, you would become hungry just as if you had gone for some time without eating. Thus, a drop in blood-sugar level is a stimulant to start eating. Conversely, a high blood-sugar level would make you want to stop eating. The latter effect is the basis for a weight-reducing diet that provides candy thirty minutes before meals. The idea is that the candy will reduce your appetite at mealtime.

Diabetics, whose problem is chronic high blood-sugar levels, still become hungry, so there must be other factors besides blood sugar involved.

Since energy is stored as fat, logically, the brain should be informed about how much reserve energy there is in storage. Dr. Mayer came up with the lipostatic theory as a complement to his glucostatic theory. The specific substances by which the body knows how much fat it has in the bank, he hypothesized, are free fatty acids, the breakdown products of stored fat. When the circulating levels of free fatty acids are high, we increase our food consumption. When they are low, indicating that fat is being stored rather than utilized, we eat less. Therefore, so the theory goes, your body knows about the level of free fatty acids because your brain's hypothalamus has sensory receptor cells that detect fatty acids just as it has sensory receptor cells that detect sugar. Working in concert with the sugar detectors, these nerve cells may activate the hunger system in your brain to make you start eating.

Both the glucostatic and the lipostatic theories are based on the idea that your body works to maintain a constant value in temperature, blood sugar, salt, and oxygen—known as *homeostasis*. Sensors in your body detect any deviations and make your body take action to recover the normal set point. Such systems operate by means of feedback from the sensors in your body to the "computer" in your brain.

## Combating Stress, Free Radicals, and Age

In addition to eating plenty of natural antioxidants in such foods as carrots, lettuce, and oranges, cutting down on fat and sugar in your diet, and easing stress in your life, what else can you do? Exercise!

Researchers at the University of Rochester School of Medicine reported at a Society for Neuroscience meeting that a prolonged high-fat, high-sugar diet exerts a chronic effect on the part of the brain related to the endocrine system, but that this effect can be retarded by moderate exercise. The affected brain region, the hypothalamus, is responsible for the production of the hormone vasopressin, which affects various heart, blood vessel, kidney, metabolic, behavioral, and immunologic functions. Vasopressin plays a part in memory and stress. These findings may be relevant to aging, since excess fat and high sugar consumption may worsen the changes that normally occur in the vasopressin system during aging.

The hormonal and autonomic nervous systems are major routes by which your brain communicates with the rest of your body.

Vasopressin may play a part in stress-induced eating and in cravings for carbohydrates. Some researchers now think that vasopressin may play a role in binge eating. Others have shown that vasopressin is affected by diets deficient in certain nutrients and that it may play an important function in the metabolic reaction to stress. Oxytocin, on the other hand, circulates in the blood and promotes the growth of fat cells, while brain oxytocin has been related to certain types of obesity. From these findings, it seems that a prolonged high-fat, high-sugar diet would hinder vasopressin and oxytocin functioning and that moderate exercise might protect against this perturbation.

Animal experiments found that prolonged high-fat, high-sugar diets substantially depleted the vasopressin content of the areas related to the neuroendocrine system, which, in turn, promoted an apparent further sugar intake. Moderate exercise was shown to retard this vasopressin activity and thereby reduce cravings for sugar.

The investigators also found that high-fat, high-sugar intake associated with obesity caused an increase in the amount of oxytocin in the blood. Because oxytocin enhances fat cell growth, the increased levels of oxytocin that accompany obesity may promote further weight gain. Exercise had no effect on oxytocin in the blood, but it did substantially increase the oxytocin content of an area of the brain involved in blood pressure regulation.

Exercise can also help your brain control your appetite. In a study reported in the journal *Metabolism,* Dr. R. Wood and F. Pi-Sunyer analyzed the effect of increased physical activity on the voluntary intake of lean women. They found that exercise burns up excess calories, promotes weight loss in the obese, and helps people control their desire to eat. The study involved both obese and lean women who normally did not exercise. The women were offered excessive amounts of food daily for three nineteen-day periods. During each period, a different level of activity was required—sedentary, mild, and then moderate. The women's voluntary food intake was monitored and records were kept of both daily food intake and prescribed exercise on a treadmill.

The caloric data showed that exercise had not significantly inhibited food intake in either the obese or the lean women. At no time was intake during exercise less than during the sedentary periods.

These data suggest that energy stores in the body may regulate eating behavior. As activity increased, the obese women in the study did not eat more food. Instead, they lost weight by using up stored fat. In contrast, the lean women maintained their weight by eating more. The researchers summarized that to maintain weight, energy output must still equal energy intake. When output exceeds intake, one loses weight. When output is lower, one gains weight and the difference is stored as fat. When you cut back on food intake, your body's natural tendency is to conserve energy, leading to as much as a 15- to- 30-percent *decrease* in basal metabolic rate. Fortunately, physical activity counteracts this diet-related decrease in metabolism, as evidenced by another recent study. Obese people on very low calorie diets had a gradual decrease in metabolic rate over a two-week period. But when they started to exercise for twenty to thirty minutes a day, their rates returned to normal within three or four days. At the end of two weeks, the rates were even higher than when they began their regimen. On the other hand, obese individuals who were on the same diet for four weeks but who did not exercise showed nearly a 20 percent decrease in basal metabolic rate.

The fat you store in your body is believed to help your brain decide your personal set point—the weight at which you stabilize. Some researchers say that if you vary too much from this set point, gaining or losing too much weight, your brain will direct your body to defend against the radical change and restore the set point. It will accomplish this by holding back or releasing stored fat and by making you want to eat or not want to eat. It has a basic "set point" that it tries to maintain even when some data input has glitches. The misinformation, however, may cause the set point to break down and result in overeating and obesity or anorexia and the progressive weight loss.

## Fat Cravers

Of the three macronutrients—sugar, fat, and protein—fat has the highest energy density and requires the least amount of energy for storage in the body. Fat ingestion leads to the release of *cholecystokinin (CCK),* which slows stomach emptying and also provides a direct satiation signal to your brain,[8] but fat is the dietary energy source most likely to lead to obesity for four reasons:

1. The body easily stores fat.
2. Overfed humans store 75 to 85 percent of excess energy from carbohydrate and 90 to 95 percent of the excess from fat.
3. Fat has a weaker effect than carbohydrate on satiety in humans.
4. Epidemiological studies show a positive correlation between high fat in the diet and obesity.

## Sugar Cravers

Carbohydrate also contributes to obesity, however. Carbohydrate cravings have been attributed to low levels of the brain neurotransmitter serotonin. This brain messenger is believed to have an inhibitory effect on the desire to eat. Neuropeptide Y, another brain chemical, has also been identified as playing a part in carbohydrate cravings.[9]

It has been reported that carbohydrates turn off "appetite" better than fats. Sugar, however, may override normal satiety because of the pleasure it gives. Researchers, however, continue to blame fat more than sugar for obesity.[10]

## Protein Power

As for protein, which provides not only energy by the building blocks of the neurotransmitters in the brain, it may cause an appetite based on the brain's need for these powerful chemicals. For some as yet unexplained reason, protein quells appetite for the next meal rather than for the one in which it is contained.[11]

The concept of set point is useful in understanding how your brain, your autonomic nervous system (which regulates automatic activities such as your breathing and heart action), neurotransmitters (which send messages between your brain cells), and hormones (which transmit messages between glands) act in unison to regulate these and other functions.

Although there is much to learn about these "on" and "off" appetite chemicals, the following brain substances are the subjects of a great deal of scientific excitement at this writing as far as eating behaviors are concerned:

- Neuropeptide Y in the hypothalamus is one of the strongest stimuli to make us eat. This peptide (chain of amino acids) has been found altered in patients with eating disorders. It is believed to regulate the desire for carbohydrates.
- Galanin is another peptide that occurs in tissues throughout the central nervous system. It is being studied for a number of disorders including Alzheimer's disease, pain, and depression as well as eating disorders. It is believed to control the desire for fat.
- Cortisol is a hormone from the adrenal glands and regulates fuel metabolism and increases the effect of neuropeptide Y. It is believed to play some role in anorexia nervosa, depression, and chronic wasting away that accompanies AIDS.
- Insulin, a hormone produced by islet cells of the pancreas gland, is essential for metabolism. It affects the need for carbohydrates.
- CCK (cholecystokinin) is one of the body's own appetite-dampening substances that acts on the nerves in the digestive system and on the brain. It is affected by fat and inhibits appetite. The body destroys CCK after its job is done so pharmaceutical companies are hoping to make a CCK product that lasts long enough to rein in appetite.
- CRH (corticotrophin-releasing hormone) is a neurotransmitter that controls the secretion of other stress-related hormones in the pituitary gland. When it is oversecreted, it is believed to contribute to decreased libido, insomnia, and decreased appetite.
- Orexin-A is a newly identified brain chemical found in the hypothalamus that is believed to stimulate appetite.
- Orexin-B is a newly identified brain chemical found in the hypothalamus that stimulates appetite.

- Estrogen increases the desire for fat and ups the amount of galanin (*see* above).
- CART, one of the latest neurotransmitters to be identified that involves satiety (*see* page 195).

As more and more is learned about these brain-body signals, more effective and safer controls of appetite will be developed. The following are some of the research projects reported involving humans with eating problems.

## Hormone Hunger

Most women know that their appetite control is affected by the time of the month and that many desire chocolate when under stress. The reason may be both physiological and psychological. While chocolate is often associated with comfort and pleasure, it does have addictive substances, including caffeine and phenyethylaminine (PEA). PEA is related to our self-made brain stimulants, tyrosine and phenylalanine. The latter has been called the "love drug."[12]

Researchers at Louisiana State University did an interesting study involving women who had a tendency to overeat sugary foods just before their menstrual period. Fifty-nine women participated in the investigation conducted by LSU associate professor of psychology, Paula Geiselman, Ph.D., and her colleagues. The subjects were selected on the basis of a test showing that they had either an above-average or below-average tendency to overeat.[13]

"The data indicate that, during the premenstrual phase, which is dominated by the production of progesterone, women who have a habitual problem with overeating are hypersensitive to the taste of food that can provoke overeating," Geiselman said.

The women were given four dishes of chocolate pudding varying in sugar and fat content to taste and rate. They were then given a dish of the high-sugar, high-fat pudding to eat. Afterward they were given a large bowl of pasta and told they could eat as much or as little as they pleased.

The study showed that women with a tendency to overeat liked the high-sugar, high-fat pudding more during the premenstrual phase and they ate more pasta.

"We found that how well the women like the taste of the chocolate food was positively and significantly associated with their eating behavior. The more they liked the pudding, the hungrier they reported they were, the more pudding they ate, the larger bites they took of it, the more they like a pasta subsequently presented to them. They ate more of the pasta at a faster rate.

"Those with a below-average tendency to overeat ate more of the pasta during the preovulatory phase than they did in the premenstrual phase. There was no difference between the two groups of women in the amount of pasta eaten in the preovulatory phase."

The study indicates that previous research on other mammals shows progesterone produces overeating and an increase in body weight. Women have twice the incidence of major weight gain as men and 40 percent of U.S. women are attempting to diet. Geiselman said, "Dieting efforts appear to be particularly dangerous in some women. Many women suffer from binge-and-purge pattern of diet in addition to other eating disorders such as anorexia and bulimia."

Yale University researchers also believe that gobbling down that handful of potato chips when you're under stress may have more to do with hormones than hunger.

The researchers examined the eating habits of 60 women and measured the levels of the hormone cortisol in their saliva. Scientists have known for some time that when people experience stress, many physiological changes occur, including a change in heart rate and a flux in cortisol levels. The question is what precipitates changes in eating patterns.

"The study was really just a first step in starting to help us untangle the biology from the psychology," said psychology professor Kelly Brownell, director of the Center for Eating and Weight Disorders at Yale.[14]

The test subjects—all healthy women ranging in age from 30 to 45—were given a variety of stressful tasks to perform with unrealistic time constraints. The tasks included counting backwards, trying to solve an unsolvable puzzle, and giving a speech.

During the tasks, the researchers periodically measured cortisol in the women's saliva. After the exercises, the women were allowed to snack without restraint on high-fat or low-fat foods.

The researchers found that the women who secreted the most

cortisol ate the most high-fat food after stress. The women who didn't eat any high-fat food had secreted the least amount of cortisol. "Cortisol is linked both to emotions and eating," researcher Elissa Epel said. "We know that during chronic stress, if we have high cortisol and high insulin, this combination tells the body to store fat to stock up resources for hard times ahead."

## Chocolate Craving

In a very interesting study on self-control, 67 undergraduate psychology students at Case Western Reserve University were put to the test. Ellen Bratslavsky, a graduate student, and Roy Baumeister, professor of psychology, found that students who were asked to refrain from eating chocolate chip cookies had less strength to complete a subsequent mental task.[15]

The researchers placed the cookies in front of the students in the first group; but instead of offering them a cookie, she asked them to chew on a radish.

Left alone with the cookies and the radish, the researchers observed through a one-way mirror that some students squirmed in their chairs as the tantalizing aroma permeated the room, others took nibbles at the radish, and some even picked up the cookies and stared longingly at the forbidden treat.

When the moment came that the students thought they could have the cookies, they were given a subsequent task of completing an unsolvable puzzle while waiting an additional 15 minutes.

The researchers found that those not permitted cookies made less than half the attempts to solve the puzzle before giving up than those who were allowed to eat the cookies immediately or were offered none at all.

The lesson learned is that self-control is a limited resource. "When people exert self-control, such as when under stress or pressure, or when dieting or coping—self-control may fail in other spheres," says Baumeister.

"Resisting temptation is often morally necessary, but it has a psychological cost," adds Bratslavsky.

# Is It All in the Liver?

Can your liver really be the source of your hunger? Your liver is a chemical-processing plant that can switch products very quickly and dramatically when you eat or fast.[16] In contrast, the supply of fuels to your brain does not seem to change that quickly. The liver is also well situated in your body to evaluate your food intake and the supply of fuels in your body.

Evidence that the liver is involved in hunger and satiety stems largely from studies showing that nutrients suppress food intake in animals more effectively when infused directly into the vein leading to the liver than when injected into veins leading elsewhere in the body. Furthermore, intravenous infusions of fructose—a sugar that is not readily utilized by the brain but is used by the liver—reduce food intake in rats, while infusions of beta hydroxybutyrate, which can be utilized by the brain and not by the liver, have little or no effect on food intake.[17]

## Gastrointestinal Distension

There are still more signals that affect your hunger. One of the earliest satiety signals proposed and still an active candidate is the filling of the stomach and intestines with non-nutritive bulk-no-calorie material that is given either before or with a meal. This is the theory behind the use of a bubble that is inserted into the stomach and inflated to cause a sensation of fullness. One model is called the Garren Edwards Gastric Bubble, developed by a husband-and-wife team of stomach specialists, Lloyd and Mary Garren of Santa Ana, California. The bubble remains in the stomach up to four months, during which three to four pounds per week are lost.

## A Matter of Timing

Preloads are substances, such as candy, that are given before meals to induce satiety.[18] Timing is important. Investigators have shown that hunger is best suppressed when the interval between the "preload" and the meal was five to thirty minutes. When the load was given simultaneously with a test meal, the amount eaten was more than when the preloads were given before the meal. This also explains why you are advised when dieting to eat slowly and put down your fork between bites. Time is needed for the chemical signals mentioned in this chapter to fully activate in your brain.[19]

Incidentally, during preload tests, it was discovered that soup was more effective in suppressing later food intake than crackers, cheese, and juice.[20]

Another interesting observation about timing concerns the period between your meals. Charles Pollak, M.D., of Cornell University Medical School's Chronobiology Center in Westchester, New York, observed patients who lived in a suite of rooms for two weeks without any time cues—no clocks, windows, or routine. Some of the people had a 30-to-40-hour day-night cycle instead of the usual 24-to-25-hour one. They would stay awake 20 hours and sleep 20 hours. They also separated their meals roughly in proportion to the day, so that the hours between meals were doubled. "They had no absolute knowledge of time. All they knew was they were hungry for lunch," Dr. Pollak says. "As far as we can tell, they were perfectly normal people."[21]

It may be that there are many of us whose meal timing is off from our true biological clocks. We eat because the clock tells us to eat, not because our brains do.

## Hypothalamic Theory of Thirst

We have described a great deal of the research that is going on to determine why we eat and stop eating. Perhaps even more important is why we drink and why we stop drinking. Your tissues require an external supply of water. Your brain must detect this need and direct you to obtain it. Your body constantly loses water through breathing, sweating, and the elimination of wastes. This water must be replaced. From eating, your body can conserve supplies of food as fat, but your body's reserves of water are scant. You could go without food for several months, but you would die if deprived of water for even a few days.

It is also possible for your tissues to be overloaded with water. Your brain must be able to direct elimination of an excess, or you would sicken and eventually die if the situation were not corrected.

There are cells in the same region of your brain associated with eating, the hypothalamus, that are called *osmoreceptors*. When these water sensors are stimulated electrically, drinking occurs. If these cells are destroyed, drinking behavior is disturbed.

A further indication that the hypothalamus is the central link for water regulation is its role in the release of *antidiuretic hormone* (ADH or vasopressin). When this hormone is released by your brain, water is retained by your kidneys. The hypothalamus releases ADH both when the water receptors in the brain indicate a fluid loss within the cells and when the pressure sensors, or *baroreceptors,* in the blood vessels indicate a fluid loss between the cells.[22]

Let's say you are working in the garden in hot weather. You sweat and lose a lot of water stored around your cells. The water in your blood pours out to replenish what you have lost. Your kidneys detect this decrease in water and secrete a chemical in your blood that is carried to your brain telling you that you are thirsty, so that you will drink and resupply your body's water. As with eating behavior, your hypothalamus contains two discrete drinking areas: a "start drinking" area and a "stop drinking" one. Electrical or chemical stimulation of the appropriate center will result in starting or stopping drinking. Surgical removal or disconnection of the appropriate area will produce an animal that will not drink or one that drinks to excess.

Thirst and hunger are not independent of each other.[23] When eating begins, a great variety of signals are produced, many of which have been implicated in making you drink. These signals include your body's release of histamine, which stimulates stomach juices, and insulin, which processes starches and sugars.

If you are deprived of food, you will consume less water. Likewise, if you are thirsty, you will eat less food. Both may be related to the ratio of the weight of food to the weight of water that you tend to keep in your stomach. Thirst and hunger also interact because many foods contain at least some water, and many liquids contain at least some nutrients; thus, eating can help satisfy thirst and drinking can help satisfy hunger. For example, you are unlikely to feel hungry after drinking a large chocolate milkshake,

and are unlikely to feel thirsty after eating large amounts of lettuce
(lettuce is 96 percent water).[24] This also explains why soup was so
effective in diminishing appetite in the preload studies described
on page 207.

## The Dry-Mouth Theory

The "dry-mouth" theory proposes that you want to drink merely
because your mouth is dry. This seems to be borne out in patients
awaiting surgery. They are not permitted to drink, but if they rinse
their mouths out with water, their thirst is often quenched. This is
called "sham drinking."

Against this premise is the fact sham drinking does not satisfy
thirst. The general consensus now is that the dry mouth is a signal
of thirst but not a cause, in the same sense that stomach contractions are a signal of hunger.[25]

*Angiotensin,* a powerful elevator of blood pressure, is believed
to be another signal for drinking. It is produced by the action of
renin, a kidney enzyme. All of the components of the renin-
angiotensin system have been found in the brain, and there are indications this system is part of the brain's mechanism for regulating
blood pressure. Water deprivation lowers blood pressure and increases salt concentration in the blood. These changes are detected
by the kidney, which then secretes renin. When renin comes into
contact with the blood, angiotensin is produced. Consequently, angiotensin levels are high in your blood when you are deprived of
water. Experiments have shown that when angiotensin is injected
into a vein or applied directly to the brain, thirst increases. Angiotensin may be the messenger between your body and brain
when your body water falls too low and you should start drinking
to replenish it.[26]

Scientists are learning more and more about how hunger, thirst,
and satiety centers in the brain work. Sometimes the investigations
are dramatic.

Take the case of Peter, a thirty-seven-year-old man who went to
two physicians because he was concerned about his habit of raiding the refrigerator three to five times every night. When Peter and
his wife went on vacation, they would place food and drink beside

the bed every night. Studies at a sleep lab over six nights showed that the nocturnal food forays coincided closely with periods of rapid-eye-movement (REM) sleep.[27] REM sleep occurs periodically during the night and is accompanied by great electrical activity in the brain. The authors linked Peter's behavior to that of babies. Research has shown that the demand for food in babies is also associated with REM activity. Infants awake periodically to be fed during the night, but adults usually suppress this rhythmic, nighttime food pattern.

An even more dramatic example of the brain's control over eating and satiety concerned a 32-year-old woman, Lucy, who was six feet tall and weighed 405 pounds. Her severe obesity posed a grave risk to her health. No conventional method helped her lose weight. Electrodes were then inserted into her brain through a hole drilled in the top of her skull. (Because the brain has no pain receptors, Lucy was conscious throughout surgery and only a local anesthetic was needed.) A battery-powered stimulator was implanted under the skin in her chest and connected to the electrodes by wires under the skin. Similar techniques to control pain and epilepsy have been used.

During the next four months at home, Lucy used the brain stimulator almost continuously. The doctors readjusted the stimulator periodically to achieve comfortable but effective levels. During this time, Lucy lost 32 pounds. She then alternated periods with the stimulator on and off. During the time it was on at high level, her caloric intake was markedly lower than when the device was turned off. There were, however, dramatic changes in brain metabolism. Sugar with a radioactive tracer was injected into her arm and a device called a PET scan was used to reveal how her brain was using the sugar. On days when the stimulator was on, overall brain metabolism was about 35 percent higher than when it was off. There were also psychologic side effects during the period of high stimulation. Lucy experienced increases in anxiety, depression, and fatigue as well as clear decreases in friendliness and vigor.[28]

The researchers said the study showed that stimulation of the VMH can be effective in reducing caloric intake. Compared to other surgical procedures, they said, it is relatively safe. However, they noted that the use of the stimulator seems to produce the same emotional problems as other types of weight-loss regimens.

As it is with many bodily processes, we can learn much from patients like Peter and Lucy and from others who have abnormal or exaggerated eating patterns. The following are descriptions of common eating disorders and new findings and theories about what happens when the brain's appetite and satiety controls go haywire.

## Self-Starvation or Bingeing

*Anorexia nervosa* is a disorder of unknown cause that occurs most often in young women who starve themselves because of a morbid fear of gaining weight. They are depressed and tend to exercise excessively. Their preoccupation with food usually prompts strange food-related rituals: crumbling food, cutting it into tiny pieces, and not eating with the rest of the family. The anorexic sometimes becomes a gourmet cook, preparing elaborate meals for others while eating low-calorie food herself. The anorexic may have trouble sleeping. As her obsession increasingly controls her life, she may withdraw from friends.

Many of the anorexic's peculiar behaviors and bodily changes are typical of any starvation victim. Thus, some functions are often restored when sufficient weight is regained. Meanwhile, the starving body tries to protect its two main organs, the brain and heart, by slowing down or stopping less vital bodily processes. Thus menstruation ceases, often before weight loss becomes noticeable; blood pressure and respiratory rate slow; and thyroid function diminishes.[29]

*Bulimia* is an eating disorder whose victims typically gorge huge amounts of high-calorie food, then purge by vomiting or the use of laxatives and diuretics, excessive exercise, and fasting. National estimates show that as many as six million Americans may be bulimic or bulimarexic, a combination of bulimic and anoretic, with as many as one out of five college-aged women experiencing the disorders.[30]

In addition to mood swings and episodes of weakness, dizziness, and headaches, bulimics suffer potassium deficiencies, stress on their hearts, loss of tooth enamel, irregular heartbeat, constipation, ruptured stomach linings, and digestive problems.

While anorexics can starve themselves to death, bulimics may have a mild or marked weight loss. About 90 percent of the anorexic and bulimic population is female.[31]

When anorexia is combined with bulimia, the degeneration can be rapid. Karen Carpenter, the singer, was a bulimarexic. She died of syrup of ipecac abuse. Ipecac is used to induce vomiting. Building up over time, ipecac irreversibly damaged her heart muscle, which eventually led to her death.

In the past, anorexia and bulimia were thought to be environmentally induced—a problem of emotional attachments and detachments. Researchers, however, are finding more and more abnormalities in the brain's chemical messenger system.

Researchers such as Walter Kaye, M.D., and his group at the University of Pittsburgh School of Medicine have measured the levels of corticotrophin-releasing factor (CRF) in the spinal fluid of patients both during anorexia and after weight gain and recovery. A significant correlation was found between the levels of CRF, which turns on the adrenal glands' release of a hormone involved in sugar metabolism, and stress and depression in these patients. CRF levels have also been found to be high in patients suffering from classical depression.[32]

Sarah Leibowitz, Ph.D., an associate professor of neuropharmacology at the Rockefeller University in New York City, and her colleagues believe that anorexics also have a problem with the brain transmitter norepinephrine.

"We believe young women with anorexia have a loss, or at least a decrease, of norepinephrine activity in the middle of the hypothalamus, where hunger is stimulated," she says. "We think that young women with anorexia may be so desperate to control their appetites, they consistently refuse to 'hear' hunger signals so that they actually end up changing their norepinephrine levels and thus the number of cell receptors on the hypothalamus. Deprived of food, their bodies may put out so much norepinephrine that the middle of the hypothalamus will hastily reduce the number of its receptors to make the 'I'm hungry' message less strident. The brain then may make more norepinephrine, the hypothalamus follows by getting rid of more receptors and eventually so much norepinephrine may be expended that the supply runs out. Or, perhaps the hypothalamus reduces its receptors so efficiently that it can no longer respond to the call for food. Whatever happens, the feeling of hunger practically vanishes."

Dr. Leibowitz maintains that we can all control our brains to some extent. Anorexics apparently teach theirs to shut off hunger signals. The Rockefeller researcher says binge eating occurs in up to 50 percent of anorexic patients. These episodes are associated with greatly increased subjective hunger and frequently are accompanied by breathlessness, sweating, heart palpitations, racing pulse, and inflated metabolic rate. All of these symptoms suggest a general increase in nervous system activity. During the binge, a large amount of food is rapidly consumed in a short time, with a specific preference for high-calorie, sweet-tasting foods. The binge is ended by stomach pain and frequently self-induced vomiting, and results in a depressed mood, feelings of guilt and remorse, and a continuation of the severely restrictive diets typical of the self-starver.

From this brief description of alternate binges and fasts, Dr. Leibowitz says, one becomes acutely aware that anorexia nervosa is not so much a disorder of appetite loss as it is one of increased desire to eat—perhaps specific foods—associated with a profound self-denial of that desire and then periodic breakdowns of the inhibition.

Dr. Leibowitz says that a variety of studies have indicated that anorexia and bulimia are associated with abnormal regulation of sugar and starch ingestion. Anorexics specifically avoid carbohydrate-rich foods, whereas bulimics focus their bingeing on high-carbohydrate foods. Drugs known to potentiate food intake and hunger in people have also been found to increase the preference for sugars and starches.

There is evidence that glucose tolerance is impaired in anorexics, Dr. Leibowitz says. Anorexics can't utilize insulin effectively, even after they regain weight.

In anorexia, disturbed hormonal rhythms have also been detected. Furthermore, in anorexics, the normal 24-hour pattern of eating behavior appears to be altered, with bingeing episodes generally occurring at night. Although the basis for these findings is unknown, it is of interest that in rats, norepinephrine and adrenal hormone levels follow a circadian rhythm and are at their peak at a time when eating behavior is normally at a maximum. For nocturnal animals such as the rat, this occurs at the beginning of the dark cycle, when carbohydrates rather than proteins are preferred.

"The relationship of these hormonal changes to the disturbed patterns of eating behavior in anorectics has not been determined," Dr. Leibowitz points out. "However, in normal human subjects, there is some evidence that the adrenal hormone, cortisol, is released at certain times during the 24-hour cycle, and must remain at normal levels for the nerve cells in the brain's hypothalamus to function properly and thus produce normal eating behavior."[33]

As described earlier, anorexia and bulimia are syndromes that involve self-starvation as a predominant feature. In contrast to true anorexics, who systematically restrict their food intake to the point of life-threatening emaciation, bulimics exhibit frequent episodes of bingeing—particularly carbohydrate-rich foods—which may alternate with periods of self-starvation.

For more information on eating disorders, contact the following:

**National Eating Disorders Organization (EDO)**
6655 South Yale Avenue
Tulsa, OK 74136
(918) 481-4044
http://www.laureate.com/

**ANRED**
http://www.ANRED.com

The latter organization provides information about anorexia nervosa, bulimia, binge eating disorder, and other less well known eating problems. All information is free but you can only access the information on the Internet.

Numerous studies, particularly in animals, show that food deprivation—which is known to release the adrenal hormone *corticosterone* and to cause a preference for carbohydrates and fats—has been shown to enhance the production of norepinephrine in the middle of the hypothalamus. The desire for sweets and fats after dieting may explain why most weight-loss regimens are failures. Our brains send out the chemical signals that overwhelm us with a desire for sweets or a cheeseburger after we've had low-caloric foods for awhile.

We asked Dr. Leibowitz if there was anything that surprised her during her more than fifteen years of research with neurotransmitters and eating behavior.

*I marvel at how potent a very small amount of these chemicals is. We can modify a whole daily pattern of feeding with a single injection. I marvel at how easy it is to disturb the neurotransmitters. We are not sure why some people become anorectic and bulimic. Stress may initiate these problems but it is not the cause.*[34]

Dr. Leibowitz points out that, ironically, it is very difficult to change human eating patterns such as a small breakfast, lunch at noon, and dinner at six.[35]

And that brings us to the most common eating disorder of all, overeating. The National Institutes of Health's definition is that "obesity is an excess of body fat frequently resulting in a significant impairment of health."[36] The NIH experts agree that an increase in body weight of 20 percent or more above desirable body weight constitutes an established health hazard.

At any one time, ten million Americans are on a diet. They spend millions of dollars for books, devices, and diet foods. Most diets work for awhile and then the regimen becomes abandoned and the weight is regained. Instead of sensing the natural hunger and satiety cues provided by their bodies, dieters follow prescribed selections of food, such as an all-fruit diet, an all-grain diet, or a rigid combination of foods, and then they stop one diet and later try another. In fact, some researchers consider this yo-yo dieting an eating disorder.

Can you really control your eating?

Should you fight your set point?

Research confirms what many obese people have been saying all along: they can just look at food and become fatter. According to Yale psychologist Judith Rodin, Ph.D., "Simply looking at or smelling food can trigger endocrine responses like those produced when the food is actually in the gastrointestinal tract."[37]

Many researchers believe that at least some obese people are more likely to eat in response to external stimuli such as television commercials or the mere sight of food. They are highly responsive to external cues.

In one set of experiments, Dr. Rodin and her colleagues divided formerly overweight subjects into two groups according to their degree of responsiveness to internal and external cues. The subjects came to the laboratory at noon, after not having eaten since the previous evening. A juicy steak was cooked in front of them, and they were told they could eat it. Blood samples that were taken while they watched the steak cooking showed that the externally responsive subjects, regardless of weight, produced significantly greater levels of insulin.

In subsequent experiments, Dr. Rodin found that the magnitude of insulin release was correlated with the palatability of the food. And the more externally responsive the subject, the more the insulin responded to the idea of the tastiness of the food.[38]

If external responders oversecrete insulin in the presence of compelling food cues, Dr. Rodin says, they are often likely to want more calories in order to balance their hormonal output. And what they do eat is more likely to be stored as fat. Externally responsive people are, in Dr. Rodin's words, "literally turned on" by food. To make matters worse, their metabolic responsiveness is even greater when they are looking at food they feel they must not eat.

Dr. Rodin points out that some physiologists believe that the body's responses when anticipating a food are, in part, reflexive and innate. However, recent research suggests that you can learn to associate the palatability and satiating power of food with the taste, texture, smell, and energy value of the food. After repeated pairings, the body responds before the food is actually digested—in effect, it anticipates the new level of energy. It is a phenomenon similar to Pavlov's dog, which salivated when a bell rang because it had learned to associate the bell with food.

## Danger of Dieting

The deprivation of dieting also is believed to underlie cravings for certain foods. While following diets that prohibit rich, high-calorie, often-favorite foods, dieters frequently report overwhelming desires for these foods. Unable to resist, they usually give in to their cravings. And once they give in, they frequently overindulge.

"Research shows that people tend to binge if they've been restricted," says Elizabeth Markley, R.D., assistant professor at the University of Connecticut. "We don't know how much of that is purely psychological—simply wanting what you can't have."

Cutting calories, furthermore, may inadvertently slow dieter's reaction times. And that effect may continue for weeks after the diet ends. U.S. Agriculture research scientists and their British colleagues found that reaction time lengthened by 11 percent in a group of 14 women volunteers who went on a strict reducing diet.

It continued to slow for three weeks after the diet ended. The scientists measured reaction times during the 21-week study by determining how long it took the women to hit the space bar on a computer keyboard after a white star appeared on the screen.[39]

The scientists are now working to determine whether the slow-down lowers dieters' alertness—and thus increases their risk of accidents—or whether the even longer term diets might increase such risk. The overweight but otherwise healthy volunteers, age 25 to 42, ate only half of the number of calories needed to maintain their beginning weight during 15 weeks of the study. They lost an average of 27 pounds. Their increase in reaction time confirms an earlier finding by British investigators, who are with the British Biotechnology Sciences Research Council.

Further study could lead to new understanding of how the body uses calories and nutrients for thought and action, the researchers concluded.

## Managing Food Cravings

How we select a diet is a complex issue. Beyond the basic issue of satisfying hunger, some of the most important physiological factors may be those of the food itself—taste, texture, color, aroma, and temperature. Whether any innate "wisdom" of the human body plays a major role in determining our food choices is unclear. But our associations with food—what particular foods signify in terms of the emotions they evoke—clearly do have great influence. "Attempting to ignore these influences, as is often prescribed in these health-conscious days, may set people up for aberrant eating behaviors, such as food cravings that result in bingeing," said Marsh Hudnall, M.S., R.D., nutrition director of Green Mountain at Fox Run, a women's weight-management facility.

"By trying to totally avoid certain foods, people instead tend to overconsume them in the end," she said.

In fact, Hudnall and other experts predict moderation will prove to be the best strategy for managing food cravings. "Eating all foods in moderation within the context of a well-balanced diet allows for the many factors that drive our food choices," she said.

If you want another excuse not to diet, British researchers may have it. Cutting calories may inadvertently slow dieters' metabolism.

In the final analysis, whether future research shows food cravings are physiologically based or psychologically based or both, blaming the specific foods for our own choices may be a mistake. Calling it "no-fault psychology," some scientists fear that people can use such beliefs as an excuse to absolve themselves of personal responsibility for their actions. In the long run, that could undermine a sense of personal control with negative effects on long-term health and well-being.

## Will the Real Diet Food Please Stand Up?

Among weight-management experts, it's a familiar story. In an attempt to avoid going off their diets, dieters literally stuff themselves with carrot and celery sticks, all the while craving ice cream, potato chips, and candy. But ice cream and the like eventually win. Further, such foods win big. Out of guilt, or with the intention that they'll go back on the diet tomorrow and have to forgo "forbidden" foods again, dieters frequently overindulge. When they do return to their diets, the vicious cycle begins again.

How can you break this cycle? Marsh Hudnall says research shows that food cravings are satisfied best by the actual substance that is craved. "Forget the carrot sticks and have a reasonable portion of ice cream, if it's ice cream that you really want," she says. "In moderation, favorite high-calorie foods can help you stay within a well-balanced diet and achieve a healthy weight."

Your appetite and eating are complicated not only by neurotransmitters sending messages between your brain and intestines but also by psychological, physical, and environmental circumstances. There has been a great deal of new research into human appetite and eating behavior, but there is still much to be learned. Many scientists now believe that obesity is a multigene disorder affected by environmental exposures.[40] In the meantime, If you want to help control your appetite, try the following:

- *Eat slowly.* Most diet programs advocate eating more slowly and putting your utensils down between bites. There is scientific evidence to back this up: it takes about twenty minutes for the signals from your stomach to reach the satiety center in your brain.

- *Use your head.* Try to become more sensitive to the feelings of satiety. Don't keep eating just because your mother always told you clean your plate or because you are watching television or talking.
- *Go for the fiber.* Vegetables, fruits, and bran provide a feeling of fullness because of their fiber content. You should not only include them in your meals but also try preloading—eat a baked potato or a few bran crackers about half an hour before your meal, and you probably will eat less when you sit down to dinner.
- *Try to have soup with your meal.* It fills you up, provides fluid, nourishment, and thus helps curb your appetite.
- *Don't eat by the clock.* Eat when you are hungry. This is often difficult to do when you are in a family or social setting, but you can manage when you are on your own.
- *Eat lettuce.* Lettuce is composed of a lot of water. It helps control hunger, has few calories, and contains plenty of vitamin C.
- *Stimulate your mind.* If you are very interested in a subject and are concentrating on it, you will not be overly concerned with food.
- *Relax and raise your serotonin levels.* You tend to eat less when you are relaxed, probably because the serotonin level in your brain is high enough to allow you to feel satiated.
- *Avoid triggers foods and drinks.* You know what yours are so keep them out of sight.
- *If you tend to binge or starve, get professional help.* Eating disorders may have a basis in hormonal and neurotransmitter imbalance.

# 10

# Nutrients to Enhance Brain Performance

What are the nutrients that might be supplements to specifically enhance your brain's performance?

There is much to be learned about the effect of what we eat in our mental abilities and there is no organization more interested in this than the United States military. The Committee on Military Nutrition Research was asked to assist a collaborative development program by evaluating the performance-enhancing effects of specific food components.[1]

"The increasing sophistication of weapon systems and the complexity of military operations places heavy demands on soldiers to effectively use these systems in military operations," Robert O. Nesheim, Ph.D., chair of the committee points out. "The U.S. Army has been led by concerns about individuals' abilities to avoid performance degradation and the need to enhance mental capabilities in highly stressful situations to an interest in devising military ration components that could enhance soldier performance."

Among the questions the Committee on Military Nutrition Research was asked to address:

- Is enhancement of physical and mental performance in "normal," healthy, young adult soldiers by diet or supplements a potentially fruitful approach or are there other methods of enhancing performance that have greater potential?
- Which food components, if any, would be the best candidates to enhance military physical and mental performance?

• Should the mode of administration be via fortification of the food in rations, supplemented via a separate food bar or beverage or administered in a pill?

The issue of mental performance that are of concern to military personnel, the committee said, in a combat setting do not differ from those in a regular workplace, with the exception of the severity of the levels and type of stress superimposed on the situation. The ability to perceive, attend to, and respond appropriately to cues, as well as make appropriate decisions, and to remain vigilant are critical in military combat settings. These areas of cognitive performance also form the basis for many physical performance tasks, such as positioning and loading artillery shells or moving through a minefield.

What are some of the food components the military and other nutrition experts believe may enhance brain function? The following are some of the major ones:

**Tyrosine.** It is an amino acid deemed nonessential because it does not seem to be necessary for growth. Tyrosine is used by the body to make neurotransmitters including norepinephrine and dopamine. Norepinephrine is an important brain chemical involved in the sleep–wake cycle, pain, anxiety, and arousal. Dopamine is involved in movement and mood. So, naturally, protection and enhancement of these brain messengers would be particularly important in a military setting. Results from several studies suggest that supplemental tyrosine does enhance dopamine and norepinephrine manufacture by the brain and reverses deficient performance.

In one study, subjects were placed in cold or high-altitude conditions. Mood and mental performance were assessed using a battery of standardized behavior tests. These adverse environmental conditions resulted in impaired cognitive performance, headache, lightheadedness, nausea, and general malaise. Tyrosine significantly reduced the severity of the symptoms and improved functioning believed to be regulated by the brain's nerve cell chemical messengers that control vigilance, alertness, and anxiety. Studies suggest strongly that single doses of tyrosine of about 100 to 150 milligrams per 2.2 pounds of body weight for an adult man—about 7 grams for a 154-pound man—can ameliorate some of the adverse effects of stress on cognitive performance in humans.[2]

The exact consequences of tyrosine administration are, as yet, unknown.

***Sweet memories—glucose.*** Glucose is a sugar that occurs naturally in blood, grapes, and corn. It is a source of energy for animals and plants. Sweeter than sucrose, table sugar, it is the main fuel for our brains. The administration of glucose—10 to 100 milligrams per 2.2 pounds of body weight—substantially blocked the impairment of accuracy in mental testing caused by cold exposure. The Committee on Military Nutrition Research concludes there are "tantalizing hints that glucose administration during cold stress and after sleep deprivation, such as could be accomplished with a candy bar, has some potential to improve memory and performance on cognition-based tasks."[3]

What about sleep deprivation that impairs alertness, cognitive performance, and mood? The ability to do useful mental work declines by 25 percent for every successive twenty-four hours an individual is awake. Early data suggest that sleep deprivation–induced degradation of performance is accompanied by decreases in brain glucose metabolism, particular in the front areas—where personality and discrimination are located. This provides a neurobiological correlate for the performance decrements. Whether the brain is less able to use glucose and hence is less able to do work, or is doing less work and hence uses less glucose, has not yet been determined.[4]

A series of studies on humans showed that ingesting a drink sweetened with glucose improves the memory performance of elderly subjects to a greater extent than does a saccharin-sweetened drink. The researchers interpret their data to suggest that aging is associated with impaired brain uptake of glucose from the blood which can be alleviated by increasing circulating blood glucose levels in these subjects.[5]

Under resting condition, glucose uptake is mainly by noninsulin-dependent pathways to the brain, blood cells, and kidneys. The blood glucose level remains quite constant being supplied by the liver. Fatty acids generated by the body fat stores are the predominant source of energy.

Dramatic changes in glucose occur when exercise begins. Rapid increases in energy demands activate the brain and nerves, which in turn stimulates both glucose production within the muscle itself and additional fat production in fatty tissues. Soon, blood flow to muscles is increased, and, as more blood is delivered, uptake of glucose by muscle is also increased.

These dramatic changes, however, are carefully regulated through a number of biochemical levels including hormone secretion and liver output of glucose. When muscle stores of glucose have been depleted and the blood glucose concentration falls, muscle glucose cannot meet the requirements and muscle fatigue rapidly ensues. Carbohydrates taken during the activity are able to maintain the blood glucose concentration above the critical level and prolong the time to fatigue during exercise of moderate intensity. The same has been shown with intense exercise.[6]

Dr. Paul Gold, a psychologist at the University of Virginia, found that when subjects were given a dose of glucose, they could think better. In one test, Gold's human subjects drank lemonade sweetened with either glucose or saccharin. They then heard a short story and were later asked what they remembered of the story. Results revealed that people given glucose tended to recall more.[7]

Gold said that glucose seemed to enhance memory even among people with cognitive disabilities like Alzheimer's. But he cautions: "It doesn't mean that I think everyone should consume large amounts of sugar so they can get smarter."

Although all the researchers say there is more research that needs to be done to determine how much supplemental glucose may be beneficial to brain and body, many lay persons have already found that a candy bar or a sugar-laden drink may help alleviate mental and physical fatigue.

**Carbohydrate edge.** Starches and sugars contain a high proportion of carbohydrates. Carbohydrates are chemicals that contain carbon, hydrogen, and oxygen and they are widely available in plants. In the body, however, carbohydrate in the blood supply is held at an almost constant level of about 0.05 to 0.1 percent.[8]

Carbohydrates are the fuel of life. Each gram of carbohydrate provides about four calories of energy—the same as protein but less than fat. Following digestion and absorption, available carbohydrates may be used to meet immediate energy needs of tissue cells, converted to glycogen, the storage form of glucose in liver and muscle for later energy needs, or converted to fat as a reserve for energy.

It is possible that relatively pure carbohydrate solutions have different effects in young and elderly individuals. Carbohydrates can act as a supplemental fuel source during exercise. The ability of carbohydrate supplements to prolong endurance during exercising is related to preventing fatigue in a physiological sense in both body and mind. The effect of carbohydrate in increasing the tryptophan ratio in blood is considered to be a possible mechanism.

HIGH NOON
Time of day differences characterize the effects of carbohydrates in the morning versus those in the early afternoon. When you eat a high-carbohydrate, low-protein lunch, fatigue increases more than after a higher protein lunch. After a high-carbohydrate, low-protein breakfast, fatigue decreases less than after a higher protein breakfast. Skipping lunch has only a modest adverse effect on performance.

Late-afternoon calorie-rich snacks enhance performance compared to consuming a low-calorie diet soda. No differences have been observed between a confectionery-type snack and yogurt when both contained at least 25 percent protein. Carbohydrate-rich, protein-poor snacks are more likely to be eaten in the late afternoon than at any other time of day except evenings. Yet no data characterize their effects on performance at that time of day. It is plausible that afternoon snacking could enhance performance, according to some studies.

Tasks involving cognitive performance including vigilance, reaction time, sorting, and arithmetic show steady improvement during the day, although the pattern is interrupted temporarily by a post-lunch slump. The bigger the lunch, the greater the cognitive performance declines. In addition, protein-poor meals have been reported to elicit large decreases in cognitive performance than protein-rich meals.

If you eat a high-carbohydrate meal that is lacking in protein, you will probably feel more fatigue than if you ate a meal higher in protein. Meals that contain a mixture of protein and carbohydrate exert more beneficial effects on cognition than do meals that are virtually protein free. Very little is known, however, of what balance between carbohydrate and protein is actually optimal for performance.

***Carbohydrate cravers.*** Carbohydrate cravers have been shown to have enhanced mood and reduced depression following carbohydrate consumption. This decreased depression has been interpreted as a consequence of the food-induced changes in the central serotonin levels.[9] Serotonin is a natural neurotransmitter in the brain. Low levels are associated with depression. The substance also plays a role in temperature regulation and sleep.

Although dietary factors certainly influence the endocrine system, there is no evidence that individual dietary components other than carbohydrates serve to alter the response patterns of the endocrine system to stress. (*see* Chapter 3 for athletics and carbohydrates.)

Even though we may crave carbohydrates, weight for weight, carbohydrate is less satiating than protein.

***Cholecystokinin (CCK) and memory.*** In Chapter 1, we described this interesting neurotransmitter that is found in both the stomach and the brain. As pointed out, one of its major duties is to tell us when we have eaten enough. Another may be to help us remember. James F. Flood, Ph.D., of the Psychobiology Research Laboratory at the Geriatric Research Center of the Veterans Administration Medical Center in Sepulveda, California, and his colleagues subjected groups of mice to different feeding routines while the mice were taught how to run a maze. One of the basic needs of even the most primitive organism is to find food. The advantage to the animal of maintaining a vivid memory of a successful hunt is obvious. The researchers reasoned that feeding animals right after a training session would enhance the animals' memories. The ability to remember the right route was best in those animals that ate voraciously after learning. The memory/eating connection was found to be linked to CCK, which is secreted during eating and is one of several neurotransmitters that carry messages to your brain to stop eating. CCK acts on the vagus nerve, which connects your stomach to your brain. When the vagus nerve was severed in the animal experiments, the memory effect of the after-learning meal was lost.

Dr. Flood speculates that the association of eating with memory may have given wild animals a survival advantage—eating caused the release of CCK, which in turn telegraphed the message along the vagus nerve to the brain. The enhanced memory of the animal, therefore, helped it to survive by filing away the successful food-hunting strategy.

So, the next time you have something to remember, study it and then eat a good meal that releases your CCK. Since the amino acids phenylalanine and tryptophan are reported to increase the amount of CCK released, that meal could include milk (high in phenylalanine) and nuts, rice, or seeds (all high in tryptophan).

*Caffeine* is a prime example of a central stimulant found in food, beverages. It has been hypothesized that supplementation with caffeine might delay the fatigue associated with endurance exercise by preventing a rise in brain serotonin levels. Again, one of the functions of serotonin, the self-made brain psychopharmaceutical, is to calm us down and make us sleepy.

Caffeine, the most common psychopharmaceutical, has been studied on cognitive performance, mood, and alertness in human subjects who had been sleep deprived. Its stimulant effects are weak when compared to other drugs, but most studies to date suggest that it tends to delay sleep, reduce the deterioration of performance associated with fatigue and boredom, and decrease steadiness of the hands, particularly when performance is already partially degraded on repetitive nonintellectual tasks.

It was concluded those large doses of caffeine from 150 to 600 milligrams in a person weighing 254 pounds reversed sleep-deprivation–induced degradation in cognitive performance, mood, and alertness without serious side effects. It has been recommended that 250-milligram tablets be made available to soldiers in their rations.

*Carnitine,* also called vitamin $B_T$, is a thyroid inhibitor found in muscle, liver, and meat extracts. Muscles, which contain approximately 98 percent carnitine, must take it up from the blood. When carnitine is deficient, muscles become weakened and the body becomes intolerant to exercise. Carnitine plays a critical role in energy metabolism. It acts as a storehouse of high-energy compounds, stimulates fatty acid oxidation, transports enzymes across membranes, and prevents accumulation of lactate (involved in muscle fatigue), and stimulates carbohydrate and amino acid utilization.

Most Americans consume 50 to 100 milligrams of carnitine in their diets per day, with some eating three times that amount. Carnitine appears to be safe, but there is little evidence that more is better in normal individuals. Basic research on the various forms of carnitine on exercise may be in order.

Peggy Borum, Ph.D., of the University of Florida at Gainesville, another member of the military nutrition panel, says that it is clear carnitine has an important metabolic role in exercising muscles. However, specific function of carnitine and acylcarnite and the effect of supplementation remain to be elucidated.[10] Carnitine has been found to be safe under most circumstances. However, more is not necessarily better, and investigation of patients with different physical ailments has indicated better results can sometimes be obtained with lower doses.

In the meantime, researchers in psychiatry at the University of Texas Houston Health Center have found that early studies with acety-L-carnitine show "some promise" in slowing the progress of the memory destroying disease, Alzheimer's.[11]

***Protein pleasure.*** Protein is substantially more satiating than carbohydrates, as pointed out. Furthermore, the satiating effect carries over until the next meal. Researchers report that intake of a high-protein meal reduces protein intake as well as total food intake in the subsequent meal.[12]

A report of improved mental performance in mental tests was measured in subjects given isoleucine, leucine, and valine in a supplement during a 30-kilometer cross-country race.[13]

Carol Greenwood, Ph.D., of the Department of Nutritional Sciences, University of Toronto Medical School, and a member of the Committee on Military Nutrition Research, notes that supplementation with certain amino acids may play a useful role under stressful conditions, but the studies are very preliminary.

She concludes that to maximize and maintain the effectiveness of supplemental amino acids, they should not be administered with meals and should be provided on an intermittent basis. She adds consumption of protein-containing foods in combination with supplemental amino acids may not produce the desired change in amino acids in the blood, especially if central nervous system uptake of the supplemented amino acids is desired.[14]

Dr. Greenwood points out, "Provision of meals high in either protein or carbohydrates may influence satiety and certain aspects of mood and performance. However, this effect of meal composition is variable and can be influenced by the age and gender of the individual. Furthermore the impact of altering meal composition on mood and behavior has not been examined under stressful conditions."

***Choline.*** Choline is a B-complex vitamin found in most animal tissues, either free or in combinations, such as lecithin or acetylcholine. Choline is an essential component of the human diet that is important for the normal functioning of all cells. Choline and choline-containing compounds are critical for a wide variety of metabolic processes within the body, including acting as a messenger within the cells and as neurotransmitters in the nervous system, controlling muscle contraction, and participating in immune response. Supplemental choline can help sustain exercise when it has been reduced by long-distance running.[15]

While the exact role and requirement of choline in the diet remains unknown, the brain is unable to make choline itself. It must be derived from the diet or from choline manufactured by the liver.[16] As far back as the September 8, 1977, issue of the *New England Journal of Medicine,* researchers from MIT reported choline supplementation could relieve the involuntary facial twitching of persons suffering from tardive dyskinesia, a brain ailment common in long-time antipsychotic-drug users.

One of the best-known functions of choline is as a component of acetylcholine, an important neurotransmitter vital to memory function. Choline is present in a wide variety of foods. Diets deficient in choline produce liver dysfunction within three weeks, resulting in massive triglyceride accumulation in the liver and also produce changes in muscle conduction. Choline is being actively studied for its effects on brain neurotransmission and memory.

In a study with normal students at West Valley College in Saratoga, California, phosphatidylcholine, a precursor of choline, was tested. Neither the researchers nor the students knew which was the choline compound and which was a placebo. The researchers reported that 3.7 grams of choline produced significant improvement in explicit memory, as measured by serial learning tasks. The major improvement was observed at 90 minutes after ingestion. A slight improvement was observed at 60 minutes.[17]

Choline, possibly because nature recognized its importance, is the only neurotransmitter that has been found that can be made from another dietary component besides protein. The amino acid serine, derived from protein, is a basic material for choline, but so is lecithin, which is found in large amounts in eggs. In addition to the lack of serine and lecithin in the diet, lack of sufficient $B_{12}$, and folic acid can also affect the formation of the brain neurotransmitter acetylcholine. Do elderly persons hampered by the lack of money to buy protein foods become deficient in choline? If so, they would lack acetylcholine to charge their brain cells and thus would probably exhibit the memory deficits so common even in "normal" aging.

There has been an effort to increase the building blocks of acetylcholine by increasing lecithin, the normal source of choline in the diet. This has been disappointing so far. Dairy products, peanuts, soybeans, and meats contain significant amounts of lecithin. The Thomas J. Lipton Company once tested a lecithin-enriched chicken noodle soup as a method of supplying large amounts of this chemical to the brain. Purified lecithin, which is more concentrated than that sold in health food stores, raises blood levels of choline, which, in turn, may aid memory. Lecithin also contains phosphatidylcholine, now being tested to see if it can help memory problems.

Animal studies suggest that increasing lecithin in the diet may prevent, not cure, memory deficits. As of this writing, a combination of lecithin and piracetam, a synthetic compound derived from alcohol, seems to affect brain energy and facilitate performance on measures of learning and retention in brain-injured and aged rats. It also appears to protect against impairment caused by lack of oxygen in animals. Piracetam is being tested on brain-injured children but seems to work better when combined with lecithin rather than either substance alone.[18] Preliminary studies in five geriatic centers suggest that some patients may respond positively to this treatment.

Supplemental choline has been used with some success in the treatment of tardive dyskinesia, abnormal grimacing and movements occurring as a side effect of some antipsychotic medications. The researchers concluded from a number of studies that choline and the cholinesterase inhibitor physostigmine were about equally effective but the choline was less toxic. Most patients exhibited some reduction in the frequency of abnormal movement, but in only a few cases as there complete cessation of movement.[19]

The concept that the impairment of the brain's system for using choline in certain diseases and in old age may be prevented or minimized by adding choline-based materials to the diet is certainly worth pursuing. Researchers agree that the importance of adequate amounts of choline or lecithin in the diet should not be minimized and that the amount probably varies greatly with age, disease, and the composition of other foods in the diet. In addition to the above, there are herbs promoted for enhancing brain function. The most prominent at this writing are:

**Ginkgo biloba.** Have you purchased any ginko biloba yet? Ginkgo is among the most popular prescription drugs in Europe. In the United States, it is sold over-the-counter as a "food."

What is ginkgo? The leaves and nuts of *Ginkgo biloba*—also called *Maidenhair*—are used in ancient Chinese remedies. The ginkgo is supposedly the oldest living tree, having survived some 200 million years. It is said to be the only tree that came through the effects of atomic radiation in Hiroshima, Japan.

Ginkgo has been reported to improve circulation, mental functioning, stop ringing in the ears, and to relieve symptoms of Alzheimer's disease, coldness, emotional depression, Raynaud's disease (a circulatory problem), arthritic disease, hardening of the arteries, dizziness, and anxiety. In recent animal studies at the University of Illinois, ginkgo protected the brains of rats to a significant degree when a toxic compound that induces oxygen damage and brain swelling was given.[20]

German researchers have reported that in patients suffering from late-onset dementia of the Alzheimer type, ginkgo biloba exerted a "positive effect." The researchers believe that ginkgo works on the membrane changes.[21]

A report in *The Journal of Urology* described a study of 60 patients suffering from impotence due to insufficient blood supply to the penis. After six months of daily treatment with an extract of ginkgo, 50 percent of the subjects were again able to achieve penile erections. Nearly 45 percent of the remaining subjects showed some improvement.

An extract of ginkgo biloba can stabilize and, in some cases, improve the cognitive function and the social behavior of demented patients for six months to one year.[22] In a report published in the *Journal of the American Medical Association,* Pierre L. LeBars,

M.D., Ph.D., from the New York Institute for Medical Research in Tarrytown, New York, and colleagues reported beneficial effects of EGb 761, a particular extract of ginkgo biloba, compared to placebo in a study of 309 demented patients with mild to moderately severe cognitive impairment caused by Alzheimer's disease, vascular dementia, or a combination of the two.

Dr. LeBars presented the findings of the research, which was a one-year double-blind, placebo-controlled, parallel-group, multicenter study.

He and his colleagues conclude: "EGb appears to stabilize and, in an additional 20 percent of cases (versus placebo), improve the patient's functioning for periods of six months to one year. Regarding its safety, adverse events associated with EGb were no different from those associated with placebo."

The researchers found that 27 percent of patients treated 26 weeks or more with EGb achieved at least a four-point improvement on the 70-point Alzheimer's Disease Assessment Scale–Cognitive subscale (ADAS-Cog), compared with 14 percent taking placebo; on the Geriatric Evaluation by Relative's Rating Instrument (GERRI), the daily living and the social behavior of 37 percent were considered improved with EGb, compared to 23 percent taking placebo.

The extract of ginkgo biloba, EGb 761, is a popular plant extract used in Europe that has recently been approved in Germany for the treatment of dementia. How EGb acts on the central nervous system is not completely understood. It contains compounds that scavenge free radicals some believe to be the mediators of the excessive lipid peroxidation and cell damages observed in Alzheimer's disease.

The study results demonstrated that EGb had a measurable beneficial effect on cognition and daily living and social behavior in patients with dementia.

The researchers stated that compared with the placebo group, the EGb group included twice as many patients whose cognitive performance improved enough to estimate a six-month delay in progression of the disease.

The researchers consider that the flavonoids acting as antioxidants might combat the cell damage from free radicals. They also think that perhaps another substance in ginkgo, terpenoids, might counteract blood clotting and inflammation.

LeBars said, however, he doubted the herb actually repaired any brain damage. "I believe as a scientist that what is lost is lost. An extract cannot generate new cells." Martin Katz, who also worked in the study, said ginkgo might be used to prevent deterioration. "When you have a drug as safe as this you can think in terms of prevention," he told a news conference.

In the meantime, if you are taking over-the-counter ginkgo, be aware that excessive use can cause itching and gastrointestinal upset. In rare instances, excessive doses can induce shortness of breath and convulsions.

***Get Hep with Hup.*** Scientists and pharmaceutical firms are excited about another ancient remedy, a tea, *Oian Ceng Ta,* brewed by elderly Chinese from the leaves of *Huperzia Serrata* (Club Moss) to improve memory. In the 1980s, scientists at the Shanghai Institute of Materia Medica and the Zhejiiang Academy of Medical Sciences isolated the active components in Huperzine (Hup A) and found that it was a remarkably potent inhibitor of acetyl-cholinesterase (AChE). Acetylcholinesterase breaks down acetyl-choline, a chemical in the brain that is vital for memory function. The Chinese have reported that Hup A is effective in treating patients with memory impairment, myasthenia gravis, and multi-infarct dementia (small clots that caused mental deterioration.)[23]

Because there is very little Hup A in the natural plant, Alan P. Kozikowski, Ph.D., at the Mayo Clinic, Jacksonville, Florida, and chemists at the Shanghai Institute have independently synthesized Hup A. The new compound has reportedly greater activity and less side effects than that of the basic extract.[24]

Alcohol, of course, is one of the oldest active beverages. It has been used since the beginning of time to cheer, calm, relieve emotional and physical pain, and to stimulate. Actually, it is a depressant that, if taken in large amounts, can destroy the brain. The Chinese have an herb to combat alcohol abuse, kudzu (*Radix puerariae*), that pesky vine now spreading unchecked throughout the southern United States. But in China, an extract from the vine was cited as a medication as early as 200 B.C. and about A.D. 600, a Chinese pharmacopeia listed the herb as having an antidrunken-ness effect.

Using Syrian golden hamsters, animals that prefer alcohol to water, two scientists from Harvard Medical School found that the extracts of the herb reduced alcohol consumption by about 50 percent.[25]

To document the use of the extract *Radix puerariae,* Dr. Wing-Ming Keung, one of the Harvard investigators, went to China and interviewed modern research scientists as well as physicians who offer traditional herbal remedies. Dr. Keung found about 80 percent of 300 alcoholics treated for two to four weeks lost their desire for alcohol and had no adverse side effects from the herb.

One of his colleagues at Harvard commented about kudzu research: "It is good to look at nature and folk medicine and realize nature has lots to teach us."

In the meantime, a Georgetown University researcher, Alan Kozikowski, Ph.D., has synthesized the active substance in the leaves of Huperzia. The synthesized substance, called Huperzine, blocks the breakdown of the chemical messenger in the brain, acetylcholine, which as pointed out a number of times is vital to the function of memory. Dr. Kozikowski says with the help of Georgetown molecular modeler Dr. Shaomeng Wang they have developed an analog that is eight times more potent than Huperzine. He says the new compound should be more targeted to affected brain tissue and should go to the brain faster than existing Alzheimer's disease medication. However, the compound must undergo clinical trials before it is available.[26]

***St. John's-wort (Hypericum perforatum)*** is also called amber, blessed, devil's scourge, God's wonder herb, grace of God, goatweed, hypericum, and klamath weed. A perennial native to Britain, Europe and Asia, it is now grown throughout North America. The plant contains glycosides, volatile oil, tannin, resin, and pectin (*see all*). It was believed to have infinite healing powers derived from the saint, the red juice representing his blood. A spray has been used for colds. It is now being studied by researchers from the National Cancer Institute and universities as a potential treatment for cancer and AIDS. The FDA listed St. John's-wort as an "unsafe herb" in 1977. The FDA issued a notice in 1992 that St. John's-wort has not been shown to be safe and effective as claimed in over-the-counter digestive-aid products. That does not mean, however, that it cannot be used for other purposes.

Hypericin, the active ingredient in this herb, has been shown in studies to inhibit the activity of monoamine oxidase, which is elevated in depressed people. People are taking as much as 200 milligrams of a 0.3-percent dosage of two to six capsules per day. It may cause sensitivity to sunlight.

Can you take St. John's-wort with prescription antidepressant medications? Be sure to ask your physician!

There are several concerns about the use of St. John's-wort. It is believed to act in part as a monoamine oxidase (MAO) inhibitor because of the active ingredient hypericin. Prescription MAO inhibitors were used clinically for many years as an antidepressant. With time it became clear that MAO inhibitors must be used with care because there is a risk of hypertensive crisis (a potentially life-threatening elevation in blood pressure) when they are taken with some over-the-counter drugs (such as decongestants and some weight-loss products) or after ingestion of foods containing high levels of tyramine (aged cheeses, sour cream, herring, wine, salami). MAO inhibitors have also caused other serious side effects, including tremors, seizures, and delirium when combined with such antidepressant as Prozac, Zoloft, and Paxil.

Because the active ingredient in St. John's-wort is an MAO inhibitor there is justifiable concern about similar interactions. The potential for life-threatening drug interactions is the reason St. John's-wort should never be taken in combination with any prescription antidepressant. Again, seek expert medical advice.

***Chervil (Anthriscus cerefolium)*** is an herb of the carrot family native to Europe. Used as a restorative for the elderly, it was called cerefolium because it was said to be a powerful brain stimulant. It is used for gout. As a poultice, it is used for arthritic pains.

***Anemone (Anemone ranunculaceae),*** also called windflower, pulsatilla, and lily-of-the-field. It is common throughout Europe. References to the small herbs can be found in Greek and Chinese ancient medicinal literature. Anemone is still used today as a homeopathic remedy for various emotional ills.

***Balm (Melissa officinalis),*** also called lemon balm and sweet balm. A sweet-tasting herb introduced into Britain by the Romans, it has been used from early times in England for nervousness.

***Berry extracts.*** Diets high in antioxidant foods appear to protect the brain against oxidative damage. In rat studies by Agriculture

Research Service and University of Denver scientists,[27] damage from oxygen is thought to lead to age-related dysfunctions such as loss of memory or motor coordination. But rats that ate extracts of strawberries, blueberries, or spinach as part of their daily diet fared far better on brain cell function tests than the animals getting chow alone. The animals were put in a high oxygen exposure which alters brain function in young rats in a manner similar to the aging process. The scientists measured the rat's response to three different types of brain function controlling memory, movement, and growth of nerve cells. In all three cases, decline in these functions due to oxygen exposure was significantly—often dramatically—reduced by strawberry extract as well as by vitamin E. Preliminary data indicate that blueberry extract provides even more protection to rat brains. Blueberries, the researchers found, have the highest antioxidant capacity of the fruits and vegetables they tested.

**Blue flag (Iris versicolor),** also called flag lily, fleur-de-lis, liver lily, poison flag, and wild iris. The rhizome contains salicylic and isophthalic acids, volatile oil, iridin, a glycoside gum, resin, and sterols (*see all in* Glossary). Herbalists use it in herbal medicines both for relaxing and stimulating.

**Brahmi (Hydrocotyle asiatica),** is an herb used in India to relieve anxiety and to treat epilepsy.

**Burdock (Actium lappa),** also called lapp, bardane, and beggar's buttons. The root, seed, and leaves contain essential oil of this common roadside plant. It contains nearly 45 percent inulin (*see* Glossary) and many minerals. Herbalists use it as a tonic. Chinese burdock is used to eliminate excess nervous energy, and the root is considered to have aphrodisiac properties.

**Chamomile (Chamomilla),** also called camomile. There are English, Roman, German, and Hungarian varieties of the plant. The daisylike white and yellow heads of these flowers contains sesquiterpene lactones, essential oil, calcium, coumarin, and tannic acid. Chamomile is widely used as a tea for digestive ills and for tranquilization and insomnia. The oil is used with crushed poppy heads as a poultice for toothaches and neuralgia. Herbalists claim that chamomile tea prevents nightmares.

*Clover, Red (Trifolium pratense)* is a perennial common through Europe and is used in medicine as a tea and sometimes combined with other herbs as a tonic. It is reputedly good for the nerves because of its sedative properties.

*Damiana (Turnera diffusa; Turnera aphrodisiaca),* also called pastorata. The leaves contain volatile oil, hydrocyanic glycoside, bitter principle, and tannin and resin (*see all in* Glossary). The drug is used by herbalists as a mild aphrodisiac for both sexes. It is reputed to be the safest of plant aphrodisiacs. It is also believed to counteract depression.

*Dill (Anethum graveolens)* is a hardy herb native to southern Europe and western Asia as well as the Americas. It was said by the ancient Greek physician Galen that it "procureth sleep." The name *dill* is derived from a Saxon word meaning "to lull." It is used by herbalists to treat symptoms of colic in children and insomnia in adults caused by indigestion. Dill in hot milk is recommended by herbalists as a drink that calms the nerves.

*Garlic (Allum sativum),* is a member of the onion family that was cultivated in Egypt from earliest times and known in China more than 2,000 years ago. Garlic contains lots of potassium, fluorine, sulfur, phosphorus, and vitamins A and C as well as 75 different sulfur compounds. In addition it contains quercetin and cyanidin and bioflavonoids (*see* Glossary). Garlic also contains selenium, which has been found to have anticancer potential. Garlic has been used since ancient times to treat all sorts of ailments, including the Great Plague in Europe and dysentery during World War I. The herb has recently been found to contain antibiotic, antiviral, and antifungal ingredients. It has also been found that aged garlic extract (AGE) can improve learning and memory, at least in older animals. A surprising result was obtained by measuring the brain size. Chronic ingestion of AGE prevented brain atrophy in elderly animals.[28] The researchers concluded that the results raise the possibility that AGE may be beneficial for age-related cognitive disorders in humans.

*Ginseng (Panax ginseng;* **Asia)** *(Panax ciquefoil;* **North America)***; Eleutherococcus senticosus* **(Siberian ginseng).** The Chinese esteem ginseng as an herb of many uses and have been using it in medicine for more than 5,000 years. The Chinese and Koreans also used it in combination with chicken soup. The word "panax" comes from the Greek *panakos,* a panacea. Among its active ingredients are amino acids, essential oils, carbohydrates, peptides, vitamins, minerals, enzymes, and sterols. In the Orient, it is esteemed for its abilities to preserve health, invigorate the system, and prolong life. It is taken in an herbal tea as a daily tonic. It is believed to be a mind/body energy booster. North American Indians used ginseng as a love potion. It has been found to normalize high or low blood sugar.

Two compounds isolated from a type of ginseng may be potent neuroprotectors, researchers from the university of Maryland School of Medicine and the Seoul National University have found.[29]

Tae H. Oh, Ph.D., professor of anatomy and neurobiology at Maryland, and Young C. Kim, Ph.D., from Seoul National University in Korea, studied the effects of extracts of ginseng, ginsenosides Rb1 and Rg3, on brain cells from rats. The compounds effectively inhibited overproduction of cell-killing nitrous oxide, which routinely follows nerve-cell poisoning by a naturally occurring amino acid byproduct called L-glutamate. They also inhibited formation of a dangerous compound called malondialdehyde, and raised diminished levels of helpful superoxide dismutase in glutamate-treated cells.

**Hops (Humulus lupulus),** also called silent night, is widely cultivated. This plant has been used in folk medicine for its calming effect on the body. It contains an estrogenlike ingredient as well as volatile oil, lupulin, bitter principle, and tannin. It is used to relieve gas and cramps and to stimulate appetite. It is used in a poultice to relieve sciatica and arthritis, toothaches, and other nerve pain. It has been used to induce sleep and as a tonic in wine. Both Abraham Lincoln and England's King George III reportedly relied on hops to promote a restful calm at bedtime. Hops flowers were listed in the USP (*see* Glossary) for 90 years.

**Hyssop (Hyssopus officinalis)** is a perennial herb native to southern Europe. It is used to calm the nerves.

**Japanese turf lily (Ophiopogon japonicus),** also called creeping lily root and dwarf lily turf, the bulbs are used by herbalists to give clients a sense of inner well-being and to relieve insomnia and fearfulness.

***Jasmine (Jasminum officinale; Gelsemium sempervirens),*** also called Carolina jessamine, gelsemium root, and yellow jessamine. For centuries the jasmine flower has been brewed in tea to aid relaxation. The rhizomes and roots contain the alkaloid gelsemine, a very potent analgesic that is used to treat the severe pain in the face known as *tic douloureux* or *trigeminal neuralgia*. Herbalists also claim that jasmine oil rubbed on the body increases sexual interest. It can be highly toxic and can cause death by respiratory arrest.

***Jujube date (Zizyhus jujuba),*** also called Da T'sao, the Chinese jujube date is commonly used in a wide variety of herbal formulas. It is found dried in most Oriental markets. It is used to enhance the taste and benefits of soups and stews and to energize the body. Chinese herbalists believe it relieves nervous exhaustion, insomnia, apprehension, forgetfulness, dizziness, and clamminess.

***Kava kava (Piper methysticum)*** is also known as kava and ava. Herbalists use the Polynesian herb's root as a remedy for insomnia and nervousness. Kava kava has been used by South Pacific islanders for centuries to relieve anxiety and elevate mood and relax muscles. A compound in kava is marketed in Europe as a mild sedative for the elderly. Other agents in kava have been shown to have antiseptic properties in the laboratory. It is also a reputedly potent analgesic and antiseptic that may be taken internally or applied directly to a painful wound. It is being sold over-the-counter in 200-milligram capsules. Since it has sedative effects, precautions should be taken. It is also a reputedly potent analgesic and antiseptic that may be taken internally or applied directly to a painful wound. Chronic use can cause diarrhea, loss of appetite, and apathy. In some cases, disorientation and hallucinations may result. It is contraindicated in pregnancy and for young children. Caution should be taken about driving or operating machinery or doing any work that requires complete alertness when taking this herb.

***Lady's slipper (Cypripedium calceoulus)*** is used to treat anxiety, stress, insomnia, neurosis, restlessness, tremors, epilepsy, and palpitations. Herbalists claim it is also useful for depression. It contains volatile oils, resins, sugars, and tannin.

**Lemon balm (Melissa officinalis).** The leaves of this herb contain essential oils, acids, and tannin (*see* Glossary). Herbalists use it to calm nervous tension and elevate mood.

**Lettuce, wild (Lactuca virosa)** is also known as lettuce opium. During the Middle Ages, lettuce was used as a valuable narcotic and its milky juice, lactuca, was used with opium to induce sleep. Herbalists use it to treat insomnia, restlessness, and anxiety, especially in children. It is also used to treat coughs, colic pains, and painful menstruation. It also reputedly eases arthritic pain.

**Lime blossom (Tilia europea),** also called linden, has flowers that contain essential oils, mucilage, flavonoids, coumarin, and vanillin (*see all in* Glossary). Herbalists used it for a relaxation from nervous tension and to lower blood pressure.

**Lovage (Ligusticum scoticum),** also known as shunis, is an ingredient in perfumery from an aromatic herb native to southern Europe and grown in monastery gardens centuries ago for medicine and food flavoring. It has a hot, sharp, biting taste. The yellow-brown oil is extracted from the root or other parts of the herb. It has a reputation for improving health and inciting love; Czechoslovakian girls reportedly wear it in a bag around their necks when dating boys.

**Passionflower (Passiflora incarnata)** is used in over-the-counter homeopathic medicines for temporary relief of simple nervous tension and insomnia. It is an extremely popular herb in Europe, where it is often used to induce relaxation and sleep. It has been shown that an extract of the plant depresses the motor nerves of the spinal cord. One of the ingredients in passionflower is serotonin, a neurotransmitter that is deficient in persons who are depressed.

**Poppy (Papaver),** also known as opium poppy, red poppy, California poppy, and papaver. Early monasteries grew poppies for use in hospitals for pain relief, and the sap was used through the Middle Ages during crude surgical operations and after serious battlefield injuries. The exudates from the poppies all contain substances with sedative and hypnotic properties. Extracts are generally used as sedatives, narcotics, and analgesics. They are used to treat diarrhea, pain, coughs, sweating, and insomnia.

*Schizandra (Schisandra chinesis),* is an herb used by Chinese women as an aphrodisiac and a youth tonic. It is a mild sedative. It is also believed to increase stamina. Schizandra has been shown in modern scientific laboratories to protect against the narcotic and sedative effects of alcohol and barbiturates. It is used as a tea. It is contraindicated in persons with high blood pressure, epilepsy, and increased pressure on the brain.

*Shanka puspi (Confolvulus mycrophyllus)* is an herb used in India to treat anxiety and mild pain.

*Sweet fern (Polypodium vulgare),* also called wood licorice, common polypody, female fern, and rock brake. The root of this fern that is distributed throughout Europe, South Africa, Siberia, Asia, and North America was used in folk medicine to treat melancholy and intestinal obstructions. The resin is considered to be useful against worms and as a purgative. It also possesses demulcent properties. Sweet fern is also reportedly useful in alleviating coughs and other lung problems as well as being a good appetite stimulant.

*Vacha (Acorus calamus)* is an herb used in India as a tranquilizer and aphrodisiac.

*Valerian (Valeriana officinalis)* is a perennial native to Europe and the United States that was reputed to be a love potion. Its vapor was found to kill the bacillus of typhoid fever after 45 minutes. The herb has been widely studied in Europe and Russia and the major constituents, the valepotriates, have been reported to have marked sedative, anticonvulsive, blood-pressure–lowering and tranquilizing effects. Valerian has been used for centuries to treat panic attacks. In Germany, valerian preparations have been used for more than a decade to treat childhood behavioral disorders, supposedly without the side effects experienced with pharmaceuticals for that purpose. It has been reported that the herb also helps concentration and energy. Prolonged use of valerian may result in side effects such as irregular heartbeat, headaches, uneasiness, nervousness, and insomnia. Very large doses may cause paralysis.

***Vervain, European (Verbena officinalis)*** is a weed of the Verbena family. Native to Europe and the Far East, it is believed the Druids introduced vervain to Rome. Hippocrates prescribed vervain for wounds, fevers, and nervous disorders. In England, vervain was used against witches. Homeopathic medicine has used it to treat nervous disorders and epilepsy. In the United States it is used as a flavoring in alcoholic beverages.

Summing it up, it has been reported that even short-term nutritional deprivation such as skipping breakfast can be detrimental to cognition. There is evidence that the nutrients mentioned in this chapter may be of some use in enhancing brain function. Anything you ingest, however, whether food, medication, or supplemental nutrients, must be taken with caution. Your body is a chemical factory that maintains an exquisite balance. You are unique and some of the supplements may be beneficial to you and some may cause adverse reactions.

As exciting research into food and nutrients and the brain continues, more edible substances to improve cognition in the healthy as well as those with deficits will be available.

# 11

# Diet for a Smart Brain

You have spent your life, thus far, with certain eating and living habits, some good and some bad. You have a measure of control over your habits—the diet you eat and the amount of exercise you get and whether you smoke cigarettes or drink alcoholic beverages. A number of the physical and mental changes you experience from day to day are influenced by your habits. Others result directly from the wear and tear of the passing years.

How many of the changes we associate with age are due to the passing of years and how many are the result of years of passing up the right foods?

Almost all experts agree that the foods we select are a big factor in maintaining the health of our brains and bodies, but there is much yet to be learned about the nutritional needs of specific ages. The RDAs are based on healthy young males, while it is now accepted that the nutritional needs of a 20-year-old, a 50-year-old, and a 70-year-old are very different.

Kidney and liver functions may decline 20 to 30 percent between the ages of 50 and 90 years. Both organs are involved in clearing drugs and foods from the body. This has been shown in the amount of time it takes to clear the drug diazepam (the muscle relaxant Valium) from the body after ingestion. On the average, it takes a 50-year-old 55 hours and an 80-year-old as long as 90 hours to clear the drug.

One change that occurs as the years pass is the rate at which your body uses energy while at rest—the basal metabolism rate—which slows down as the total amount of lean body tissue decreases and the amount of total body fat increases. But how much of the slowed metabolism is due to aging and how much is due to too much fat and sugar in the diet? How much does stress or exercise affect how you process food?

Edward Schneider, M.D., of the National Institutes of Health and his colleagues point out that on the one hand, a cut in calories has been recommended for us as we grow older, to adjust for our slowed metabolism and our decrease in physical activity. The slower metabolism results in a reduction in lean body mass. On the other hand, an increased intake of calcium has been recommended for older women, to counter the age-associated decline in bone mass. The recommended changes in intake are based on the assumption that the age-related declines in muscle and activity levels are normal and harmless, but that the declines in bone mass is abnormal. However, researchers such as Dr. Schneider now suggest that many of the age-related disabilities of the brain and body might be decreased if lean body mass and physical activity were maintained rather than diminished in older persons.[1]

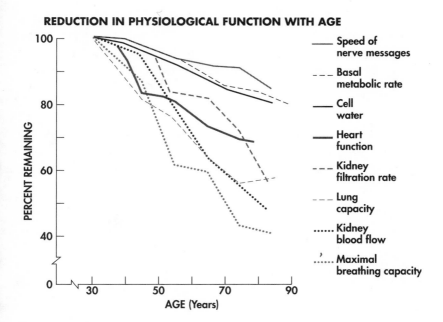

Graph adapted from B. L. Strohler, "Origin of the Effects of Time and High-Energy Radiation on Living Systems," *Quarterly Review of Biology,* (1959) 34: (2), 117–42.

## Protein Power for Your Brain

All through this book we have described the importance of amino acids, the building blocks of protein, and brain function. Twenty percent of your body's inner energy is spent on processing protein. Proteins form the major cell structure of your body. They are biochemical workers and are vital to regulate gene function. They are the chief nitrogen-containing constituents of our bodies—the essential constituents of every living cell. They are complex but by weight contain about 50 percent carbon, 20 percent oxygen, 15 percent nitrogen, 7 percent hydrogen, and some sulfur. Some proteins also contain iron and phosphorus. How much protein do you need in your diet? Does protein need vary greatly with age?

For babies, the standard amino acid pattern of human milk is used. The RDA for adults has been set at 600 to 800 milligrams per kilogram of protein. Many bodybuilders and marathon runners believe that increasing their intake of protein will enable them to achieve greater stamina. The results have been equivocal. Some studies say that higher than normal intake of protein increased muscle mass, while other studies have shown no benefit.[2]

Do we need to decrease protein as we age?

Jeff Blumberg, Ph.D., assistant director of the Tufts Center on Nutrition and the Aging, says,

> We're questioning the basic assumption that older people require smaller amounts of nutrients because their bodies are slowing down and because they're less active. While their calorie requirements may be diminished because they are less active, their nutrient requirements are the same or may be even greater than they were. Perhaps if elderly people get more of certain nutrients, the aging process may slow down.[3]

Therefore, one of the nutrients in our diet that we may need to increase or at least maintain as we grow older is protein. Lean body mass declines with age, it is believed, because of changes in protein absorption or metabolism or both. Therefore, older people may need more protein, not only for lean body mass but because their brains' neurotransmitters are made from protein bases.

As we grow older, most of us begin to have problems with our memories: Where did I put those keys? What is her name? Why did I open the refrigerator door? In fact, such problems are so common that they are called "benign senile forgetfulness." (Then, of course, there is the devastating brain degenerative disease that affects more than two million Americans and their families—Alzheimer's—in which the loss of memory is severe.)

What happens to the brain and its memory function as we age, and what part does protein play? Remember that old belief that fish is brain food? There may be some truth to it, because fish contains high levels of choline, as do meat and eggs. Choline in the food we eat is taken from our digestive tracts by our blood and carried to our brains where it becomes acetylcholine, the brain chemical very important to memory function.

As we age, the capability of transferring information from one cell to another or to a target organ is markedly reduced. In part, this is due to the amount of acetylcholine and in part to the ability to use what is there. An enzyme used to produce acetylcholine is *N-acetyltransferase*. Interestingly, it has been discovered that stress depresses the amount of acetyltransferase. We've all experienced difficulty when trying to think under stress—blame your acetyltransferase.

One of the most consistent neurochemical findings is the reduced activity of choline acetyltransferase in the aged human brain and its markedly reduced activity in the brains of Alzheimer's victims.

**Protein** (*two servings per day*): Choose a fish like flounder, instead of chicken, and you'll ingest half the fat and calories. Fresh fish, chicken, turkey, legumes, lean veal, fat-trimmed flank steak, and fat-trimmed leg of lamb are all good choices. Below are some samples of protein-rich foods.

## EXAMPLES OF PROTEIN IN COMMON FOODS

| Food | Amount | Protein grams |
|---|---|---|
| Flounder (baked) | 1 slice | 30 |
| Tuna | 1 can | 28.8 |
| Swordfish (broiled) | 3½ ounces | 28.0 |
| Club steak | 1 portion | 16.0 |
| Hamburger | 1 patty | 21.8 |
| Lamb (ground) | 3½ ounces | 22.4 |
| Chicken (canned) | 1 portion | 21.7 |
| Canadian bacon | 1 slice | 38.9 |
| Veal cutlet | 1 portion | 27.1 |
| Brie cheese | 1 portion | 28.8 |
| Milk (whole) | 1 glass | 3.3 |
| Milk (low-fat) | 1 glass | 3.3 |
| Oatmeal | 1 portion | 14.2 |
| Wheat germ (toasted) | 1 ounce | 6.2 |
| Egg | 1 | 12.1 |
| Yogurt, plain | 1 cup | 5.3 |
| Swiss cheese | 1 slice | 28.4 |
| Soybean flour | 3½ ounces | 34.8 |
| Soybean miso | 3½ ounces | 10.5 |
| Ham (fresh) | 2 slices | 39.6 |

## Carbohydrate Cresting

Many athletes believe that to increase endurance high-carbohydrate drinks or food gives them the edge. During strenuous exercise, the body may take extra sugar from the muscles' reserves. If a high-carbohydrate drink of about 5 grams per 2.2 pounds of weight is taken three hours prior to exercising, runners have found it allows them to keep going 17 percent longer than those who did not "carb up." Other runners have tried to eat 70 grams of carbohydrates—for example, oatmeal—one hour before race time and they were found to run a faster time or exercise longer than those who did not eat the carbohydrates. This means that if you are 150 pounds and eat three hours before racing, you should consume 225 grams of carbohydrates.

| EXAMPLES OF CARBOHYDRATES IN COMMON FOODS | | |
|---|---|---|
| Food | Amount | Carbohydrates (grams) |
| Orange juice | 12 ounces | 46 |
| Tuna fish | 12 ounces | 39 |
| Bagel | 1 medium | 30.9 |
| Cranberry juice | 12 ounces | 54 |
| Dry cereal | 2 ounces | 50 |
| Cooked cereal | ½ cup | 15 |
| Yogurt with fruit | 1 cup | 43 |
| Banana | 1 | 27 |
| Rice | 1 cup cooked | 50 |
| Jelly | 1 tablespoon | 13 |
| High-carbohydrate beverage | 16 ounces | 80–100 |
| Spaghetti with tomato sauce | 7 ounces | 26 |

## Fat and Fact

Some dietary fat is needed for good health. Fats supply energy and essential fatty acids and promote the absorption of the fat-soluble vitamins A, D, E, and K.

One of the main nutrients in food that supply energy, fat consists of a group of compounds made of glycerol and fatty acids. It also makes food taste good and carries flavor. It gives a smooth texture to foods like ice cream and peanut butter. Fat tenderizes, adds moisture, holds in air so baked foods are light, and affects the shape. Furthermore, a 1998 report of a twenty-year study found that a high-fat diet was associated with fewer strokes. Researchers said the explanation may be that brain arteries responsible for strokes have a much different architecture than heart arteries and some fats may protect brain arteries even if they clog arteries in the heart.

One thing seems certain—a high-fat diet drives up blood cholesterol and promotes heart disease. However, another study adds some fuel to the fire. Cholesterol-lowering drugs may significantly reduce the risk of dying from a heart attack but they may dull your mental and physical performance. Stome studies have found that those who lower their cholesterol seem more likely to die in tragedies such as car accidents and suicide, while other research has found no such link.[4]

In a new study presented at the American Heart Association meeting in Orlando, November 10, 1997, researchers at the University of Pittsburgh said they were the first to give psychological tests to people taking cholesterol-lowering drugs. Dr. Matthew Muldoon, who led the study, speculated that the drugs could reduce mental functioning in several ways. For instance, cholesterol particles in the bloodstream are known to carry nutrients such as vitamin A. Further lowering cholesterol could reduce the brain's supply of chemicals it needs to manufacture signal-carrying proteins.

Other researchers have surmised that cholesterol-lowering drugs might preserve mental function by preventing small strokes in the brain.

The answers are not in yet, but even Dr. Muldoon advises, "Even if the medicines truly do impair performance—and this is not yet proven beyond doubt—their benefits on the heart are still likely to outweigh any possible risks."

In the meantime, knowledge and moderation are the keys. Below are the various forms of fat.

**Fatty acids** are the basic chemical units of fat. They can be either saturated, monounsaturated, or polyunsaturated, depending on how many hydrogen atoms they hold. All dietary fats are a mixture of three types of fatty acids but vary in the amount of each they contain. Fatty acids are a molecular chain proven to inhibit production of prostaglandins, hormones that, among other things, play a part in inflammation. Since 1985, when a study in the *New England Journal of Medicine* showed that a group of people in the Netherlands who ate about an ounce of fatty fish a day reduced heart disease by 50 percent, omega-3 fatty acids have been used to help reduce cholesterol and are now being studied as a possible treatment for other prostaglandin-related disorders, such as rheumatoid arthritis and multiple sclerosis.

Netherlands studies also showed that a high intake of polyunsaturated fatty acids such as linoleic, or a low intake of antioxidants, may increase cognitive impairment. High intake of omega-3 polyunsaturated fatty acids and their main source, fish, however, may reduce the risk of blood clots. Little is known, however, the researchers said, about the relationship between these dietary factors and cognitive function.[5]

Omega-3 fatty acids are highly concentrated in our brains and may help signals flow smoothly among brain cells, according to psychiatrist Joseph Hibbeln, M.D., of the National Institute of Alcohol Abuse and Alcoholism. This is why he thinks low omega-3 levels may be related to higher risk of depression.[6]

All dietary fats are mixtures of three types of fatty acids, but vary in the amount of each they contain. The following are the three types of fatty acids that influence cholesterol levels in our blood:

**Saturated fatty acids** tend to raise blood cholesterol levels. They are found in the largest amounts in meat and dairy products, but also in some vegetable oils, including coconut and palm kernel oil.

**Monounsaturated fatty acids** are found in varying amounts in both plant and animal fat. Olive oil, peanut oil, some margarines, and vegetable shortening tend to be high in monounsaturated fatty acids. Research has shown that substituting monounsaturated fat for saturated fat reduces blood cholesterol.

**Polyunsaturated fatty acids** tend to lower blood cholesterol levels. They are found mainly in foods from plants. Safflower, sunflower, corn, soybean, and cottonseed oils contain large amounts of polyunsaturated fatty acids.

**Cholesterol** is a fatlike substance found in all foods of animal origin (meat and dairy products) but not in foods from plants. Some cholesterol is needed by the body, but too much can build up in the arteries and lead to heart disease, heart attack, or stroke.

- Don't overdo the restrictions of fat and cholesterol. Cholesterol isn't all bad. In fact, it is essential for producing new cells and manufacturing certain hormones. It is especially important that the adult low-cholesterol diet not be given to children without medical advice because children need cholesterol for the growth of their brain. The National Institutes of

Health National Cholesterol Education Program
Guidelines say:

1. Total cholesterol should be below 200 milligrams per deciliter of blood.
2. LDL (bad form of cholesterol) should be 100 milligrams per deciliter if you have heart disease or two or more risk factors. (It can be 130 if you have no coronary artery disease or risk factors.)
3. HDL cholesterol should be 45 milligrams per deciliter or higher for men and 55 or higher for women.

- In many European countries, fat accounts for 40 to 50 percent of total energy in the diet. In the United

## FATS, BIOTIN, AND CHOLINE IN COMMON FOODS

| Food (3.5 ounces) | Calories | Total Fat (grams) | Saturated Fat (grams) | Polyunsaturated Fat (grams) |
|---|---|---|---|---|
| Egg (whole) | 158 | 11.1 | 3.4 | 1.5 |
| Swiss cheese | 334 | 25 | 16 | 0.6 |
| Whole wheat bread | 61 | 1.1 | | |
| Oatmeal | 133 | 6.1 | | 0.6 |
| Watermelon | 25 | 0.7 | | |
| Turkey pot pie | 237 | 13.5 | 4.0 | |
| Pizza w/cheese & sausage | 282 | 13.3 | 3.4 | |
| Chicken fricassée | 161 | 9.3 | 3.0 | |
| Margarine | 720 | 81 | | 14.8 |
| Corn oil | 884 | 100 | 12.7 | 58.4 |
| Whole milk | 64 | 3.7 | 2.3 | 0.1 |
| Butter | 717 | 81.1 | 50.5 | 3.0 |
| Yogurt (plain) | 61 | 3.3 | 2.1 | 0.1 |
| Peanut butter | 581 | 49.4 | 10.5 | 5.1 |
| Hamburger (cooked) | 286 | 20.3 | 9.5 | 2.8 |

States, fat intakes are between 30 to 40 percent, and, in Asia, 14 to 25 percent of energy. A widely held premise is that fat contributes to heart disease, cancer, diabetes, and obesity. This has caused experts to recommend a diet in which fat is less than 30 percent.

• Eat more fish, particularly sardines, mackerel, lake trout, salmon, and herring (if you are not taking medications that inhibit MAO; *see* Glossary). Also, flaxseed oil and canola oil contain the same substance that is contained in fish—omega-3 fatty acids.

However, nutrition expert Scott M. Grundy, M.D., Ph.D., of the Center for Human Nutrition, University of Texas Southwestern Medical

| Oleic Acid (grams) | Linoleic Acid (grams) | Cholesterol (milligrams) | Biotin (micrograms) | Choline (milligrams) |
|---|---|---|---|---|
| 4.1 | 1.2 | 274 | 10.8 | 527 |
| 5.9 | 0.3 | 85 | 1.1 | |
| | | | 6.0 | 101 |
| | | | 4.0 | 101 |
| | | | 4.0 | |
| 7.0 | 1.0 | 31 | | |
| 4.7 | 1.2 | 0.6 | | |
| 4.0 | 2.0 | 40 | | |
| 41.4 | 22.2 | | | 5.0 |
| 24.6 | 57.4 | | | 5.0 |
| 0.9 | 0.1 | 14 | | 7.6 |
| 20.4 | 1.8 | 219 | | 4 |
| 0.7 | 0.1 | 13 | 2.7 | |
| 23.1 | 15.1 | | | 145.0 |
| 9.1 | 0.6 | 94 | | |

**FATS, BIOTIN, AND CHOLINE IN COMMON FOODS**

School, points out that fat is a major nutrient and an important source of body fuel.

And then there are the conflicting reports about diet that drive consumers crazy. In the 1960s, doctors told us to eat margarine instead of butter to lower our cholesterol levels and protect our hearts. The amount of butter consumed by Americans is now half of what it was in 1961.[7] In 1992, reports from the United States Department of Agriculture researchers and other scientific institutions in Europe stated that margarines, which develop trans fatty acids during the processing to form "sticks," may be as bad or worse for our cholesterol levels and our hearts.[8] The sale of margarine immediately plummeted after publicity about the research.[9] Joseph T. Judd at the United States Department of Agriculture (which funded the million-dollar margarine study) then said: "At this point, we really do not have all of the evidence to relate trans fatty acids to heart disease because in cardiovascular disease there are many factors. . . . And we don't know the effect of trans fatty acids in these other risk factors, all we're looking at is blood cholesterol."[10]

A fat that may be beneficial to body and brain is omega-3. A University of Chicago study isolated omega-3 fatty acids in fish, believed to be the heart-protecting ingredients in the Eskimos' diet. Fatty fish and marine mammals are excellent sources of omega-3 fatty acids, proven to inhibit production of prostaglandins, hormones that, among other things, modulate cell metabolism. A 20-year study of the effects of fish consumption on the health of 852 middle-aged men in Zutphen, the Netherlands, found that death from coronary heart disease was more than 50 percent lower for those men who ate 30 grams (1 ounce of fish per day) than among those who did not eat fish.[11]

The Zutphen study supports the findings of a previous study in which the low death rate from coronary heart disease among Greenland Eskimos was attributed to an average per capita fish consumption of 400 grams per day.

Since the publication in 1985 of the Zutphen study in the *New England Journal of Medicine* omega-3 fatty acids have been used to help reduce cholesterol and are now being studied as a possible treatment for such other prostaglandin-related disorders as rheumatoid arthritis and multiple sclerosis.[12]

Your mother may have told you that fish is brain food. A number of studies have now shown that fish contains compounds that can:[13, 14]

- Decrease blood pressure in persons with normal and moderately high blood pressure
- Decrease blood viscosity
- Decrease blood vessel leakage in insulin-dependent diabetics
- Decrease blood triglycerides
- Decrease vascular response to norepinephrine, a hormone that stimulates
- Decrease irregular heartbeats
- Decrease cardiac toxicity of cardiac glycosides (sugars)
- Decrease platelet stickiness
- Increase platelet survival

The consumption of as little as one or two fish dishes per week may be of preventive importance in relation to coronary heart disease.[15] Fish oil supplements, on the other hand, do carry a small but potentially serious risk of bleeding complications and can cause gastrointestinal side effects, such as nausea and diarrhea, so they should not be taken in large amounts or over a long period of time without medical supervision.

Flaxseed oil is also rich in omega-3 fatty acids.

One of the problems with our eating habits is not what we are eating but how big a portion we are ingesting. The following may give you some clues:

## WHAT COUNTS AS A SERVING?

**Bread, Cereal, Rice & Pasta**

| 1 slice bread | 1 ounce of ready-to-eat cereal | ½ cup cooked cereal, rice, and pasta |
|---|---|---|

**Vegetables**

| 1 cup raw leafy vegetable | ½ cup other vegetables— cooked, chopped, or raw | ¾ cup vegetable juice |
|---|---|---|

| **What Counts As a Serving?** *(cont.)* | | |
|---|---|---|
| **Fruit** | | |
| 1 medium apple, banana, orange | ½ cup chopped, cooked, or canned fruit | ¾ cup fruit juice |
| **Milk, Yogurt, and Cheese** | | |
| 1 cup milk or yogurt | 1½ ounces natural cheese | 2 ounces processed cheese |
| **Meat, Poultry, Fish, Dry Beans, Eggs, and Nuts** | | |
| 2–3 ounces of cooked lean meat, poultry, or fish | | ½ cup cooked dry beans, 1 egg or 2 tablespoons peanut butter count as 1 ounce of lean meat |

In a study of long-distance runners who ran for 60 minutes, the runners consumed 12 grams milk protein, 29 grams carbohydrate, and 10 grams amino acid (branched chain) 90 minutes before running. (It was suggested that the branched chain amino acids in conjunction with relatively intense exercise can modify hormonal release and perhaps reduce some catabolic effects of exercise.)[16]

You know that old joke about the elderly man who exclaimed, "If I had known I was going to live so long, I would have taken better care of myself"? Well, we are living longer, but we also want to live better—that is, we want to keep our brains and bodies in the best shape possible. As far as protecting your brain is concerned, you can't do anything about your heredity, but you can do something about your diet.

# The Golden Rules of Healthy Eating

The following are the basics for a balanced, varied diet: You should have daily at least two servings of dairy products such as cottage cheese, yogurt, or milk; two servings of high-protein foods such as lean meat, poultry, fish, eggs, beans, nuts, or peanut butter; four servings of fruits and vegetables, including citrus fruits or juice and a dark green, leafy vegetable; and four servings of bread or cereal products made with whole grain or enriched flour, rice, or pasta.

**General Meal Percentages Recommended by U.S. Government and Other Agencies (may not be good for you, personally, if you have special needs).**

- Complex carbohydrates such as pasta, bread, cereal, and starch should make up 50 to 60 percent of your calories
- Protein should constitute about 15 to 20 percent
- Fats should be 20 to 30 percent of your calories, with two-thirds to three-quarters polyunsaturated or monounsaturated (*see* Glossary)

**Protein passion.** As pointed out through the book, neurotransmitters in the brain are made from the amino acid building blocks of protein. Best sources of protein are milk, beef, poultry, cheese, and liver. While animal proteins contain all nine of the essential amino acids, plant proteins—with the exception of soy—are often deficient in one or another. Amino acids, from which the brain's neurotransmitters are made, come from protein in the diet, as mentioned previously. There is a lot of emphasis in the lay and medical literature on complex carbohydrates, but the older you get, the more protein you may need. In fact, the RDA of protein is 56 grams for adult men and 45 grams for women, but some people may need as much as 80 to 90 grams of protein per day, depending on their physical condition. For others with kidney or liver problems, protein in their diet may need to be reduced. Check with your physician.

**Shake the salt habit.** Americans are the salters of the earth. They love salt. Despite strong evidence in favor of an association between salt intake and blood pressure, the debate continues. The evidence supporting a general reduction of salt intake is strong and is based on epidemiological, interventional, genetic, migration, treatment, and animal studies. For example, the InterSalt study, a comparison of more than 10,000 people in 52 countries, showed that populations that eat less salt had lower blood pressure than populations who eat more salt. Researchers say that reduction in salt use would greatly lower the rate of strokes.[17] If you have a normal blood pressure and no heart disease, you could try to stay with the FDA's recommendation of 2,000 milligrams per day. If you have high blood pressure, there are many good books on cooking and living well without salt.

***Try a meatless alternative for a few meals per week.*** Vegetables with beans and legumes can give you needed protein as well as the other benefits described throughout this book.

***Cultured carbohydrates.*** Your body can easily convert carbohydrates—sugars and starches—to blood sugar, the only fuel your brain can use. (The other organs can burn protein and fats as well.) Try to get most of your sugar from fructose in fruits and vegetables because it is metabolized slowly, it does not cause the drop in blood sugar and the consequent two-hour later "rebound" effects of lethargy and irritability associated with table sugar. You may need a quick boost from carbohydrates before a test of either mental or physical ability, but go easy on the sugar. As we get older, our tolerance for sugar in the blood may be lower. Cut down on sugar and skip sodas and imitation fruit drinks containing only 10 percent fruit because they are very high in sugar and coloring. Four servings of bread or cereal products is the usual recommended daily intake. Among good selections are whole wheat, rye, pumpernickel, raisin breads; cornmeal; whole wheat pasta; brown rice; potatoes (sweet are best), pumpkin, beans, lentils; grits; wheat germ; oatmeal; puffed rice; low-salt crackers.

***Don't forget fat.*** Fats in fish and most oils are a good choice. Junkets, puddings, or shakes made with skim milk; angel food cake; popsicles; sherbet; gelatin ice; hard and jelly candies; and no-salt pretzels are good choices for low-fat treats. Dairy nonfat fortified milk, skim milk, ice milk, low-fat yogurt, margarine, buttermilk (made with skim milk), low-fat cottage cheese; cheeses containing less than one percent butterfat are also recommended.

***Change your oil.*** Choose liquid vegetable oils that are highest in unsaturated fat such as canola, safflower, sunflower, corn, olive, sesame, and soybean oils in cooking and in salads.

***Get enough tryptophan.*** This is the least abundant amino acid in our diets. It increases levels of the neurotransmitter serotonin in the brain. As a result, there is lowered sensitivity to pain, increased calm, and it makes it easier to fall asleep. The best sources of tryptophan are peanuts, oatmeal, bananas, a glass of chocolate milk, a peanut-butter-and-banana sandwich as an evening snack.

***Eat some of your vegetables and fruits raw.*** If your digestive apparatus permits, eat as much as half of your fruits and vegetables raw. Processing causes many fruits and vegetables to lose some of their vitamins. Freezing kills vitamin E, for example, and storage depletes the vitamin C in orange juice. Raw foods may be more filling and satisfying than highly processed foods, and the fiber aids elimination. Two to four servings per day of vegetables are recommended; choose from broccoli, cabbage, carrots, tomatoes, cauliflower, watercress, lettuce, corn, and green peppers for optimal benefits.

Among the super vegetables is the *cruciferous* family of plants characterized by flowers and fruits that bear a cross. This family includes Brussels sprouts, cauliflower, and broccoli. These vegetables contain large qualities of substances that have been shown to inhibit chemically induced cancer in animals.

Also of value are the *phytoestrogens,* the female hormones in plants. These also may fight cancer and replace animal estrogen on receptors and may prove therapeutic to the brain, as estrogen has been shown to delay the progression of Alzheimer's disease.

***Add vegetables to your stews.*** You have learned that aging and heart disease and many other ailments we suffer are the result of the oxidation of fats and tissues in our bodies. It is not unlike the rust of metals or rancidity of fat, both caused by oxidation. Scientists have known for some time that another natural antioxidant exists that can be found in onions, garlic, peppers, soybeans, and many green leafy plants. Professor Dan Pratt of Purdue University's foods and nutrition department is testing plant compounds for their antioxidant properties. Oxidation is a problem for foods such as meat, oil, salad dressing, shortening, nuts, butter, cereal, and many novelty and commercial foods.

Says Dr. Pratt: "We knew, for example, that if you take two beakers of stew meat, one with vegetables and one without, that spoilage will occur first in the one without the vegetables. But few researchers focused on determining what within the plants was doing the work." Dr. Pratt adds: "In a lot of cases, it's not the edible part of the plant that is high in antioxidants. For example, the seed of the pepper is much higher in antioxidants than the pepper pod; the skin of the potato has more than the inside of the potato."

A number of researchers now believe that including antioxidants in your diet can prevent or slow brain cell damage from oxidized fat.

***Find joy in soy.*** Cooked soybeans contain 23 percent of the RDA of folacin, 22 percent of the RDA for calcium, and 49 percent for phosphorus, all of which are particularly important to brain function. Dried soybeans are also a good value. A half-cup serving of cooked dried soybeans contains the protein in two ounces of meat, the iron equivalent of three eggs, and the calcium equivalent of a half-cup of milk. Soybeans are also high in $B_6$ and $B_{12}$, which are necessary for optimal brain function (*see* Chapter 8). They also are high in lecithin, which is the precursor for the manufacture of the brain chemical acetylcholine, so important in memory.

***Eat your oatmeal.*** Rich in amino acids—valine, tryptophan, tyrosine, cysteine—vitamins, iron, magnesium, and zinc, real oatmeal takes only a few minutes to prepare. The "instant" varieties often contain added sugar and salt. Check the label and choose wisely.

***Catch a fish.*** Eat fish at least twice a week. Choose a deep-water fish which is especially rich in the fish oils that help prevent clogged arteries and strokes. Researchers believe fish oil works by curtailing production of the body agents called leukotrienes that promote inflammation. In addition to helping to keep blood from clogging blood vessels, a number of studies have shown fish oil eases joint pain and stiffness after 6 to 12 weeks of use.[18] Fish is also rich in choline found in most animal tissues, either free or in combination such as lecithin or acetylcholine. Choline is being actively studied for its effects on memory via its involvement in the transmission of messages between nerve cells in the brain.

***Top banana.*** A small banana contains just 80 calories, is 99.8 percent fat-free, and is made up of protein, carbohydrates, calcium, phosphorus, potassium, lots of vitamin A, vitamin C, tyrosine, serotonin, and tryptophan. Obviously, it is a good food choice.

***Go for fiber.*** Fruits and vegetables and grains will give you the fiber that can help lower cholesterol and provide other benefits.

***Be sure you get enough of the B vitamins.*** The B vitamins are vital to the nerves and brain. As we get older, we may have more trouble absorbing these vitamins. (See Chapter 3 for foods that are high in B vitamins.) You may need $B_{12}$ or $B_6$ by injection because you are not absorbing enough by mouth. Ask your physician.

***Be sure you get enough vitamins A, C, and E.*** These antioxidant vitamins can help protect your cells against the wear and tear that occurs with age. (See Chapter 3 for foods that are rich in these vitamins.) It is best to get vitamin A from beta-carotene, vitamin A's precursor in vegetables. It also is wise to obtain vitamins C and E from food, but supplementary vitamins C and E can't hurt and may help significantly.

***Check marginal vitamin deficiencies.*** A gradual depletion of these nutrients—often hard to detect—can result in depression, anxiety, irritability, and loss of appetite, sleepiness, or insomnia. Older people may develop problems absorbing vitamins, even when their diets contain sufficient amounts. Their ability to absorb vitamins may be compromised due to physical conditions and/or interference from medicines taken to combat those conditions. Estrogens, for example, may interfere with the body's use of folic acid and vitamin $B_{12}$. Overuse of antacids containing calcium carbonate may lower magnesium while even aspirin can cause a depletion in iron. Check with a physician about supplements.

***Avoid vitamin depleters.*** Alcohol, tobacco, and estrogen pills are among the depleters. Too much fiber can also interfere with the absorption of minerals. Oxalates in spinach, wheat, beef, and cocoa may block calcium absorption. Tannin found in tea and red wine may reduce available iron, protein, and vitamin $B_{12}$.

***Eat local produce.*** You are more likely to get fresher fruits and vegetables that still contain many of their vitamins.

***Substitutes can help.*** If you are vulnerable to heart problems, substitute low-fat or nonfat yogurt for sour cream in recipes or as toppings and substitute low-fat sour creams, mayonnaise, and margarines for the regular versions. Check with your physician or nutritionist.

***Eat as many simple, unprocessed foods as possible.*** Food
processing prevents the growth of germs and decay-producing organisms, but it uses heat, refrigeration, freezing, radiation, separa-
tion methods, gas, alterations in water content, fermentation
processes, and packaging, all of which may affect nutrients.
Canned vegetables, for example, contain only 30 to 50 percent of
the vitamin C present in the fresh product and may lose up to 20
percent of the vitamin A and thiamine. Part of the loss occurs during blanching before canning. Once a food is canned and stored,
there are few changes in its nutritional quality if the product is
stored below 70 degrees Fahrenheit. Approximately 25 percent of
the vitamin C, however, is lost during one year of storage at 70 to
80 degrees Fahrenheit.

***Frozen foods,*** because they are not treated by heat, have a nutritional quality close to that of the fresh product, except for the loss
of 10 to 20 percent of vitamins C, E, and A which occurs during
blanching before the freezing process. But factors such as loss of
flavor, textural changes, and loss of nutritional value allow only an
intermediate shelf life—nine months to one year—for many frozen
fruits and vegetables. In dried foods, the essential amino acid lysine
is unavailable for absorption. Browning is a result of the reaction
between reducing sugars such as fructose and available amino acid
groups found in proteins, as Rockefeller University's Dr. Cerami
points out in Chapter 10. Since increasing amounts of high-fructose
corn syrups are being used as sweeteners in processed foods, this
type of browning may prove to be more of a problem.

***Fruits and fruit juices.*** For your two to four recommended daily
servings, choose fresh, when possible, or canned in their own
juices, from the following: apples, apricots, bananas, berries, cherries, grapes, oranges, peaches, plums, citrus fruit, fresh fruit juices
without added sugar, fruit ice.

***Condiments.*** Low fat and/or low salt products help protect your
brain. Therefore, choose natural herbs and spices such as garlic
powder and pepper instead of high fat and/or highly salted taste
enhancers. Lemon juice and fresh onions, for example, can perk up
a dish and give you a nutrient boost as well. Select low-salt, low-
fat salad dressings (or make your own) with safflower, corn, olive,
or cottonseed oil.

***Treats.*** Choose fresh fruits and vegetables; dried fruits; low-fat yogurt; frozen yogurt; popcorn; homemade oatmeal cookies; raw apples; raisins; ice milk; almonds, walnuts, and peanut butter. Downing one drink of alcohol or devouring a single candy bar is not going to hurt your brain if you do it infrequently and are in reasonably good health.

***Don't succumb to the single-eater syndrome.*** Many people in our society live alone. The tendency for single eaters is to not fuss with meals and to gulp down whatever is handy in the refrigerator or on the shelf. Instead, make sure your meals are attractive and balanced. You need protein, fresh fruits and vegetables, and carbohydrates even if you dine alone. Treat yourself as you would a guest. An attractively set table with flowers or other decorations can help nourish your brain as well as your body.

***Boost your senses.*** Your taste and smell sensitivity may need a boost. If you find that your food tastes too bland, use more herbs and spices. Tart foods may enhance flavors. Orange juice, lemonade, vinegar, and lemon juice used as seasonings may help. Many foods taste better if they are either cold or at room temperature. Try new taste treats. There are a lot of ethnic foods, and if they are novel to you they may spark your taste buds and capture your interest. If you find you have a problem with the ability to taste or smell, consult your physician. You may benefit from a zinc supplement.

***Take your vitamins and supplements.*** Certain vitamin supplements are good for your brain, particularly the Bs. Supplements such as ginkgo may be beneficial for your brain, but before you swallow any vitamins or supplements in large doses, consult your physician and your pharmacist. There may be interactions with the medications you are taking or you may have a condition which would preclude the supplement. Almost everyone should take a multivitamin each day for insurance.

***Talk a walk.*** Numerous studies have shown that exercise aids metabolism and is good not only for the body but also for the brain. Walking is probably the most beneficial since it doesn't stress the joints or injure the shoulders or neck, as many popular exercises may do. If you do nothing more than park the car a little farther from the store than you usually do and walk that extra distance, you will benefit. Walking in place can be fun if you do it to the beat of your favorite music.

***Don't bring your troubles to the table.*** You may be having work or family problems, but make it an unbreakable rule to leave them out of the dining area. Stress inhibits digestion and keeps you from obtaining the proper nourishment for your brain.

***Variety and moderation.*** Reduce or moderate your fat (especially animal and other saturated fats), cholesterol, and salt intake and eat more whole grains, vegetables, and fruits. If food choices are limited because of availability, preferences, and abnormal digestion or metabolism, seek expert help. Your physician or local hospital dietitian may be able to advise you.

***Use your brain to motivate yourself.*** Anyone over age thirty-five usually has special physical conditions that may warrant more of some things in the diet and less of others. By now, you've read this book and probably many other books and articles on nutrition. You *know* what you should and should not eat. Make promises to yourself about how you are going to change your diet for the better. Write down those promises. Post them on your refrigerator. You may not keep all of them, but they may help you make some improvements. And before you eat something when you are not hungry or that you know is not good for you, ask yourself, Do I really want to eat this? Ask yourself five times. If the answer is still yes, do it, but don't do it too often!

## How Can You Buy Wisely? What Should You Eat?

You may have special needs, depending on your heredity, your health, and your lifestyle, so the following is merely a general menu from which to choose. The safest bet for most people—both in terms of health and effectiveness—is a well-balanced, varied, low-calorie diet.

A rough way to estimate your personal calorie needs is to estimate your basal metabolism rate (BMR), the rate at which you burn energy at rest. Multiply your current weight by 10. If, for example, you are a woman who weighs 130 pounds, your BMR calorie needs are 1,300. The second calculation you need to make is how many calories you burn a day through your various activities. Because most of us are sedentary, some experts believe you can figure only 30 percent of BMR for activity calories. Thus, unless you are a physically active 130-pound woman, you should add only another 390 calories (30 × 1,300) to the 1,300-calorie basic level for a total of 1,690 calories to maintain your current weight.

Once you know the daily calorie intake that keeps you at your present weight, you can lose weight by creating a "negative energy balance." Specifically, to lose one pound of fat you need to consume about 3,500 calories less than you use each week. If you cut back 500 calories a day, you'll lose a pound a week.

The main feature of a balanced diet is that although calories are limited you can still choose from a variety of foods—breads and other starches, fruits, vegetables, dairy products, and protein sources such as lean meat and poultry. For your body and brain, a balanced diet emphasizing more carbohydrates and less protein is recommended.

This book has been about the "free will" to select a nutritious diet for your brain to protect it and maintain it in the best condition possible based on your "hard-wired" heredity and your malleable lifestyle. There is increasing evidence that certain foods do have an effect on your brain, and we have tried to explain and analyze some of the many factors involved in those interactions. We have reported current research on such questions as how lifestyle, age, sex, culture, and economic and social influences affect food choices and what the cause and effect of eating habits may be.

In a recent forum on "Keeping Americans Healthy Into the 21st Century," it was pointed out that we want short-term solutions. "Comfort foods," convenience and the need to relieve stress and anxiety are taking primary focus/attention away from weight management, nutrition, and health. "Stop-gap" convenience foods are replacing home cooking. We want real convenience products that address health, nutrition, and good taste at the same time.[19]

A survey by the newspaper USA Today found that 70 percent of the time consumers eat out because they don't have time, desire, or know-how to cook. Two decades ago, American consumers spent about 63 cents of every food dollar on food eaten at home. Today, that's down to 52 cents—down by a dime in 20 years. To the food industry, the loss of that dime is equivalent to about $60 billion in annual at-home food sales. The trend is also toward prevention rather than cure of diseases. Emotional and spiritual well-being as well as physical health are part of the new directions in health promotion. We are also looking for information to enable, empower, take personal responsibility, and do the right thing. People want to know "How can I do better on my own?"

We have described the possible effects that salt, sugar, fat, alcohol, additives, and allergens in the food may have on your brain. We have pointed out the interaction of food and medication on the brain, and we presented some of the research reports concerning food, learning, and memory. The information is drawn from many scientific fields because research into food and the brain spans many disciplines—from neurosciences to nutritional science to advertising psychology.

> *The brain is, after all, an organ, like the kidney, the heart, or the liver, and organs are known to fail because of hereditary factors as well as environmental ones. The answer is probably that to many people the brain is much more than an organ; it is the center of the poetry, the sophistication, the special qualities that make human beings an order of magnitude more complex than the closest related species. To believe that the brain is merely a series of chemical reactions is to denigrate free will, to remove the humans from the responsibility for their actions, to eliminate the relation between sin and guilt. Moreover, the recent findings are just the beginning; many other behavioral characteristics have been analyzed by studies of adopted children and identical twins and by biochemical approaches. Those who dread complexity will try to reduce the new evidence to the old confrontation of extremes: chemistry versus free will, heredity versus environment, fate versus responsibility. In fact, the neurobiological evidence indicates that part of the brain is "hard-wired" in advance of birth and part is designed to be plastic and learn from experience.*
> *—Daniel E. Koshland, Jr.*

## What Is Smart Food for Your Brain?

You are a unique human being with your own genetic, social, and medical history, and one of the major purposes of this book is to help you make informed choices for yourself. The time is approaching, however, when meals may be especially designed for you. As research continues to determine the interaction among brain, body, and food, genetic engineering and a wide choice of foods will make it possible to obtain the nourishment you need. The only problem is will you eat what is good for *you?* As you can determine from this book, there is much that is already known about food and the brain.

The adage "you are what you eat" applies not just to heart muscles and bone but to the brain as well. Food fuels your brain and powers its control over your body. Neurotransmitters, those chemical messengers between your nerve cells, are made directly or indirectly from the nutrients you ingest. Carbohydrates can jumpstart your brain as can caffeine. Fats give you energy and taste. Next time you select your meals at a supermarket or in a restaurant, use your brain to feed your brain.

# Glossary

**Acetylcholine:** A neurotransmitter that is released by nerve cells and acts on either other nerve cells or muscles and organs throughout the body. This neurotransmitter has been found to be essential to memory function.

**ACTH:** Adrenocorticotropic hormone, a hormone controller.

**Action potential:** An electric burst that travels the length of the nerve cell and causes the release of a neurotransmitter.

**Adrenal glands:** Each about the size of a grape, your two adrenal glands lie on top of each of your kidneys. Each adrenal gland has two parts. The first part is the medulla, which produces epinephrine and norepinephrine, two hormones that play a part in controlling your heart rate and blood pressure. The second part of the adrenal cortex produces three groups of steroid hormones that help convert carbohydrates, or starches, into energy-providing glycogen in your liver. Hydrocortisone is the main hormone in this group. The third group consists of the male hormone androgen and the female hormones estrogen and progesterone.

**Aerobic exercise:** Aerobic exercise refers to the kind of fast-paced activity that makes you "huff and puff." It places demands on your cardiovascular apparatus and, over time, produces beneficial changes in your respiratory and circulatory systems.

**Agonist:** A compound or drug that activates or facilitates a receptor on the post-synaptic cell.

**Allergen (food allergen):** A food allergen is the part of a food that stimulates the immune system of food-allergic individuals. A single food can contain multiple food allergens, the majority of which are likely to be proteins, not carbohydrates or fats.

**Allergy (food allergy):** A food allergy is any adverse reaction to an otherwise harmless food or food component that involves the body's immune system. To avoid confusion with other types of adverse reactions to foods, it is important to use the terms "food allergy" or "food hypersensitivity" only when the immune system is involved in causing the reaction.

**Alzheimer's disease:** A deterioration of the brain with severe memory impairment.

**Amino acids:** Building blocks of proteins and neurotransmitters.

**Anemia:** Anemia is a condition in which a deficiency in the size or number of erythrocytes or the amount of hemoglobin they contain limits the exchange of oxygen and carbon dioxide between the blood and the tissue cells. Most anemias are caused by a lack of nutrients required for normal erythrocyte synthesis, principally iron, vitamin $B_{12}$, and folic acid. Others result from a variety of conditions, such as hemorrhage, genetic abnormalities, chronic disease states, or drug toxicity.

**Angiotensin:** A powerful elevator of blood pressure, angiotensin is produced by the action of renin, an enzyme made in the kidney. All of the components of the renin-angiotensin system have been found in the brain, and there are indications that they are part of the brain's mechanism for regulating blood pressure as well as for telling you when you should or should not drink fluid.

**Anorexia nervosa:** An eating disorder characterized by refusal to maintain a minimally normal weight for age and height. The condition includes weight loss leading to maintenance of body weight 15 percent below normal; an intense fear of weight gain or becoming fat, despite the individual's underweight status; a disturbance in the self-awareness of one's own body weight or shape; and in females, the absence of at least three consecutive menstrual cycles that would otherwise be expected to occur.

**Antagonist:** A compound or drug that blocks or inhibits the effects of a neurotransmitter on receptor activation in the post-synaptic cell.

**Anticholinergic:** The blocking of acetylcholine receptors, which results in the inhibition of nerve impulse transmission.

**Antioxidant:** May be used in conjunction with currently defined claims for "good source" and "high" to describe a nutrient scientifically shown to be absorbed in a sufficient quantity such as vitamin E to inactivate free radicals (*see in dictionary*) or prevent free radical-initiated chemical reactions in the food.

**Aspartame:** Aspartame is a low-calorie sugar substitute used to sweeten a variety of foods and beverages and as a tabletop sweetener. It is about 200 times sweeter than sugar. The calories in foods can be substantially reduced, and in many products be almost eliminated, by using aspartame in place of sugar. Joining two protein components, aspartic acid and phenylalanine, and a small amount of methanol makes aspartame. Aspartic acid and phenylalanine are building blocks of protein and are found naturally in all protein-containing foods, including meats, grains, and dairy products. Methanol is found naturally in the body and in many foods such as fruit and vegetable juices. Upon digestion, aspartame breaks down into its basic components and is absorbed into the blood. Phenylketonurics should check with their physicians before using aspartame products.

**Aspartic acid:** A nonessential amino acid which provides amino groups that help to conserve the body's supply of protein. Also, it is involved in the formation of urea and other compounds in the body.

**Atherosclerosis:** Too much cholesterol can build up in the blood and accumulate in the walls of the blood vessels, a condition known as atherosclerosis.

**Attention Deficit Hyperactivity Disorder (ADHD):** Commonly called "hyperactivity," Attention Deficit Hyperactivity Disorder is a clinical diagnosis based on specific criteria. These include excessive motor activity, impulsiveness, short attention span, low tolerance to frustration, and on-set before seven years of age.

**Autonomic nervous system:** The division of the nervous system that regulates the involuntary vital functions, such as the activity of the heart and breathing.

**Axon:** The principal fiber of a nerve.

**Bioflavonoids:** Vitamin P. A group of water-soluble, brightly colored substances that are often found with vitamin C in fruits and vegetables. They contain citrin, hesperidin, rutin, flavones, and flavonols. Bioflavonoids are essential for the utilization of vitamin C. The bioflavonoids reportedly have an antihistamine action, and reduce the fragility of blood vessels. There is no Recommended Daily Allowance (RDA) (*see* page 284) for bioflavonoids.

**Biotechnology:** The simplest definition of biotechnology is "applied biology," the application of biological knowledge and techniques to develop products and services. It may be further defined as the use of living organisms to make a product or run a process. By this definition, the classic techniques used for plant and animal breeding, fermentation and enzyme purification would be considered biotechnology. Some people use the term only to refer to newer tools of genetic science. In this context, biotechnology may be defined as the use of biotechnical methods to modify the genetic materials of living cells so they will produce new substances or perform new functions. Examples include recombinant DNA technology, in which a copy of a piece of DNA containing one or a few genes is transferred between organisms or "recombined" within an organism.

**Blood-brain barrier:** The blood-brain barrier is a selectively permeable membrane made up of capillaries more tightly packed than throughout the rest of the body. These closely packed capillaries supply blood to the brain and spinal cord. Large molecules cannot permeate the narrow spaces; however, fat-soluble (lipophilic) molecules can dissolve through the capillary cell membranes and be absorbed into the brain.

**Bulimia nervosa:** This is an eating disorder characterized by rapid consumption of a large amount of food in a short period of time, with a sense of lack of control during the episode and self-evaluation unduly influenced by body weight and shape. There are two forms of the condition, purging and nonpurging. The first type regularly engages in purging through self-induced vomiting or the excessive use of laxatives or diuretics. Alternatively, the nonpurging type controls weight through strict dieting, fasting, or excessive exercise.

**Caffeine:** Caffeine is a naturally occurring substance found in the leaves, seeds, or fruits of over sixty-three plant species worldwide and is part of a group of compounds known as methylxanthines. The most commonly known sources of caffeine are coffee and cocoa beans, cola nuts, and tea leaves. Caffeine is a pharmacologically active substance and, depending on the dose, can be a mild central nervous system stimulant. Caffeine does not accumulate in the body over the course of time and is normally excreted within several hours of consumption.

People differ greatly in their sensitivity to caffeine. Research indicates individuals tend to find their own acceptable level of daily caffeine consumption. Those people who feel unwanted effects tend to ease off their caffeine consumption; those who don't continue to consume caffeine at their own normal levels.

**Calcium messenger system:** As calcium ions increase in the cell, a specific receptor protein, calmodulin, interacts with other proteins to initiate cell responses such as smooth muscle contraction. The calcium messenger system is believed to play a part in learning.

**Calorie:** A calorie is the amount of energy required to raise the temperature of one milliliter (ml) of water at a standard initial temperature by one degree centigrade.

**Carbohydrate:** Carbohydrates are organic compounds that consist of carbon, hydrogen, and oxygen. They vary from simple sugars containing from three to seven carbon atoms to very complex polymers. Only the hexoses (six carbon sugars) and pentoses (five carbon sugars) and their polymers play important roles in nutrition. Plants manufacture and store carbohydrates as their chief source of energy. The glucose synthesized in the leaves of plants is used as the basis for more complex forms of carbohydrates. Classification of carbohydrates relates to their structural core of simple sugars, saccharides. The principal monosaccharides that occur in food are glucose and fructose. Three common disaccharides are sucrose, maltose, and lactose. Polysaccharides of interest in nutrition include starch, dextrin, glycogen, and cellulose.

**Catecholamines:** A group of self-made chemicals, such as neurotransmitters and hormones, which can be made synthetically. Among the major catecholamines are dopamine, norepinephrine, and epinephrine. The catecholamines are involved in the regulation of blood pressure, heart rate, muscle tone, metabolism, and central nervous system function.

**CCK:** *see* Cholecystokinin.

**Chinese Restaurant Syndrome (CRS):** Manifested by anxiety, flushed face, and pressure in the chest, CRS has been shown to be caused by eating large amounts of the flavor enhancer MSG. Sulfite preservatives are now known to have the potential to cause a serious attack of asthma and even death.

**Cholecystokinin (CCK):** A hormone produced by the small intestine during movement of food from the stomach into the intestine, CCK causes the contraction of the gall bladder, thus releasing bile into the small intestine where the enzymes and other components of bile aid digestion. This hormone has also been found in the brain and may help to stop eating.

**Cholesterol (dietary):** Cholesterol is not fat, but rather a fatlike substance classified as a lipid. Cholesterol is vital to life and is found in all cell membranes. It is necessary for the production of bile acids and steroid hormones. Dietary cholesterol is found only in animal foods. Abundant in organ meats and egg yolks, cholesterol is also contained in meats, chicken, and shellfish. Vegetable oils and shortenings are cholesterol-free.

**Cholesterol (serum, or blood):** High blood cholesterol is a risk factor in the development of coronary heart disease. Most of the cholesterol that is found in the blood is manufactured by the body, at a rate of about 800 to

1,500 milligrams a day. By comparison, the average American consumes 300 to 450 milligrams daily in foods. Cholesterol travels through the blood via particles called lipoproteins—combinations of lipids and proteins. Too much cholesterol can build up in the blood and accumulate in the walls of the blood vessels, a condition known as atherosclerosis. This can ultimately reduce the flow of blood in major arteries, leading to heart attack. Blood cholesterol reflects the amount of three major classes of lipoproteins: very-low density lipoprotein (VLDL); low-density lipoprotein (LDL), which contains most of the cholesterol found in the blood; and high-density lipoprotein (HDL). LDL seems to be the culprit in coronary heart disease and is popularly known as the "bad cholesterol." By contrast, HDL is increasingly considered desirable and known as the "good cholesterol."

Diet is just one factor influencing blood cholesterol levels. For some people at risk, heredity is a stronger predictor of cholesterol levels than diet. Age, race, and gender are other risk factors for high cholesterol levels.

**Choline:** It is found in most animal tissues, either free or in combinations such as lecithin or acetylcholine. Choline is being actively studied for its effects on brain neurotransmission and memory.

**Cholinesterase:** This is the enzyme that processes the neurotransmitter acetylcholine. There is a great deal of scientific interest in this enzyme, particularly in the study of Alzheimer's disease, because it is believed to be involved in poor memory function.

**Chromosomes:** These are the threadlike components in the cell that contain DNA and proteins. Genes are carried on the chromosomes.

**Clinical trials:** Clinical trials undertake experimental study of human subjects. Trials may attempt to determine whether the finds of basic research are applicable to humans, or to confirm the results of epidemiological research. Studies may be small, with a limited number of participants, or they may be large intervention trials that seek to discover the outcome of treatments on entire populations. The "gold standard" clinical trials are double-blind, placebo-controlled studies which employ random assignment of subjects to experimental and control groups.

**Control group:** The group of subjects in a study to whom a comparison is made in order to determine whether an observation or treatment has an effect. In an experimental study it is the group that does not receive a treatment. Subjects are as similar as possible to those in the test group.

**Controlled experiment:** In this type of research, study subjects (whether animal or human) are selected according to relevant characteristics, and then randomly assigned to either an experimental group, or a control group. Random assignment ensures that factors known as variables, which may affect the outcome of the study, are distributed equally among the groups and therefore could not lead to differences in the effect of the treatment under study. The experimental group is then given a treatment (sometimes called an intervention), and the results are compared to the control group, which does not receive treatment. A placebo, or false treatment, may be administered to the control group. With all other variables controlled, differences between the experimental and control groups may be attributed to the treatment under study.

**Correlation:** An association, or when one phenomenon is found to be accompanied by another. A correlation does not prove cause and effect. Correlation may also be defined statistically.

**CRF:** *see* CRH.

**CRH (corticotrophin-releasing hormone) or CRF (corticotrophin-releasing factor):** CRH or CRF, a type of neurotransmitter, controls the secretion of other stress-related hormones in the pituitary. Evidence exists that indicates that CRF is oversecreted in depression, perhaps contributing to some of the symptoms of depression such as decreased libido, insomnia, and decreased appetite, and CRF also may be involved in anxiety disorders. Neurogen is developing CRF antagonists to block the effects of CRF that may underlie several diseases.

**Cyanidin:** Found in many fruits and flowers such as cherries and cornflowers, herbalists use it to treat night blindness.

**Cysteine:** A nonessential amino acid.

**Cystine:** A product of cysteine, produced by oxidation.

**Dendrites:** Spiderlike projections from the cell body that receive and send messages between nerve cells.

**Diabetes:** Diabetes is the name for a group of medical disorders characterized by high blood-sugar levels. Normally when people eat, food is digested and much of it is converted to glucose—a simple sugar—which the body uses for energy. The blood carries the glucose to cells where it is absorbed with the help of the hormone insulin. For those with diabetes, however, the body does not make enough insulin, or cannot properly use the insulin it does make. Without insulin, glucose accumulates in the blood rather than moving into the cells. High blood-sugar levels result.

The number of Americans with diabetes is 8,700,000. Diabetes is the leading cause of adult blindness in the United States, the leading cause of end-stage renal disease, and a leading cause of nontraumatic amputation. So far there is no cure, but diabetes can be controlled through diet, exercise, and medication. Unfortunately, the disease often escapes diagnosis.

**Diuretic:** A drug that promotes the excretion of urine.

**DNA:** Also known as deoxyribonucleic acid. This is the molecule that carries the genetic information for most living systems. The DNA molecule consists of four bases (adenine, cytosine, guanine, and thymine) and a sugar-phosphate backbone, arranged in two connected strands to form its characteristic double helix.

**Dopamine:** A neurotransmitter of the catecholamine family, which also includes norepinephrine and epinephrine. Dopamine is involved in emotional behavior, and at least five receptor subtypes have been identified. Excess levels of dopamine are thought to cause schizophrenia, while low dopamine levels result in the shaking and lack of motor control seen in Parkinson's disease.

**Double-blind, placebo-controlled study:** In a double-blind, placebo-controlled study, neither the researchers nor the participants in the study are aware of which subjects receive the treatment under study and which subjects receive the placebo—until after the study is completed. The study design is intended to remove bias on the part of both researcher and study subject.

**Endorphins:** Self-made tranquilizers and painkillers. Each endorphin is composed of a chain of amino acids and acts on the nervous system to reduce pain.

**Enkephalins:** Self-made painkillers to which endorphins belong.

**Enteric nervous system:** Our digestive systems also are chemical factories. In the linings of the esophagus, stomach, small intestine, and colon, there are millions of nerve cells that send out stop-and-go messages to our brains. The components of this digestive control center are lumped under the title *enteric* (from the Greek *entera,* meaning "bowels)" *nervous system.* Current thinking among a number of scientists is that there is a "brain" in the gut, independent from the brain encased in the skull and that the *enteric nervous system* may be able to learn and remember independently of the *central nervous system.*

**Epidemiology:** The study of distribution and determinants of diseases or other health outcomes in human populations. It seeks to expose potential associations between aspects of health (such as cancer, heart disease, etc.) and diet, lifestyle, habits, or other factors within populations. Epidemiological studies may suggest relationships between two factors, but do not provide the basis for conclusions about cause and effect. Possible associations inferred from epidemiological research can turn out to be coincidental.

**Epinephrine (adrenaline):** The major hormone of the adrenal gland, epinephrine increases heart rate and contractions, relaxation and contraction of the blood vessels, relaxation of the muscles in the lungs and smooth muscles in the intestines and the processing of sugar and fat.

**Fats (dietary fats):** Fats are referred to in the plural because there is no one type of fat. Fats are composed of the same three elements as carbohydrates—carbon, hydrogen, and oxygen; however, fats have relatively more carbon and hydrogen and less oxygen, thus supplying a higher fuel value of nine calories per gram (versus four calories per gram from carbohydrates and protein). One molecule of fat can be broken down into three molecules of fatty acids and one of glycerol. Thus fats are known chemically as triglycerides. Fats are a vital nutrient in a healthy diet. Fats supply essential fatty acids, such as linoleic acid, which is especially important to childhood growth. Fat helps maintain healthy skin, regulate cholesterol metabolism, and is a precursor of prostaglandins, hormone-like substances that regulate some body processes. Dietary fat is needed to carry fat-soluble vitamins A, D, E, and K and to aid in their absorption from the intestine.

The body uses whatever fat it needs for energy, and the rest is stored in various fatty tissues. Some fat is found in blood plasma and other body cells, but the largest amount is stored in the body's adipose, or fat cells.

These fat deposits not only store energy, but also are important in insulating the body and supporting and cushioning organs.

**Fatty acid:** A fat molecule is made up of three molecules of fatty acids and one of glycerol. Thus fats are known chemically as triglycerides. Fatty acids are generally classified as saturated, monounsaturated, or polyunsaturated. These terms refer to the number of hydrogen atoms attached to the carbon atoms of the fat molecule. In general, fats that contain a majority of saturated fatty acids are solid at room temperature, although some solid vegetable shortenings are up to 75 percent unsaturated. Fats containing mostly unsaturated fatty acids are usually liquid at room temperature and are called oils. *See also* Hydrogenation.

**FDA (Food and Drug Administration):** The U.S. Food and Drug Administration is part of the Public Health Service of the U.S. Department of Health and Human Services. It is the regulatory agency responsible for ensuring the safety and wholesomeness of all foods sold in interstate commerce except meat, poultry, and eggs (which are under the jurisdiction of the U.S. Department of Agriculture). The FDA develops standards for the composition, quality, nutrition, safety, and labeling of foods including food and color additives. It conducts research to improve detection and prevention of contamination. It collects and interprets data on nutrition, food additives, and pesticide residues. The agency also inspects food plants, imported food products, and mills that make feeds containing medications or nutritional supplements that are destined for human consumption. And it regulates radiation-emitting products such as microwave ovens. The FDA also enforces pesticide tolerances established by the Environmental Protection Agency for all domestically produced and imported foods, except for foods under USDA jurisdiction.

**Fiber:** Dietary fiber generally refers to parts of fruits, vegetables, grains, nuts, and legumes that can't be digested by humans. Meats and dairy products do not contain fiber. Studies indicate that high-fiber diets can reduce the risk of heart disease and certain types of cancer. There are two basic types of fiber—insoluble and soluble. Soluble fiber in cereals, oatmeal, beans, and other foods has been found to lower blood cholesterol. Insoluble fiber in cauliflower, cabbage, and other vegetables and fruits helps move foods through the stomach and intestine, thereby decreasing the risk of cancers of the colon and rectum.

**5-A-Day:** Refers to the dietary recommendation to consume five servings of fruits and vegetables every day. The tagline 5-A-Day became a promotional message in campaigns to increase fruit and vegetable consumption.

**Folic acid:** Folic acid, folate, folacin, all form a group of compounds functionally involved in amino acid metabolism and nucleic acid synthesis. Good dietary sources of folate include leafy, dark green vegetables, legumes, citrus fruits and juices, peanuts, whole grains and fortified breakfast cereals. Recent studies show that if all women of childbearing age consumed sufficient folic acid (either through diet or supplements), 50 percent to 70 percent of birth defects of the brain and spinal cord could be prevented, according to the U.S. Centers for Disease Control and

Prevention (CDC.) Folic acid is critical in the first four to six weeks of pregnancy when the neural tube is formed. This means adequate diet or supplement use should begin before pregnancy occurs. Recent research findings also show low blood folate levels can be associated with elevated plasma homocysteine and increased risk of coronary heart disease.

**Food Guide Pyramid:** The Food Guide Pyramid is a graphic design used to communicate the recommended daily food choices contained in the Dietary Guidelines for Americans. The information provided is developed and promoted by the U.S. Department of Agriculture and the U.S. Department of Health and Human Services. The Food Guide Pyramid shows at its wide base what should form the foundation of a healthful diet—6 to 11 servings daily from the bread, cereal, rice, and pasta group. The next level up the tapered pyramid is divided between the vegetable group, 3 to 5 servings daily, and the fruit group, 2 to 4 servings daily. The next level up the narrowing pyramid is divided between the milk, yogurt, and cheese group, 2 to 3 servings daily, and the meat, poultry, fish, dry beans, eggs, and nuts group, 2 to 3 servings daily. The top level, the smallest part of the pyramid, shows the fats, oils, and sweets in the diet that should be used sparingly.

This pyramid is designed to provide a guide to daily food choices based on the 1995 Dietary Guidelines for Americans. These state:

## Food Guide Pyramid: A Guide to Daily Food Choices

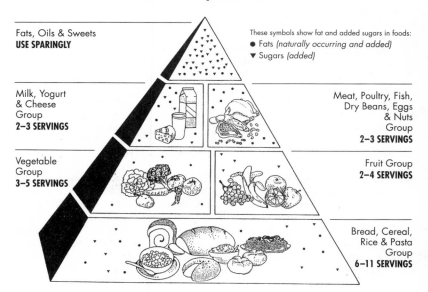

Fats, Oils & Sweets
**USE SPARINGLY**

These symbols show fat and added sugars in foods:
● Fats (naturally occurring and added)
▼ Sugars (added)

Milk, Yogurt & Cheese Group
**2–3 SERVINGS**

Meat, Poultry, Fish, Dry Beans, Eggs & Nuts Group
**2–3 SERVINGS**

Vegetable Group
**3–5 SERVINGS**

Fruit Group
**2–4 SERVINGS**

Bread, Cereal, Rice & Pasta Group
**6–11 SERVINGS**

- Eat a variety of foods.
- Balance the food you eat with physical activity—maintain or improve your weight.
- Choose a diet with plenty of grain products, vegetables, and fruits.
- Choose a diet low in fat, saturated fat, and cholesterol.
- Choose a diet moderate in sugars.
- Choose a diet moderate in salt and sodium.
- If you drink alcoholic beverages, do so in moderation.

**Foodborne disease:** Disease, usually gastrointestinal, caused by organisms or their toxins carried in ingested food. Also commonly known as "food poisoning."

**Free Radicals:** Molecules that are "single" and looking for a partner. The most commonly and potentially hazardous free radicals are oxygen singles that look for a mate by stealing someone else's partner by attaching themselves to a couple. They damage cells lining blood vessels and arteries. They are also believed to play a role in the development of cancer and in aging.

**Fresh:** Signifies a food that has not been heat processed or frozen and contains no preservatives.

**Fructose:** Fructose is a monosaccharide found naturally in fruits, as an added sugar in a crystalline form, and as a component of high-fructose corn syrups (HFCS). HFCS formulations generally contain 42 percent, 55 percent, or 90 percent fructose (the remaining carbohydrate being primarily glucose), depending on the product application—such as soft drinks or cake mixes. Crystalline fructose is 1.2 to 1.8 times as sweet as sucrose. It is produced from cornstarch in a process called isomerization. When used in combination with other sweeteners, including intense sweeteners, a synergistic effect results and the sweetening power of both sweeteners is enhanced.

**Fruit:** Fruit is the usually edible reproductive body of a seed plant, especially one having a sweet pulp associated with the seed.

**Functional foods:** Foods that may provide health benefits beyond basic nutrition.

**GABA (gamma aminobutyric acid):** An inhibitory neurotransmitter which when at lower than normal levels may be responsible for some types of anxiety. Evidence for this is given by the fact that antianxiety drugs such as the benzodiazepines Valium and Librium bind to the receptor and increase its response to GABA.

**Galanin:** Galanin is a neuropeptide neurotransmitter whose receptors are found in areas of the brain responsible for feeding, as well as for learning and memory. It is theorized that a small-molecule drug which blocks the effects of galanin might be useful in reducing the body's appetite for fatty food, as well as modulating acetylcholine, a neurotransmitter implicated in Alzheimer's disease.

**Gastronomy:** The study and appreciation of good food and good eating, and a culture's culinary customs, style, and lore. Any interest or study of culinary pursuits as relates essentially to the kitchen and cookery, and to the higher levels of education, training, and achievement of the professional chef and the chef apprentice.

**Genome:** The total hereditary material of a cell, containing the entire chromosomal set found in each nucleus of a given species.

**Glucagon:** A neurotransmitter involved in glucose metabolism and hunger.

**Glutamate:** Glutamate is an amino acid. It is necessary for metabolism and brain function, and is manufactured by the body. Glutamate is found in virtually every protein food we eat. In food, there is "bound" glutamate and "free" glutamate. Glutamate is used to enhance flavors in foods when it is in its free form and not bound to other amino acids in protein. Some foods have greater quantities of glutamate than others. Foods that are rich in natural glutamate include tomatoes, mushrooms, Parmesan cheese, milk, and mackerel. (*See* Chinese Restaurant Syndrome.)

**Glutamic acid:** A nonessential amino acid.

**Glycine:** A nonessential amino acid usually derived from gelatin.

**Grains:** Within the Dietary Guidelines for Americans, grain foods include items such as bread, cereal, rice, and pasta. Grains are the seeds or fruits of various food plants, including cereal grasses. Wheat, corn, oats, barley, rye, and rice comprise a partial list.

**GRAS (Generally Recognized as Safe):** The regulatory status of food ingredients that were not evaluated by the prescribed testing procedure and were already in use when the 1959 Food Additives Amendment was enacted.

**High or Excellent Source of:** Contains twenty percent or more of the Daily Value (*see* page 310) for a particular nutrient in a serving.

**High or Source of:** Denotes the beneficial presence of a nutrient such as fiber or vitamins.

**High potency:** Describes a nutrient in a food that is 100 percent or more of the RDI (*see* page 310) established for that product. The term may also be used with multi-ingredient products if two-thirds of the nutrients are present at 100 percent of the RDI.

**Hydrogenation:** The process of adding hydrogen molecules directly to an unsaturated fatty acid such as a vegetable oil to convert it to a semisolid form such as margarine. Hydrogenation contributes important textural properties to food. The degree of hydrogenation influences the firmness and spreadability of margarines, flakiness of piecrust and the creaminess of puddings. Hydrogenated oils are sometimes used in place of other fats with higher proportions of saturated fatty acids such as butter.

**Hyperactivity:** *See* Attention Deficit Hyperactivity Disorder (ADHD).

**Hypertension:** Hypertension is the persistently elevated arterial blood pressure. It is the most common public health problem in developed countries. Emphasis on lifestyle modifications has given diet a prominent role for both the primary prevention and management of hypertension.

**Hypoglycemia:** Abnormal decrease of sugar in the blood—the opposite of diabetes.

**Hypothalamus:** Brain control area involved in emotion, movement, and eating. Less than the size of a peanut and weighing a quarter of an ounce, this small area deep within the brain also oversees appetite, blood pressure, sexual behavior, sleep, and emotions, and sends orders to the pituitary gland.

**Insecticide:** A class of crop protection and specialty chemicals used to control insects on farms and in forests, as well as nonagricultural applications such as residential lawns, golf courses, and public tracts of land.

**Intense sweeteners:** Intense sweeteners are nonnutritive sweeteners, also referred to as low-calorie sweeteners. Intense sweeteners can replace nutritive sweeteners in most foods at a caloric savings of approximately 16 calories per teaspoon. Thus caloric reduction may be achieved when low-calorie sweetened foods and beverages are substituted for their full-calorie counterparts. Examples of intense sweeteners in use in the U.S. food supply are saccharin, aspartame, and acesulfame K.

**International Units (I.U.s):** A quantity measurement of vitamins that are fat-soluble (do not mix with water and need fat for proper absorption). Vitamins A, E, D and K are usually measured in I.U.s.

**Inulin:** Soluble natural dietary fiber which replaces fat and improves mouthfeel in low-fat food systems, providing textural properties to food products and health benefits to consumers.

**Lean and Extra Lean:** Describes the fat content of meats, poultry, seafood, and game meats. Lean = fewer than five grams of fat per serving. Extra lean = fewer than five grams of fat per serving.

**Less:** Means a product contains twenty-five precent less of a nutrient or twenty-five percent fewer calories than the reference food. For example, pretzels that have twenty-five percent less fat than potato chips could carry a "less" claim.

**Light or Lite:** Signifies a product contains one third fewer calories or one half the fat of the comparison food. "Light in sodium" may be used on food in which the sodium content has been reduced by at least fifty percent.

**Low cholesterol:** Signifies twenty milligrams or less per serving.

**Low fat:** Three grams or less per serving.

**Low saturated fat:** Means one gram or less per serving.

**Lycopene:** Lycopene is a carotenoid related to the better-known beta-carotene. Lycopene gives tomatoes and some other fruits and vegetables their distinctive red color. Nutritionally, it functions as an antioxidant. Research shows lycopene is best absorbed by the body when consumed as tomatoes that have been heat-processed using a small amount of oil. This includes products such as tomato sauce and tomato paste (*Also see* Functional foods.)

**MCG (microgram):** A metric measurement that is 1/1000 part of a milligram.

**MG (milligram):** A metric measurement that is 1/1000 part of a gram.

**Monoamine:** Containing one amine group.

**Monoamine oxidase inhibitors (MAOIs):** A group of drugs that is used in the treatment of depression and that elevates the level of neurotransmitters by preventing their destruction by enzymes.

**Monounsaturated fats:** Found in varying amounts in both plant and animal fat. Olive oil, peanut oil, some margarines, and vegetable shortening tend to be high in monounsaturated fatty acids. Research has shown that substituting monounsaturated fat for saturated fat reduces blood cholesterol.

**Morbid obesity:** This is a state of adiposity or overweight in which body weight is 100 percent above the ideal and a body mass index of 45 or greater.

**More:** Means a product contains at least ten percent more of the Daily Value (*see* page 310) for a desirable nutrient, such as fiber, than the regular food.

**MSG (monosodium glutamate):** MSG is the sodium salt of glutamic acid. Glutamic acid, or glutamate, is one of the most common amino acids found in nature. It is the main component of many proteins and peptides, and is present in most tissues. Glutamate is also produced in the body and plays an essential role in human metabolism. Virtually every food contains glutamate. It is a major component of many protein-rich food products such as meat, fish, milk, and some vegetables. In the early 1900s scientists isolated MSG as an ingredient in plants that was responsible for greatly enhancing flavor. In the early part of the century, MSG was extracted from seaweed and other plant sources. Today, MSG is produced in many countries through a fermentation process of molasses from sugar cane or sugar beets as well as starch and corn sugar. When present in its "free" form—not bound together with other amino acids in protein—glutamate has a flavor-enhancing effect in foods.

**National Health and Nutrition Examination Survey (NHANES):** A series of surveys that include information from medical history, physical measurements, biochemical evaluation, physical examination, and dietary intake of population groups within the United States. The U.S. Department of Health and Human Services conducts the NHANES approximately every five years.

**Nerve growth factor (NGF):** The subject of a great deal of scientific interest, it is believed to maintain and repair nerves in the brain.

**Neural tube defect (NTD):** In simple terms, a neural tube defect is a malformation of the brain or spinal cord (neurological system) during embryonic development. Infants born with spina bifida, where the spinal cord is exposed, can grow to adulthood but usually suffer from paralysis or other disabilities. Babies born with anencephaly, where most or all of the brain is missing, usually die shortly after birth. These NTDs make up about 5 percent of all U.S. birth defects. If all women of childbearing age consumed sufficient folic acid (either through diet or supplements), 50 percent to 70 percent of birth defects of the brain and spinal cord could be prevented, according to the U.S. Centers for Disease Control and Prevention. Folic acid is critical in the first four to six weeks of pregnancy when the neural tube is formed. This means adequate diet or supplement use should begin before pregnancy occurs. A leading CDC authority refers to folic acid as "the sleeping giant of preventive medicine" for its potential to eliminate much of the risk of NTDs—if only it were consumed in the right quantities by the right people at the right time.

**Neuron:** The nerve cell that serves as the information processing and transmitting element of the nervous system. It is made up of the soma, or cell body, dendrites which receive messages via neurotransmitters from other neurons across the synapse, and the axon which transmits the message from one cell across the synapse to another cell.

## Glossary    281

**Neuropeptide Y (NPY):** NPY is a peptide from the pancreatic polypeptide family, with at least six NPY receptor subtypes and in differing concentrations throughout the brain. Researchers have shown that NPY is a potent stimulator of eating by injecting NPY into the ventricles of the brain, whereby it stimulates eating to the point of obesity in several laboratory species by making an antagonist drug that blocks the binding of NPY to a receptor.

**Neurotensin:** A peptide of thirteen amino acid derivatives that helps regulate blood sugar by its effects on a number of hormones, including insulin and glucagon. It is also thought to play a part in pain suppression.

**Neurotransmitter:** A chemical that is secreted by the terminal buttons of an axon into a synapse and produces an excitatory or inhibitory postsynaptic electrical charge in the specific receptors in the membrane of the postsynaptic, or receiving, cell. Neurogen is developing drugs that work with the GABA, dopamine, neuropeptide Y, corticotrophin-releasing factor, and other neurotransmitter systems.

**Nitrite:** Nitrite is a food additive that has been used for centuries to preserve meats, fish, and poultry. It also contributes to the characteristic flavor, color, and texture of such processed meats as hot dogs, bacon, and salami. Because nitrite safeguards cured meats against the most deadly foodborne bacterium of all, *Clostridium (C.) botulinum,* its use is supported by the public health community. In the 1970s, there were concerns about a potential cancer risk from a digestive reaction-product of nitrite called nitrosamines. A subsequent FDA-commissioned study conducted by the National Academy of Sciences concluded that nitrite levels in cured meat have not been linked to the development of human cancers and the report noted nitrite's beneficial antimicrobial activity. Nitrates consumed in foods such as carrots and green vegetables are converted to nitrite during digestion.

**Nitrosamines:** Nitrosamines are a digestive reaction-product of nitrite, a food additive used to preserve meats, fish, and poultry. They are potential cancer-causing agents. (*Also see* Nitrite *above.*)

**Norepinephrine (noradrenaline):** A hormone released by the adrenal gland possessing the ability to stimulate, as does epinephrine, but with minimal inhibitory effects. It has little effect on the lungs' smooth muscles and metabolic processes and differs from epinephrine in its effects on the heart and blood vessels.

**Nutraceuticals:** A term used to describe substances in or parts of a food that may be considered to provide medical or health benefits beyond basic nutrition, including disease prevention. (*Also see* Functional foods.)

**Obesity, or overweight:** Although precise definitions vary among experts, overweight has been traditionally defined as 10 percent to 20 percent above an optimal weight for height derived from statistics. Some scientists argue that the amount and distribution of an individual's body fat is a significant indicator of health risk and therefore should be considered in defining overweight. Abdominal fat has been linked to more adverse health consequences than fat on the hips or thighs. Thus calculations of waist-to-hip ratio are preferred by some health experts to help determine if an individual is overweight.

**Osteoporosis:** Osteoporosis is a skeletal disease in which the bones lose mass and density, the pores in bones enlarge, and the bones generally become fragile. Osteoporosis often is not diagnosed until a fracture occurs, most commonly in the spine, hip, or wrist. The National Osteoporosis Foundation says about 1.5 million such fractures occur each year in the United States, at an estimated annual cost of $14 billion in 1995.

**Parasympathetic nervous system:** A group of nerve fibers that leave the brain and spinal cord and extend to nerve cell clusters (ganglia) at specific sites. From there they are distributed to blood vessels, glands, and other internal organs. Parasympathetic nerves are involved in the heart rate, stimulating digestion, and contracting bronchioles in the lungs, pupils in the eyes, and the esophagus. The parasympathetic nervous system works in conjunction with the sympathetic nervous system. (*Also see* Sympathetic nervous system.)

**Peptidase:** An enzyme that splits simple peptides or their derivatives.

**Peptide:** Two or more amino acids combined in head-to-tail links. Generally larger than simple amino acids or the monoamines, the largest peptides discovered thus far have forty-four amino acids. Neuropeptides signal the body's endocrine glands to balance salt and water. Opiate peptides can help control pain and anxiety. The peptides work with amino acids. A peptide is present at two ten-thousandths of its partner amino acid or one hundredth of a monoamine.

**Percent fat free:** Used only to describe food that qualify as low fat.

**Pesticide:** A broad class of crop protection chemicals of four major types: insecticides used to control insects; herbicides used to control weeds; rodenticides used to control rodents; and fungicides used to control mold, mildew, and fungi. In addition, consumers use pesticides in the home or yard to control termites and roaches, clean mold from shower curtains, stave off crab grass on the lawn, kill fleas and ticks on pets, and disinfect swimming pools, to name just a few "specialty" pesticide uses. Some pesticides are immediately toxic to humans; others take a long time to produce cancer and other illnesses.

**Pharmacokinetics:** Pharmacokinetics examine the effects of the drug on a body, specifically examining issues such as how quickly a drug is absorbed into the blood and how different dosages affect the absorption, how the drug is distributed into organs or tissues of the body, how the body metabolizes the drug, and whether what the drug is changed into by the body is active, as well how long it takes the body to metabolize half of the drug (the drug's half-life), and how long it takes the drug to clear the body and be excreted.

**Pharmacology:** Pharmacology examines the effects of the drug on the body, looking at such issues as how the drug works, its safety, whether it affects one organ or area of the body more than another, and what common adverse experiences (AEs) are associated with its use.

**Phytochemical:** Phytochemicals are substances found in edible fruits and vegetables that may be ingested by humans daily in gram quantities and that exhibit a potential for modulating the human metabolism in a manner favorable for reducing the risk of cancer.

**Pituitary gland:** The pea-sized gland situated at the base of the brain, once thought to be the master gland that gave "orders" to other glands. It is now known that the pituitary gland takes its orders from the hypothalamus (*also see* Hypothalamus). The pituitary then sends out orders to the other glands in your body. The frontal lobe of the gland produces six hormones: growth hormone, which regulates growth; prolactin, which stimulates the breasts and has other functions as yet not clearly understood; and four other hormones that stimulate the thyroid, adrenals, ovaries in women, and testes in men. The back lobe of the pituitary produces two hormones: antidiuretic hormone, which acts on the kidneys and regulates urine output, and oxytocin, which stimulates contractions of the womb during childbirth.

**Placebo:** Sometimes casually referred to as a "sugar pill," a placebo is a treatment with an innocuous or inert substance that seems identical to the real treatment in a study. Placebo treatments are used to eliminate bias that may arise from the expectation that a treatment should produce an effect.

**Polyunsaturated fats:** Tend to lower blood cholesterol levels. They are found in mainly in fat of foods from plants. Safflower, sunflower, corn, soybean, and cottonseed oils contain large amounts of polyunsaturated fatty acids.

**Prevalence:** The number of existing cases of a disease in a defined population at a specified time.

**Prospective study:** Epidemiological research that follows a group of people over a period of time to observe the potential effects of diet, behavior, and other factors on health or the incidence of disease. In general, this is considered a more valid research design than retrospective research.

**Protein:** Chemically, a protein is a complex nitrogenous compound made up of amino acids in peptide linkages. Dietary proteins are involved in the synthesis of tissue protein and other special metabolic functions. In anabolic processes they furnish the amino acids required to build and maintain body tissues. As an energy source, proteins are equivalent to carbohydrates in providing 4 calories per gram. Proteins perform a major structural role in all body tissues and in the formation of enzymes, hormones and various body fluids and secretions. Proteins participate in the transport of some lipids, vitamins, and minerals and help maintain the body's homeostasis.

**Quercetin:** A bioflavonoid believed to reduce allergic process due to its ability to stabilize mast cells and basophils, thereby inhibiting release of histamine and its ability to inhibit certain enzymes and leukotriene involved in the inflammatory response. Rheumatoid arthritis is characterized by substantially increased numbers of mast cells in the fluid and membranes around the joints. These cells release destructive enzymes believed to be major factors in the tissue destruction in arthritis. Quercetin is a potent inhibitor of mast cell enzyme release.

**Random sample:** A random sample is a procedure to select subjects for a study in which all individuals in a population being studied have an equal chance of being selected. Using a random sample allows the results of the study to be generalized to the entire population. The term *random* also applies to assignments within controlled studies, or the division of subjects into groups. Random assignment ensures that all subjects have an equal chance of being in the experimental and control groups, and increases the probability that any unidentified variable will systematically occur in both groups with the same frequency. Randomization is crucial to control for variables that researchers may not be aware of or that they cannot adequately control, but which could affect the outcome of an experimental study.

**(RDA) Recommended Daily Dietary Allowance:** The RDA was started in the 1940s to safeguard the public's health. The RDAs set at the time were estimates of the nutritional needs of adults and children, and were developed by the Food and Drug Administration (FDA) to be used as the legal standards for labeling foods in regards to nutritional content.

## U.S. RDA (RECOMMENDED DAILY ALLOWANCES)

### Adults & Children (4 years and over)

| | |
|---|---|
| Vitamin A* | 5,000 I.U. |
| Vitamin C (ascorbic acid)* | 60 mg |
| Vitamin $B_1$ (thiamine)* | 1.5 mg |
| Vitamin $B_2$ (riboflavin)* | 1.7 mg |
| Niacin* | 20 mg |
| Calcium* | 1.0 g |
| Iron* | 18 mg |
| Vitamin D | 400 I.U. |
| Vitamin E | 30 I.U. |
| Vitamin $B_6$ | 2.0 mg |
| Folic Acid | 4 mg |
| Vitamin $B_{12}$ | 6 mcg |
| Phosphorus | 1.0 g |
| Iodine | 150 mcg |
| Magnesium | 400 mg |
| Zinc | 15 mg |
| Copper | 2 mg |
| Biotin | 3 mg |
| Pantothenic acid | 10 mg |

*These nutrients *must* appear on nutrition labels. The other nutrients *may* appear.

**Receptor:** Found in the postsynaptic side of the synapse, a receptor consists of a protein molecule embedded in the membrane of the cell, which contains active sites that bind to a particular chemical or neurotransmitter. When a receptor is stimulated, changes take place either at the receptor through chemically gated ion channels, which change the electrical potential of the cell, or within the cell using transmembrane transduction, which activates second messengers to carry out secondary effects.

**Receptor subtypes:** A receptor is made up of folded protein sections, or subtypes, forming the central pore of the receptor which opens and closes as the receptor is stimulated. Each subtype may have active binding sites which change the activity of the receptor through its response to other neurotransmitters.

**Recombinant DNA (rDNA):** The DNA formed by combining segments of DNA from different organisms.

**Reliability:** Whether a test or instrument used to collect data, such as a questionnaire, gives the same results if repeated on the same person several times. A reliable test gives reproducible results.

**Reduced:** Means a product has been nutritionally altered and contains at least 25 percent less of a nutrient (such as fat) or 25 percent fewer calories than the regular product.

**Research design:** How a study is set up to collect information or data. For valid results, the design must be appropriate to answer the question or hypothesis being studied.

**Retrospective study:** Research that relies on recall of past data, or on previously recorded information. Often this type of research is considered to have limitations, due to the number of variables that cannot be controlled, and because memory is not infallible.

**Risk:** A term encompassing a variety of measures of the probability of an outcome. It's usually used in reference to unfavorable outcomes such as illness, accident, or death. Be certain to distinguish between absolute and relative risk.

**RNA (ribonucleic acid):** RNA is a molecule similar to DNA that functions primarily to decode the instructions carried by genes for protein synthesis.

**Saccharin:** Saccharin, the oldest of the nonnutritive sweeteners, is currently produced from purified, manufactured methyl anthranilate, a substance occurring naturally in grapes. It is 300 times sweeter than sucrose, heat stable, and does not promote dental caries. Saccharin has a long shelf life, but a slightly bitter aftertaste. It is not metabolized in the human digestive system, is excreted rapidly in the urine, and does not accumulate in the body. There is some history of controversy surrounding saccharin. In 1977, the FDA proposed banning the sweetener after animal studies implicated it as a weak carcinogen. Public opposition to the ban led Congress to pass a law allowing continued use of saccharin with a product warning label. In 1991, Congress extended the saccharin ban moratorium for the fifth time, effective through 1997. Then in December 1991, the FDA withdrew its proposed ban. The warning label remains in effect.

**Serotonin:** A neurotransmitter thought to play a role in temperature regulation, migraine headaches, mood, and sleep.

**Sodium free:** Less than 5 milligrams per serving.

**Spina bifida:** Spina bifida is a birth defect in which the infant is born with the spinal cord exposed. These children can grow to adulthood, although they often suffer from paralysis and other disabilities. (*Also see* Neural tube defects [NTDs].)

**Substance P:** Substance P is a neurotransmitter believed to carry pain messages from the body to the brain, and vice versa.

**Sucrose:** Sucrose, a type of sugar, is a diglyceride composed of glucose and fructose. (*Also see* Carbohydrates.)

**Sugar:** Although the consumer is confronted by a wide variety of sugars—sucrose, raw sugar, turbinado sugar, brown sugar, honey, corn syrup—there is no significant difference in the nutritional content or energy each provides, and therefore no nutritional advantage of one over another. There also is no evidence that the body can distinguish between naturally occurring or added sugars in food products.

**Sympathetic nervous system:** The sympathetic nervous system consists of nerve fibers that leave the brain and spinal cord, pass through the nerve cell clusters (ganglia), and are distributed to the heart, lungs, intestine, blood vessels, and sweat glands. In general, sympathetic nerves dilate the pupils, constrict small blood vessels, and increase heart rate. The system also involves circulating substances produced in the adrenal glands.

**Synapse:** The minute space between two neurons or between a neuron and an organ across which nerve impulses are chemically transmitted.

**Thyroid gland:** A butterfly-shaped gland located in the neck with a "wing" on either side of the windpipe. The gland produces thyroxine, which controls the rates of chemical reactions in the body. Generally, the more thyroxine, the faster the body works. Thyroxine needs iodine to function.

**Time release (slow release):** When a vitamin or mineral has a time-release factor, it means that the ingredients have been scientifically coated and calibrated in tiny "memory granules" that are released over a period of 2 to 6 hours. The advantage of time release is it gives the body the vitamin or mineral gradually instead of all at one time.

**Trans fatty acids:** Trans fatty acids occur naturally in beef, butter, milk, and lamb fats and in commercially prepared, partially hydrogenated margarines and solid cooking fats. The main sources of trans fatty acids in the American diet today are stick margarine, shortening, commercial frying fats, and high-fat baked goods. Partially hydrogenated vegetable oils were developed in part to help displace highly saturated animal and vegetable fats used in frying, baking and spreads. However, trans fatty acids, like saturated fatty acids, may raise blood LDL cholesterol levels (the so-called bad cholesterol), but not as much as the saturates do. At high consumption levels they may also reduce the HDL, or "good," cholesterol levels.

**USDA:** The United States Department of Agriculture. The agency is involved in research, educational, and nutritional programs. It shares responsibility for food safety with the FDA.

**Vagus nerve:** Literally the "wandering nerve" because it has such a wide distribution in the body, the vagus nerve connects the stomach to the brain

# Glossary    287

and is involved in other autonomic functions such as breathing and heart rate.

**Variable:** Any characteristic that may vary in study subjects, such as gender, age, body weight, diet, behavior, attitude, or other attribute. In an experiment, the treatment is called the "independent variable"; it is the factor being investigated. The variable that is influenced by the treatment is the "dependent variable"; it may change as a result of the effect of the independent variable.

**Vasoactive intestinal peptide (VIP):** A neurotransmitter present in both the gut and the brain. Its peripheral effects include lowering blood pressure by causing vasodilation, suppressing the secretion of stomach acid, and stimulating secretion in the small intestine and colon. VIP stimulates the release of a number of pituitary hormones, including growth hormone and prolactin, and may thus help to regulate the hormone-producing glands.

**Vector:** The agent used to carry new DNA into a cell (ex., plasmid or virus).

**Vegetarian:** According to the Vegetarian Resource Group, less than 1 percent of Americans are true vegetarians. Such people never eat meat, fish, or poultry, although they may eat foods derived from animals, such as dairy products and eggs. There are even fewer vegans, strict vegetarians who avoid all animal-derived foods—even honey.

**Very Low Sodium:** Less than 35 milligrams per serving.

**Vitamins:** Vitamins are organic compounds that are nutritionally essential in small amounts to control metabolic processes and cannot be synthesized by the body. Vitamins are usually classified by their solubility, which to some degree determines their stability; occurrence in food stuffs; distribution in body fluids; and tissue storage capacity. Each of the fat-soluble vitamins, A, D, E, and K, has a distinct and separate physiologic role. Several are among those supporting antioxidant efforts to depress the effects of metabolic byproducts called free radicals, which are thought to cause degenerative changes related to aging. Most of the water-soluble vitamins are components of essential enzyme systems. Many are involved in the reactions supporting energy metabolism. These vitamins are not normally stored in the body in appreciable amounts and are normally excreted in small quantities in the urine. Thus a daily supply is desirable to avoid depletion and interruption of normal physiologic functions.

**Water:** Although deficiencies of other nutrients can be sustained for months or even years, a person can survive only a few days without water. Experts rank water second only to oxygen as essential for life. In addition to offering true refreshment for the thirsty, water plays a vital role in all bodily processes. It supplies the medium in which various chemical changes of the body occur, aiding in digestion, absorption, circulation, and lubrication of body joints. For example, as a major component of blood, water helps deliver nutrients to body cells and removes waste to the kidneys for excretion. Average adults need about 64 ounces of fluid each day for optimal health. Although experts generally advise drinking several glasses of water a day, the need for fluid can also be met by consuming a variety of foods and beverages.

# Notes

## Introduction

1. Richard Mattes, Ph.D., R.D., "Physiologic responses to sensory stimulation by food: Nutritional Implications," *Journal of the American Dietetic Association* (1997); 97: 406–10, 413.

## 1. Your Brain–Belly Connection

1. Michael Gershon, professor of anatomy and cell biology, Columbia-Presbyterian Medical Center, New York, personal communication with authors, May 6, 1998.
2. John E. Morley et al., "Neuropeptides and Appetite: Contribution of Neuropharmacological Modeling," *Federation Proceedings* 43(14): 2903–07.
3. "Hypothalamic Link with GI Tract," *Science News,* 13 September 1980, 165.
4. "Weight Control Drugs In the FDA Pipeline," *www.loop.com/~bkrentzman /media/upmeds.html* 6/1/97.
5. John E. Morley et al., "Effects of Peripheral Hormones on Memory and Ingestive Behaviors," *Psychoneuroendocrinology* (1992 August); 17 (4): 391–9.
6. S. F. Leibowitz and C. Rossakis, *Neuropharmacology* (1986); 17: 691–702.
7. Ibid.
8. Ibid.
9. John E. Morley and A. S. Levine, "Appetite Regulation: Modern Concepts Offering Food for Thought," *Postgraduate Medicine* (1985 February 15); 77(3): 42–8, 52–4.
10. Jeffrey Friedman, M.D., Ph.D., professor and associate investigator. "Report scientists from the Howard Hughes Medical Institute (HHMI) at the Rockefeller University find Leptin gene." In February 15 *Nature,* 1996.

## 2. Food and Medicines of the Mind

1. Raymond Bartus, personal communication with authors, April 15, 1985.
2. P. Ferro et al., "A Brain Octadecaneuropeptide Generated by Tryptic Di-

gestion of DBI Functions as a Proconflict Ligand of Benzodiazepine Recognition Sites," *Neuropharmacology* (1996): 23(11); 1359–62.
3. M. A. Diamond et al., "Treatment of Idiopathic Postural Hypotension with Oral Tyramine and Monoamine Oxidase Inhibitor," *Journal of Clinical Research* (1986); 17:237.
4. Brian L. G. Morgan, *Food and Drug Interaction Guide* (New York: Simon & Schuster, 1986), 271.
5. G. B. Raiczyk and J. Pinto, "Troublesome Combinations and Susceptible Patients," *Biochemical Pharmacology* (1988): 85–105.

## 3. From Table to Able—Amino Acids

1. Andrew Mebane, "L-glutamine Mania," *American Journal of Psychiatry,* 141 Oct. 10, 1984, 1302–03.
2. "The Case of Too Much Amino Acids," *Tufts University Diet and Nutrition Letter,* 4 (3): 7.
3. K. A. Smith, C. G. Fairburn, and P. J. Cowen, "Relapse of depression after rapid depletion of tryptophan," *Lancet,* Vol. 349, March 29, 1997, 915–19.
4. John Fenstrom et. al, "Diurnal Variations in Plasma Concentration of Tryptophan and Other Neutral Amino Acids: Effects of Dietary Protein Intake," *American Journal of Clinical Nutrition,* 32, September 1979, 1912–22.
5. E. Reynolds, "Folic Acid, S-Adenosyl Methionine and Affective Disorders," *Psychological Medicine* (1985); 13 (4): 705010.
6. M. Fava et al., "Rapidity of Onset of the Antidepressant Effect of Parenteral S-adenosyl-L-methionine," *Psychiatric Research,* 1995 April 28; 56(3): 295–97.
7. H. Volkmann et al., "Double-Blind, Placebo-Controlled Cross-over Study of Intravenous S-adenosyl-L-methionine in Patients with Fibromyalgia," *Scandinavian Journal of Rheumatology* (1997); 26 (3): 206–11.
8. Arthur Winter, "New Treatment for Multiple Sclerosis," *Neurological and Orthopedic Journal of Medicine and Surgery,* April 1984, 39–43.
9. Food and Agriculture Organization of the United Nations, Food Policy and Food Science Service, Nutrition Division, *Amino Acid Content of Foods and Biological Data on Proteins* (Rome Food and Agriculture Organization of the United Nations), 1980.
10. L. Vazelli et al., "On the Significance of Tryptophan Content of Foods," *Research Communications in Psychology, Psychiatry and Behavior* (1990); 7(4): 485–88.
11. Ernest Hartmann and C. L. Spinweber, "Sleep Induced by L-tryptophan: Effect of Dosages Within the Normal Dietary Intake," *Journal of Nervous and Mental Diseases,* 167 (1979): 497–99.
12. Michael Yogman, "Nutrients and Newborn Behavior: Neurotransmitters as Mediators?" *Nutrition Reviews Supplement,* 44 (May 1986): 74–75.
13. Vaselli, L., *op. cit.*
14. Elaine Nemzer et al., "Amino Acid Supplementation as Therapy for Attention Deficit Disorders," *Journal of the American Academy of Child Psychiatry,* 25 (July 1986): 509–13.
15. M. B. Yunus et al., "Plasma Tryptophan and Other Amino Acids in Primary Fibromyalgia: A Controlled Study," *Journal of Rheumatology,* 1992,

19:90–4; S. Jacobsen et al., "Single Cell Morphology of Muscle in Patients with Chronic Muscle Pain," *Scandinavian Journal of Rheumatology,* 20 (5) 336–343; D. S. Bell et al., "Primary Juvenile Fibromyalgia Syndrome and Chronic Fatigue Syndrome in Adolescents," *Clinical Infectious Diseases,* 1994, 18 (suppl) 521–3.

16. "Eating Away Your Pain," *Science News,* 19 February 1983, 125.
17. B. Birmaher et al., "Neuroendocrine Response to 5-hydroxy-L-tryptophan in Prepubertal Children at High Risk of Major Depressive Disorder," *Archives of General Psychiatry,* 1997 December; 54 (12): 1113—19.
18. M. A. Ellenbogen et al., "Mood Response to Acute Tryptophan Depletion in Healthy Volunteers: Sex Differences and Temporal Stability," *Neuropsychopharmacology,* 1996 November; 15 (5): 465–74.
19. "Clinical Spectrum of Eosinophilia-Myalgia Syndrome," *Morbidity and Mortality Weekly Report* (Centers for Disease Control) 39, No. 6 (February 16, 1990): 1–3.
20. "Beefy Boosters for Ailing Immune System," *Medical World News,* 16 February 1981, 34.
21. R. L. Prior et al., "Conditions Altering Plasma Concentrations of Urea Cycle and Other Amino Acids in Elderly Human Subjects," *Journal of the American College of Nutrition,* 1996 June, 15 (3): 237–47.
22. A. J. Gelenberg et al., "Tyrosine for the Treatment of Depression," *American Journal of Neural Transmission,* 47 (1980); 1014–15.
23. E. Melamed et al., "Plasma Tyrosine in Normal Humans: Effects of Oral Tyrosine and Protein-Containing Meals," *Journal of Neural Transmission,* 47 (1980) 1014–15.
24. D. F. Neri et al., "The Effects of Tyrosine on Cognitive Performance During Extended Wakefulness," *Aviation Space Environmental Medicine,* 1995 April; 66 (4): 313–19.
25. Carol Ballentine, "The Essential Guide to Amino Acids," *FDA Consumer,* 19 (1986) (7): 23–24.
26. C. Wayne Callaway, "Nutrition," *Journal of the American Medical Association,* (1987) 256 (15): 2097–98.
27. John Fenstrom, "Acute and Chronic Effects of Protein and Carbohydrate Ingestion on Brain Tryptophan Levels and Serotonin Synthesis," *Nutrition Reviews Supplement,* 44 (May 1986): 25–35.
28. *National Institute of Mental Health Science Reporter,* March 1984, S-3.
29. Paul Teychenne, *Questions and Answers About Parkinson's Disease and Its Treatment* (East Hanover, NJ: Sandoz Pharmaceutical Co., 1985), 20.
30. J. H. Pincus, and K. M. Barry, "Dietary Methods for Reducing Fluctuations in Parkinson's Disease," *Yale Journal of Biological Medicine,* (1986) 60 (2): 133–37.
31. Ibid.
32. "Changes in Diet for Victims of Parkinson's Disease," *Tufts University Diet and Nutrition Letter,* 5 (4) 1986.
33. Ibid.
34. "Potato Dilemma: To Bake or Fry?" *Science News,* 4 February 1984, 125.
35. Michael Trulson, (paper presented to the 95th Annual Meeting of the American Psychological Association, New York, 31 August 1987).

## 4. Mood and Food: Brain and Blood Sugar

1. Massachusetts General Hospital, Department of Dietetics, *Energy Modification Diet Reference Manual* (Boston: Little Brown, 1984), 41–61.
2. "Hypoglycemia—Fact or Fiction," *Harvard Medical School Health Letter,* 5 (1):1.
3. Ruth Winter, "Do You or Don't You Have Hypoglycemia?" *Glamour,* December 1980, 244–45.
4. National Institutes of Health, "Special Report on Aging," NIH Pub. No. 80-2135 August 1980, 10.
5. M. A. Nauck et al., "Glucagon-like peptide 1 inhibition of gastric emptying outweighs its insulinotropic effects in healthy humans," *American Journal of Physiology,* 1997 Nov; 273 (5Pt.1): E981–8; J. Gromada et al., "Glucagon-like peptide 1 (7-36) amide stimulates exocytosis in human pancreatic beat cells by both proximal and distal regulatory steps in stimulus-secretion coupling," *Diabetes* 1998 January; 47 (1): 57–65.
6. Ibid.
7. Larry Christensen, paper presented at the 95th Annual Meeting of the American Psychological Association, New York, 31 August 1987.
8. Robin Kanarek and Robin Marks-Kaufman, *Nutrition and Behavior: New Perspectives* (New York: Van Nostrand Reinhold, 1991), 3.
9. E. Pollitt et al., *American Journal of Clinical Nutrition,* 34 (1981): 1526–33.
10. Anita Lewis, Ph.D., University of Texas at Houston (1983), *Dissertation Abstracts International,* 43 (11).
11. Michael J. Murphy, Ed.D., et al., "School Breakfast Participation Leads to Academic, Psychological Improvements," *Archives of Pediatric and Adolescent Medicine* (September 1998): 124.
12. Bonnie Spring et al., study done at Health Sciences/Chicago Medical School, 1991 but as yet unpublished. Communication with author, February 18, 1998.
13. Vicky Rippere, "Dietary treatment of chronic obsessional ruminations," *British Journal of Clinical Psychology* (1983): 314–16.
14. Betty Li and Priscilla Schumann, "Sugar Content of Breakfast Cereals," *Agriculture Research* ( January–February) 1980:15.
15. Angus Craig, "Acute Effects of Meals on Perceptual and Cognitive Efficiency," *Nutrition Reviews Supplement,* 44 (May 1986): 163–71.
16. B. Spring et al., "Effects of Carbohydrates on Mood and Behavior," *Nutrition Reviews Supplement,* 44 (May 1986): 51–60.
17. B. Spring et al., "Dietary Distress Inventory Scale," *Journal of Psychiatric Research,* 17 (1982/83): 155.
18. B. Spring et al., "Psychobiological Effects of Carbohydrates," *Journal of Clinical Psychiatry,* 1989 May; 50 Suppl: 27–33; discussion 34.
19. Craig, *op.cit.,* 165.
20. M. L. Wolraich, S. D. Lindgren, and P. J. Stumbo, et. al., "Effects of Diets High in Sucrose or Aspartame on the Behavior and Cognitive Performance of Children," *The New England Journal of Medicine,* 330:5: 301–07, February 3, 1994.
21. Ronald Prinz and David Riddle, "Associations Between Nutrition and Behavior in Five Year Old Children," *Nutrition Reviews Supplement,* 44 (May 1986): 151–57.

## 292   Notes

22. Keith C. Conners, "Carbohydrates and Sucrose: Psychological, Cognitive and Behavioral Effects" (paper presented at the 95th Annual Meeting of the American Psychological Association, New York, 31 August 1987).
23. Ibid.
24. Judith Rapoport, "Diet and Hyperactivity," *Nutrition Reviews Supplement,* 44 (May 1986): 158–62.
25. Bonnie Spring, "Carbohydrate Craving: Clinical Implications" (paper presented at the 94th Annual Meeting of the American Psychological Association, Washington, D.C., 23 August 1986).
26. Judith Wurtman, "Carbohydrate Craving in Obesity" (paper presented at the 94th Annual Meeting of the American Psychological Association, Washington, D.C., 23 August 1986).
27. Ibid.
28. C. Zacchia et al., "Effect of Sucrose Consumption on Alcohol-Induced Impairment in Male Social Drinkers," *Psychopharmacology* (1991); 105 (1): 49–56.
29. Neal Grunberg and Deborah Bowen, "Carbohydrate Craving in Bulimic Individuals" (paper presented at the 94th Annual Meeting of the American Psychological Association, Washington, D.C., 23 August 1986).
30. Ibid.
31. Norman E. Rosenthal et al., "Carbohydrate and Protein Meals: Acute Effects on Mood and Performance" (paper presented at the 94th Annual Meeting of the American Psychological Association, Washington, D.C., 23 August 1986).
32. P. J. Andreason et al., "Regional cerebral glucose metabolism in bulimia nervosa," *American Journal of Psychiatry* (November 1992); 149(11): 1506–13.
33. June Chiodo, "Carbohydrate Craving in Bulimic Individuals" (paper presented at the 94th Annual Meeting of the American Psychological Association, Washington, D.C., 23 August 1986).
34. John Bantle et al., "Postprandial Glucose and Insulin Responses to Meals Containing Different Carbohydrates in Normal and Diabetic Subjects," *New England Journal of Medicine* (1986) 309 (1): 7–12.
35. Ibid.
36. *Rockefeller University Research Profiles,* Spring 1987, 1–4.
37. "Nutritive Value of Brown, Raw, and Refined Sugar," *Journal of the American Medical Association,* 221(2): 201.
38. Richard Bernstein, *Diabetes,* "The Glucograph Method of Normalizing Blood Sugar" (Los Angeles: J. P. Tarcher, 1981), 154.
39. Ibid.
40. Norman Ertel, *Diabetes Care* (May–June 1985); 8: 279–83.
41. Bernstein, *op.cit.*
42. Ibid.
43. Ruth Winter, *A Consumer's Dictionary of Food Additives* (New York: Crown, 1984), 224.
44. Phyllis Crapo, "Theory vs. Fact: Glycemic Response to Food," *Nutrition Today,* 19(2): 6–12.
45. Ibid.
46. Gina Kolata, "Diabetics Should Lose Weight, Avoid Diet Fads," *Science,* 9 January 1987, 235.

47. Gina Kolata, "High Carbohydrate Diets Questioned," *Science,* 9 January 1987, 162. "Diabetics Should Lose Weight, Avoid Diet Fads," *Science,* 9 January 1987, 235.
48. Sugar Organization Statistics, *www.sugar.org/scoop/scoopfaq.htm.* February 19, 1998.
49. R. E. Hodges and W. H. Krehl, "The Role of Carbohydrates in Lipid Metabolism," *American Journal of Clinical Nutrition,* 17 (1965): 334–46.
50. Hans Fisher and Eugene Boe, *The Rutgers Guide to Lowering Your Cholesterol* (New Brunswick, NJ: Rutgers University Press, 1985), 85.

## 5. Food Allergies, Your Brain, Body, and Behavior

1. T. Uhlig, A. Merkenschlager, R. Brandmaier, and J. Egger, "Topographic mapping of brain electrical activity in children with food-induced attention deficit hyperkinetic disorder," *European Journal of Pediatrics* (July 1997); 56(7): 557–61.
2. Food Allergy Organization Website: *http://foodallergy.org/facts,* 3/31/97.
3. Richard Thompson, "Food Allergies Separating Fact from Hype," *FDA Consumer,* June 1986, 25–26.
4. Joan Arehart-Treichel, "Migraines: Unmasking The Causes," *Science News,* 11 October 1980, 237.
5. W. R. Shannon, "Irritation of the nervous system due to allergic reactions," *American Journal of Diseases of Children,* 124 (1922): 89–94.
6. E. B. Nasr et al., "Concordance of Atopic and Affective Disorders," *Journal of Affective Disorders,* 3 (1981): 291; and H. J. Ossofsky, "Affective and Atopic Disorders and Cyclic AMP," *Comparative Psychiatry,* 17 (1976), 335.
7. Academy of Allergy and Immunology, "Adverse Reactions to Foods," 72–74.
8. "Childhood Autism Linked to Brain Allergy," *Science News,* 27 November 1982, 340.
9. Kevin Murray, Report on Allergy, Asthma & Immunology Online, Website of the American College of Allergy, Asthma & Immunology *(http:/allergy.mcg.edu.),* November 14, 1995; S. Gupta et al., "Dysregulated Immune System Children with Autism: Beneficial Effects of Intravenous Immune Globulin on Autistic Characteristics," *Journal of Autism Developmental Disorder,* 4 (26 August 1996): 439–52.
10. Benjamin Wolozin et al., "A Neuronal Antigen in the Brains of Alzheimer Patients," *Science,* 12 May 1986, 648–50.
11. John Crayton, "Adverse Reactions to Foods: Relevance in Psychiatric Disorders," *Journal of Allergy and Clinical Immunology,* 78 (July 1986), 243–47.

## 6. Protecting Yourself from Brain Toxins

1. Bernard Weiss, Ph.D., University of Rochester School of Medicine, *Nutrition Update,* Vol. 1, 1983, 21–38.
2. Charles Vorhees and R. E. Butcher, *Developmental Toxicology,* ed. K. Snell (London: Croom Helm, 1982), 247–98.
3. Ibid.

## 294    Notes

4. Bernard Weiss et al., "Behavioral Response to Artificial Colors," *Science*, 8 March 1980, 1487–89.

5. FDA government website www.fda.gov, NCTR Research Projects, February 26, 1998.

6. Thomas J. Sobotka, Ph.D., "Revisions to the FDA's Redbook Guidelines for Toxicity Testing: Neurotoxicity," *Critical Reviews in Food Science and Nutrition*, (1992) 32(2): 165–171.

7. *The Concise Encyclopedia of Foods & Nutrition*, ed. by Audrey Ensminger, M. E. Ensminger, James Konlande, and John Robson (Boca Raton, FL: CRC Press, 1994), 860.

8. Ibid.

9. National Institutes of Health Press Packet, December 1986.

10. George Augustine, Jr., and Herbert Levitan, "Neurotransmitter Release from a Vertebrate Neuromuscular Synapse Affected by a Food Dye," *Science*, 28 March 1980, 1489–90.

11. "Alzheimer's Research Aims at Aluminum," *Advertising Age*, 23 June 1986, 12.

12. "Aluminum in Water Tied to Alzheimer's," *American Medical News*, March 3, 1989, 2.

13. Ralph Garruto et al., "Intraneuron Co-localization of Silicon with Calcium and Aluminum in Amyotrophic Lateral Sclerosis and Parkinsonism with Dementia on Guam," *New England Journal of Medicine*, 11 September 1986, 315.

14. Anabel Hecht, "Searching for Clues to Alzheimer's Disease," *FDA Consumer*, November 1985, 23–24.

15. Russell L. Blaylock, *Excitotoxins, the Taste That Kills* (Santa Fe, NM: Health Press, 1997).

16. L. J. Flier and L. D. Stegink, "Report of the proceedings of the glutamate workshop, August 1991." *Critical Reviews in Food Science and Nutrition*, 34(2): 159–174, 1994.

17. Institute of Food Technologists' Expert Panel on Food Safety and Nutrition. "Monosodium Glutamate," *Food Technology*, 441(5): 143–45, 1987 (a).

18. Federation of American Societies for Experimental Biology.

19. *FDA Backgrounder*, October 1991, Washington, D.C.

20. S. S. Schiffman, "Taste and smell perception in elderly persons," in J. E. Fielding & Frier Hill, eds, *Nutritional Needs of the Elderly* (New York: Raven Press, 1991), 61–73.

21. Federation of American Societies for Experimental Biology (FASEB). "Analysis of Adverse Reactions to Monosodium Glutamate (MSG)." Prepared by the Life Sciences Research Office, FASEB, for the Center for Food Safety and Applied Nutrition, U.S. Food and Drug Administration, Bethesda, MD, FASEB 1995; D. Daniels, F. Joe, and G. Diachenko, "Determination of free glutamic acid in a variety of foods by high-performance liquid chromatography," "Food Additives and Contaminants" (1995) 12 (1): 21–29.

22. J. W. Olney, "The Toxic Effects of Glutamate and Related Compounds," the Opthalmic Communication Society, presented at the Symposium on Nutrition Pharmacology and Vision sponsored by the Committee on Vision, National Research Council, National Academy of Sciences, Washington D.C., November 16–17, 1981.

23. S. L. Taylor, "Irritation of the nervous system due to allergic reactions," *op.*

Notes    295

*cit.;* H. A. Sampson and D. D. Metcalfe, "Food Allergies," *Journal of the American Medical Association,* 268: (1993) 2840–44.

24. American Council on Scientific Affairs, "Aspartame: Review of Safety Issues," *Journal of the American Medical Association,* 254 (1985), 400–02.

25. "Aspartame Hearing Rejected," *American Medical News,* 27 February 1984, 23–24.

26. "Aspartame Critics Persist: Recommend Avoidance During Pregnancy," *Medical World News,* 27 February 1984, 23–24.

27. Ibid.

28. National Research Council. National Academy of Sciences, subcommittee report on safety and suitability of MSG and other substances in baby foods, Washington, D.C., 1970: J. W. Olney, *Neurotoxicology,* 2 (1080); 163–92.

29. L. D. Stegink, L. J. Filer, G. L. Baker et al., "Plasma glutamate concentrations in 1-year-old infants and adults ingesting monosodium L-glutamate in consommé," *Pediatric Residents* (1986) 20:53–58.

30. S. A. Lipton et al., "Neurotoxicity Associated with Dual Actions of Homocysteine at the N-methyl-D-aspartate Receptor," *Proceedings of the National Academy of Science USA,* 1997 May 27; 94 (11): 5923–28; M. V. Johnson, "Hypoxia and Ischemic Disorders of Infants and Children (lecture of 38th meeting of Japanese Society of Child Neurology, Tokyo, Japan, July 1996); *Brain Development,* 1997 June, 19 (4): 235–9, review article; R. Lappalainen and R. S. Riikonen, "High Levels of Cerebrospinal Fluid Glutamate in Rett Syndrome," *Pediatric Neurology,* 1996 October; 15 (3):213–16.

31. P. D'Eufemia, R. Finocchiaro et al., "Erythrocyte and Plasma Levels of Glutamate and Asparate in Children Affected by Migraine," *Cephalalgia,* (1997 October); 17 (6); 652–57.

32. R. Dawson et al., "Attenuation of Leptin-mediated Effects by Monosodium Glutamate–induced Arcuate Nucleus Damage," *American Journal of Physiology* (1997 July); 273 (1 pt 1): E202–06.

33. M. E. Spurlock, K. J. Hahn, and J. L. Miner, "Regulation of Adipsin and Body Composition in the Monosodium Glutamate (MSG)–treated Mouse," *Physiological Behavior* (1996 November); 60 (5): 1217–21.

34. L. J. Flier, "Public Forum, Analysis of Adverse Reactions to Monosodium Glutamate," (paper presented at meeting of the Federation of American Societies for Experimental Biology, April 1993, Washington, D.C.).

35. R. M. Pitkin, W. A. Reynolds, L. D. Stegink et al., "Glutamate metabolism and placental transfer in pregnancy," in L. J. Filer, S. Garattini, M. R. Kare, et al. (eds.), *Glutamic Acid: Advances in Biochemistry and Physiology:* (New York: Raven Press, 1979), 103–10.

36. T. Yu, Y. Zhao et al., "Effects of material oral administration of monosodium glutamate at a late stage of pregnancy on developing mouse fetal brain," *Brain Research,* 1997 February 7; 747 (2) 195–206.

37. Joint FAO/WHO Expert Committee on Food Additives, "L-Glutamic acid and its ammonium, calcium, monosodium and potassium salts," in *Toxicological Evaluation of Certain Food Additives and Contaminants,* WHO Food Additives Series No. 22, (New York: Cambridge University Press, 1988), 97–161; J. E. Steiner, "What the Neonate Can Tell Us About Umami," in Y. Kawamura and M. R. Kare (eds.), *Umami: A Basic Taste.* (New York: Marcel Dekker, Inc., 1987), 97–123.

## 296   Notes

38. L. J. Flier and L. D. Stegink, "Report of the proceedings of glutamate workshop, August 1991," *Clinical Reviews in Food Science and Nutrition* (1994); 34(2): 159–74.
39. R. H. M. Kwok, "Chinese Restaurant Syndrome," *New England Journal of Medicine* (1968); 17:796.
40. G. R. Kerr, M. Lee Wu, M. El-Lozy et al., "Prevalence of the Chinese Restaurant Syndrome," *Journal of the American Dietetic Association,* 75: 29–33.
41. Centers for Disease Control, Report on foodborne disease, 1975–1981, CDC Surveillance Annual Summary, April 1981; Centers for Disease Control, Foodborne disease outbreaks, five-year summary, 1983–87. CDC Surveillance Summaries, Vol. 39, No. SS-1, March 1990, 15–59.
42. Federation of American Societies for Experimental Biology (FASEB), *Analysis of Adverse Reactions to Monosodium Glutamate* (MSG), prepared by the Life Sciences Research Office, FASEB, for the Center for Food Safety and Applied Nutrition, U.S. Food and Drug Administration. (Bethesda, MD: FASEB, 1995.)
43. R. A. Kenney and C. S. Tidball, "Human susceptibility to oral monosodium L-glutamate," *The American Journal of Clinical Nutrition* (1972); 25: 140–46. R. A. Kenney, "Chinese Restaurant Syndrome," *The Lancet* (1980) 8163: 311–12; R. A. Kenney, "The Chinese Restaurant Syndrome: An Anecdote Revisited," *Food and Chemical Toxicology,* (1986) 24(4): 351–54.
44. T. Beaudette, *Adverse Reactions to Food.* Chicago, the American Dietetic Association, 1991, 27–32.
45. Federation of American Societies for Experimental Biology (FASEB), *Analysis of Adverse Reactions to Monosodium Glutamate (MSG),* prepared by the Life Sciences Research Office, FASEB, for the Center for Food Safety and Applied Nutrition, U.S. Food and Drug Administration (Bethesda, MD: FASEB, 1995).
46. S. Yamaguchi and C. Takahashi, "Interactions of Monosodium Glutamate and Sodium Chloride on Saltiness and Palatability of a Clear Soup," *Journal of Food Science* (1995) 49 (1): 21–29.
47. National Academy of Sciences, National Research Council, *The 1977 Survey of the Industry on the Use of Food Additives: Estimates of Daily Intake,* Vol. 3 (Washington, D.C.: National Academy Press, 1979).
Federation of American Societies for Experimental Biology (FASEB), *Analysis of Adverse Reactions to Monosodium Glutamate (MSG),* prepared by the Life Sciences Research Office, FASEB, for the Center for Food Safety and Applied Nutrition, U.S. Food and Drug Administration. (Bethesda, MD: FASEB, 1995).
American Medical Association's Council on Scientific Affairs, Report D of the Council on Scientific Affairs on Food and Drug Administration Regulations regarding the inclusion of added L-glutamic acid content on food labels. Report adopted at proceedings of the American Medical Association's House of Delegates Meeting. June 1992. U.S. Food and Drug Administration. FASEB Issues Final Report on MSG, FDA Talk Paper T95-44, August 1995.
48. L. Reif-Lehrer, "A Questionnaire Study of the Prevalence of Chinese Restaurant Syndrome," *Federal Proceedings,* 36 (1977), 1617–23; H. Ghadimi et al., "Studies on Monosodium Glutamate Ingestion: Biochemical Explo-

rations of Chinese Restaurant Syndrome," *Biochemical Medicine,* 5 (1971), 44–56.

49. W. H. Yang, M. A. Drouin et al., "The monosodium glutamate symptom complex: assessment in a double blind, placebo-controlled, randomized study," *Journal of Allergy and Clinical Immunology* (1997 June); 99 (6 Pt l), 757–62.

50. Russell Blaylock, M.D., *Excitotoxins: The Taste That Kills.* (Santa Fe, NM: Health Press, 1997), 120.

51. J. A. Yesavage, and V. O. Leirer, "Hangover effects on aircraft pilots 14 hours after alcohol ingestion: a preliminary report," *American Journal of Psychiatry* (1986 December); 143 (12): 1546–50.

52. "The Alcoholic's Shrinking Brain," *Science News* (7 February 1987), 87.

53. Constance Holden, "Alcoholism and the Medical Cost Crunch," *Science* (6 March 1987), 132–33.

54. J. M. Graziano and C. Henneken, of Harvard Medical School, "Moderate Alcohol Use Lowers Risk of Deadly Second Heart Attack," paper presented at the American Heart Association's 70th Scientific Session, Orlando, Florida, November 12, 1997.

55. National Institute on Alcohol Abuse and Alcoholism, "Alcohol Health and Research World," U.S. Department of Health and Human Services, Pub. No. ADM 85–151 (1985), 44.

56. Ibid.

57. U.S. Department of Health and Human Services, *Phobias and Panic,* DHHS Pub no. ADM86-1472 (1986): 20.

58. Thomas Uhde, "Biological Issues in Panic," paper presented at National Conference on Phobias and Relaxed Anxiety Disorders, New York, 17 October 1986.

59. Carol Mithers, "The Caffeine, Coffee, Cola, and Chocolate Debate," *Self,* August 1979, 10.

60. Richard Gilbert, "Caffeine: History, Habits, Health," *The Journal of Addiction Research Foundation,* Ontario, 1 October 1984, 5.

61. P. W. Curatolo, and D. Robertson, "The Health Consequences of Caffeine," *Annals of Internal Medicine,* 98 (5): 64–53.

62. Morris Shorofsky and Norman Lamm, *New York State Journal of Medicine,* February 1977, and R. Gilbert "Caffeine," *op. cit.,* 528.

63. Thomas Sobotka, "The Regulatory Perspective of Diet-Behavior Relationships," *Nutrition Reviews Supplement,* 44 (May 1986): 241–43.

64. Hugh Tilson, personal communication with authors, 3 May 1987.

## 7. Smart Food for Smart Children

1. "Fetal Distress from Something Mother Ate," *Emergency Medicine,* 15 April 1985, 87.

2. J. A. Miller, "Brain Already Busy While In the Womb," *Science News,* 20 October 1984.

3. Ibid.

298    Notes

4. R. Balaza et al., *Human Growth,* Vol. 2, *Neurobiology and Nutrition,* ed. F. Falkner and J. M. Tanner (New York: Plenum Press, 1979), 415–80.

5. R. W. Smithells et al., "Further Experience of Vitamin Supplementation for Prevention of Neural Tube Defect Recurrences," *The Lancet* (May 7, 1983): 1027–31.

6. Godfrey Oakley, Jr., M.D. M.P.H., director of the Birth Defects and Developmental Disabilities Division of CDC, International Food Council Information Bureau, Internet Posting 1/28/98 www.lficinfo.health.org. Washington, D.C., June 1997.

7. Ibid.

8. R. Balaza et al., *Human Growth,* vol. 3. *Neurobiology and Nutrition,* ed. F. Falkner and J. M. Tanner (New York: Plenum Press, 1979), 415–80.

9. Ibid.

10. Audrey Ensminger, *Concise Encyclopedia of Foods and Nutrition,* First Edition, M. E. Ensminger, J. Konlande, and John Robson, (Boca Raton, FL: CRC, 1994) 713.

11. Harold Sandstead, "Nutrition and Brain Function: Trace Elements," *Nutrition Review Supplement* (May 1986): 37–41.

12. Ibid.

13. Carl Pfeiffer and Eric Braverman, "Zinc, the Brain and Behavior," *Biological Psychiatry,* 17 (4): 513–19.

14. H. Sanstead, "Nutrition and Brain Function," *op. cit.,* 37–41.

15. M. W. Miller, "The Time of Origin of Neurons in Rat Motor Cortex in Experimental Fetal Alcohol Syndrome" (paper presented at the 16th Annual Meeting of the Society for Neuroscience, Washington, D.C., November 1986).

16. "Study Notes Alcohol Use Can Affect Birth Weight," *American Medical News,* 19 September 1986, 7.

17. "Booze and Pregnancy: the Pickled Brain," *Science News,* 17 January 1980.

18. Statement of the American Academy of Pediatrics, 1 October 1986.

19. B. Frieder and V. E. Grimm, "Prenatal Caffeine Causes Long Lasting Behavior and Neurochemical Changes" (paper presented at the 16th Annual Meeting of the Society for Neuroscience, Washington, D.C., November 1986).

20. H. D. Vlajinac et al., "Effect of caffeine intake during pregnancy and birth weight," *American Journal of Epidemiology,* 1997 February 15; 145 (4): 335–38.

21. M. Huisman et al., "Nicotine and Caffeine: Influence on Prenatal Hemodynamics and Behavior in Early Twin Pregnancy," *Journal of Reproductive Medicine,* 1997 November, 42 (11) 731–34.

22. H. M. Barr and P. Streissguth, "Coffee Use During Pregnancy and Childbirth Outcome and a 7 Year Prospective Study," *Neurotoxicology and Teratology,* 1991 July–August 13 (4), 441–48.

23. H. Gerster, "The Importance of vitamin $B_6$ for development of the infant," *Ernahrungswiss,* 1996 December, 35 (4): 309–17.

24. U.S. Department of Health and Human Services, "The Neural Basis of Psychopathology: The Neuroscience of Mental Health," DHHS Pub. 9 (1985), 96–97.

25. R. Morley, "The Influence of early diet on later development," *Journal of Biosocial Science* (1996 October); 28 (4): 481–87.

26. Marvin Eiger and Sally Wendkos Olds, *The Complete Book of Breast Feeding* (New York: Workman, 1987), 59–60.
27. S. A. Richardson et al., *American Journal of Mental Deficiency,* 77 (1973): 623.
28. Z. A. Stein et al., *Famine and Human Development: the Dutch Hunger Winter of 1944–45* (New York: Oxford University Press, 1975).
29. Merrill Read, "Malnutrition and Behavior," *Applied Research in Mental Retardation,* 3 (1982), 279–91.
30. J. Cravioto, "Nutrition, Stimulation, Mental Development and Learning," *Nutrition Today,* September/October 1981, 4–15.
31. Ellen Hale, "Good Nutrition for Your Growing Child," *FDA Consumer,* April 1987, 21.
32. A. M. Mauer and H. S. Dweck, "Toward A Prudent Diet for Children," *Pediatrics,* 71 (1): 78–79.
33. Ellen Hale, "Good Nutrition For Your Growing Child," *FDA Consumer,* April 1987, *op cit.*
34. M. Pugliese and F. Lifshitz, "Parents Misconceptions on Diet, Health Can Delay Growth of Their Infants," news release, American Academy of Pediatrics, 5 August 1987.
35. B. Watkins and B. Hennig, paper published as a chapter in *Lipids in Infant Nutrition,* the American Oil Chemists' Society, Washington, D.C., January 1998.
36. Gina Kolata, "Obese Children: A Growing Problem," *Science,* 4 April 1986.
37. S.I. Gortmaker, W. H. Dietz et al., "Television viewing as a cause of increasing obesity among children in the United States 1986–1990," *Archives of Pediatric and Adolescent Medicine* (1996 April); 150(4): 356–62.
38. A. W. Logue, *The Psychology of Eating and Drinking* (New York: Freeman, 1986), 99.
39. D. Behar et al., "Sugar Challenge Testing with Children Considered Behaviorally 'Sugar Reactive,'" *Nutritional Behavior,* 1 (1984): 279–88.
40. R. J. Prinz and David Riddle, "Associations Between Nutrition and Behavior in Five Year Old Children," *Nutrition Reviews Supplement,* 44 (May 1986), 151–57.
41. M. L. Wolraich, S. D. Lindgren, and P. J. Stumbo et. al., "Effects of Diets High in Sucrose or Aspartame on the Behavior and Cognitive Performance of Children," *The New England Journal of Medicine,* 330:5: 301–07, February 3, 1994. "Position of The American Dietetic Association: Use of Nutritive and Non-Nutritive Sweeteners," *Journal of the American Dietetic Association,* 93:7: 816–21, July 1993.
42. Alan Leviton, M.D., "Behavioral Correlates of Caffeine Consumption by Children," *Clinical Pediatrics,* vol. 31, December 1992, 749–47.
43. "New Harvard Research Shows School Breakfast Program May Improve Children's Behavior and Performance," PRN Newswire, 3/02/98.
44. Stephen Schoenthaler et al., "The Testing of Various Hypotheses as Explanations for the Gains in National Test Scores in the 1978–83 New York City Nutrition Policy Modification Project," *International Journal of Biosocial Research,* 8 (2): 198–99.
45. Jane Hersey, personal communication with authors, 8 May 1987.
46. Bernard Weiss et al., "Behavioral Response to Artificial Colors," *Science,* 8 March 1980, 1487–89.

47. C. M. Carter et al., "Effects of new food diet in attention deficit disorder," *Archives of Diseases of Children,* 1993 November, 69(5): 564–68.
48. National Institute of Diabetes, Digestive and Kidney Diseases, "Helping Your Overweight Child," http://www.niddk.nih.gov/health.nutrit/pubs/helpchild.htm.
49. Ibid.
50. Doris Pertz and Lillian Putnam, "The Reading Teacher," 35 (March 1982): 702–06.
51. R. J. Prinz and David Riddle, "Associations Between Nutrition and Behavior in Five Year Old Children," *Nutrition Reviews Supplement,* 44 (May 1986), 151–57.

## 8. Vitamins, Minerals, and Your Mind

1. "Niacin (Nicotinic Acid) Deficiency," in *Merck Manual,* 14th ed., ed. Robert Berkow (Rahway, NJ: Merck, 1982), 900–02.
2. Herman Baker, Ph.D., personal communication with authors, 13 February 1987.
3. Frederick C. Goggans, "A Case of Mania Secondary to Vitamin $B_{12}$ Deficiency," *American Journal of Psychiatry,* (1984) 141 (2): 300–01.
4. Frank Press (Chairman, National Research Council), letter to Dr. James Wyngaarden (Director, National Institutes of Health), 7 October 1985; made public by the National Research Council, 7 October 1985, Washington, D.C.
5. Jess Thoene, Herman Baker et al., "Biotin-Responsive Carboxylase Deficiency Associated with Subnormal Plasma and Urinary Biotin," *New England Journal of Medicine,* 304 (April 1981): 817–20; and personal communication with authors, 13 February 1987.
6. Baker, personal communication.
7. M. Brin, "Dilemma of Marginal Vitamin Deficiency," in *Proceedings of the Ninth International Congress on Nutrition,* 4 (Basel, Switzerland: S. Karger, 1975), 102–15.
8. Ibid.
9. Ibid.; and M. Brin, "Erythrocytes as a Biopsy Tissue in the Functional Evaluation of Thiamine Status," *Journal of the American Medical Association,* 187 (1964): 762.
10. Baker, personal communication.
11. Ibid.
12. H. Baker and O. Frank, *Clinical Vitaminology: Methods and Interpretation* (New York: J. Wiley, 1968).
13. Jonathan Alpert, M.D., Ph.D., and Maurizio Fava, M.D., Harvard Medical School, *Medscape mental health* 2 (1), 1997.
14. Baker, personal communication.
15. Ibid.
16. Ibid.
17. Richard F. Macko, M.D.; co-authors include Steven Kittner, M.D., M.P.H., Dorothy Kimberly Cox, B.S., Anne Epstein, M.S., and Mary Sparks, R.N., University of Maryland School of Medicine; Helga Refsum, Ph.D., and Per Ueland, Ph.D., University of Bergen, Norway; and Constance Johnson,

M.D., and Robert Wityk, M.D., Johns Hopkins University School of Medicine. Baltimore Veterans Administration Medical Center and assistant professor of neurology and geriatrics at the University of Maryland presented here today at the American Heart Association's 23rd International Joint Conference on Stroke and Cerebral Circulation, Orlando, FL., February 7, 1998.

18. M. Tsacopoulos et al., "The Nutritive Function of Glia is Regulated by Signals Released by Neurons," *Glia*, (1997 September); 21(1): 84–91; G. Lenaz et al., "Mitochondrial Complex I Defects in Aging," *Molecular Cell Biochemistry*, (1997 September); 174(1–2): 329–33; H. Zimmerman, "Biochemistry, localization and functional roles of ectonucleotidases in the nervous system," *Progress in Neurobiology*, (1996 August); 49(6): 589–618.

19. J. Greenwood et al., "Thiamine, Malnutrition, and Alcohol-related Damage to the Central Nervous System," *Progress in Alcohol Research*, Vol. 1, (Utrecht, The Netherlands: VNU Press, 1985), 287–310.

20. R. Finlay-Jones, "Should Thiamine Be Added to Beer?" *Australian and New Zealand Psychiatric Journal*, (1986) 20(1), 3–6.

21. P. F. Nixon et al., "How Does Alcohol Cause Brain Damage?" Report of the Medical Research Advisory Committee to the Australian Associated Brewers, February 1986, 19–24.

22. Vichai Tanphaichitr and Beverly Wood, "Thiamine," in *Present Knowledge in Nutrition*, 5th ed. (Washington, D.C.: Nutrition Foundation, 1984), 273–83.

23. R. J. Harrell, "Mental Response to Added Thiamine," *Journal of Nutrition*, 31 (1946): 283.

24. J. Brozek, "Physiological Effects of Thiamine Restriction and Deprivation in Young Men," *American Journal of Clinical Nutrition*, 26 (1973): 150.

25. Ibid.

26. M. Brin, "Erythrocyte as a Biopsy Tissue in the Functional Evaluation of Thiamine Status," *Journal of the American Medical Association*, 187: 762.

27. M. Brin, "Examples of Behavioral Changes in Marginal Vitamin Deficiency in the Rat and Man" (Paper delivered at the International Nutritional Conference, Washington D.C., 30 November to 2 December 1977), National Institutes of Health Pub No. 79, 1906.

28. Richard Rivlin, "Riboflavin," in *Present Knowledge in Nutrition*, 5th ed. (Washington, D.C.: International Life Sciences Institute, 1997), 167–72.

29. B. S. Narasinga Rao and C. Gopalan, "Niacin," in *Present Knowledge in Nutrition*, 5th ed., 1984, 318–31.

30. J. R. Wittenborn, "A Search for Responders to Niacin Supplementation," *Archives of General Psychiatry*, 31 (1974): 547.

31. L. M. Henderson, "Vitamin $B_6$," in *Present Knowledge in Nutrition*, 5th ed., 1984, 303–17.

32. H. Schaumburg et al., "Sensory Neuropathy from Pyridoxine Abuse," *New England Journal of Medicine*, 34, 1983 (suppl 1): 137.; A. R. Berger H. H. Schaumburg et al., "Dose response, coasting, and differential fiber vulnerability in human toxic neuropathy: a prospective study of pyridoxine neurotoxicity," *Neurology*, 1992 July; 42 (7): 1367–70.

33. Victor Herbert, "Vitamin $B_{12}$," in *Present Knowledge in Nutrition*, 5th ed., 1984, 347–64.

34. Ibid.

## 302    Notes

35. Godfrey Oakley, International Food Council Information Bureau, Internet Posting, 1/28/1998 *http://www.lficinfo.health.org.*
36. Council for Responsible Nutrition Press Release, February 5, 1998, Washington, D.C.
37. V. P. Sydenstricker et al., "Observations on the 'Egg White' Injury in Man and Its Cure with a Biotin Concentration," *Journal of the American Medical Association,* 118 (1983): 1199–1200.
38. William Gottlieb, "Encyclopedia of Vitamins," *Source Book on Food and Nutrition* (Chicago: Marquis Academy Media, 1982), 89.
39. Ibid.
40. Robert E. Olsen, "Pantothenic Acid," in *Present Knowledge in Nutrition,* 5th ed. (1984): 377–92.
41. G. Milner, "Ascorbic Acid in Chronic Psychiatric Patients—A Controlled Trial," *British Journal of Psychiatry,* 109 (1963): 294–99; and N. Subramanian, "On the Brain Ascorbic Acid and Its Importance in the Metabolism of Biogenic Amines," *Life Sciences,* 20 1980 (9): 1479–84.
42. David Agus, M.D. and David Golde, M.D., "Vitamin C Shown to Cross the Blood Brain Barrier, Findings May Be Useful To Slow Progression of Some Brain Disorders," *Journal of Clinical Investigation,* November 30, 1997.
43. Sloan-Kettering release, November 11, 1997.
44. *Merck Manual,* 14: 871.
45. William Gottlieb, "Encyclopedia of Vitamins," *op. cit.,* 86.
46. "Hypervitaminosis A," in Berkow, *Merck Manual,* 14: 891.
47. L. E. Shambles, E. Shahar, J. F. Toole, "Association of transient ischemic attack/stroke symptoms assessed by standardized questionnaire and algorithm with cerebrovascular risk factors and carotid artery wall thickness: The ARIC Study, 1987–1989," *American Journal of Epidemiology,* 1996 November 1; 144(9): 857–66; *Newswire,* Winston Salem, North Carolina, October 30, 1996.
48. Stephen Kritchevsky, Ph.D., Tomoko Shimakawa, Sc.D., et al., "Dietary Antioxidants and Carotid Artery Wall Thickness: The ARIC Study," *Circulation* (1995); 92:2142–50.
49. Mary Sano, Ph.D., "Vitamin E Supplementation Appears to Slow Progression of Alzheimer's Disease," *New England Journal of Medicine,* April 24, 1997.
50. James Anderson, M.D., and Maury Breecher, M.P.H., Ph.D., *Dr. Anderson's Antioxidant, Antiaging Health Program* (New York: Carroll & Graf Publishers, 1996), 78.
51. J. L. Cadet et al., "Free Radicals in Tardive Dyskinesia," *Trends in Neuroscience,* (1986); 9:107–8; J. D. Grimes et al., "Antioxidant Therapy in Parkinson's Disease, *Canadian Journal of Neurology* (1987), 14:483–487.
52. S. Fahn, "The endogenous toxin hypothesis of the etiology of Parkinson's disease and a pilot trial of high-dose antioxidants in an attempt to slow the progression of the illness," *Annals of the New York Academy of Science,* (1989); 570:186–96.
53. J. B. Lohr et al., "Alpha tocopherol in tardive dyskinesia," *Lancet,* (1987), 1: 913.
54. The Parkinson Study Group, "The Effects of Tocopherol and Deprenyl on the Progression of Disability in Early Parkinson's Disease," *New England Journal of Medicine,* January 21, 1993; 328:176–83.

55. The Parkinson Study Group, *op. cit.*

56. D. P. Muller, "Vitamin E—its role in neurological function," *Postgraduate Medicine* (1986), 62: 107–12.

57. *NAS–NRC Recommended Dietary Allowances,* 10th ed., (Washington D.C.: National Academy of Sciences, 1989), 102–04.

58. Masayuki Yasui et al., "Effects of low calcium and magnesium dietary intake on the central nervous system tissues of rats and calcium-magnesium–related disorders in the amyotrophic lateral sclerosis focus in the Kii Peninsula of Japan," *Magnesium Research* (1997), 10, 1: 39–50.

59. "Calcium and Short-Term Memory," *The Harvard Mahoney Neuroscience Institute Letter on the Brain,* Vol. 4, Number 1/Calcium.html. 1998.

60. J. S. Dittman and W. G. Regher, "Mechanisms and kinetics of heterosynpatic depression at a cerebellar synapse," *Journal of Neuroscience,* 1997 December 1; 17(23): 9048–59.

61. Sally Schuette and Helen Linkswiler, "Calcium," in *Present Knowledge in Nutrition,* 5th ed. (1984): 408.

62. Kaymar Arasteh (paper presented at the 95th Annual Meeting of the American Psychological Association, New York, 31 August 1987).

63. "Natural Absorbable Calcium," http://www.herbcare.com/prod/nac.htm; J. A. Gilbride et al., "Nutrition and health status assessment of community-residing elderly in New York City: a pilot study," *Journal of the American Dietetic Association* (1998 May); 98(5): 554–58.

64. *Merck Manual,* 14:872, *op cit.*

65. F. Xavier Pi-Sunyer and Esther Offenbacher, "Chromium," in *Present Knowledge in Nutrition,* 5th ed. (1984): 571–86.

66. E. P. Novikova, "Effect of Different Amounts of Dietary Cobalt on Iodine Content of Rat Thyroid Gland," *Federal Proceedings,* 23 (1963): 1459–60; and R L Blokhima, "Trace Elements Metabolism in Animals," ed. C. F. Mills (Edinburgh: Livingston 1970), 426–32.

67. Eric Underwood, "Cobalt," in *Present Knowledge in Nutrition,* 5th ed. (1984): 528.

68. Ronald J. Amen, "Trace Minerals as Nutrients," *Nutrition for Food Executives,* October 1973, 751–56.

69. "Copper on the Brain," the *Harvard Mahoney Neuroscience Institute Letter, On The Brain,* Fall 1994, Vol. 3, No. 4, 2.

70. E. DeMaeyer et al., "The Prevalence of Anemia in the World," World Health Statistics, 1985, Q 38:302–16.

71. Joel Beard, "Nutrient Status and Central Nervous System Function," *Present Knowledge in Nutrition,* 7th ed., eds. Ekhard Ziegler and L. J. Filer, Jr. (Washington, D.C.: ILSI Press, 1996).

72. Ibid.

73. J. R. Connor, "Proteins of Iron Regulation in the Brain in Alzheimer's Disease," *Iron and Human Disease,* ed. R. B. Lauffer (Ann Arbor, MI: CRC Press, 1992), 365–93.

74. E. Sofic et al., "Increased Iron and Total Iron Content in Postmortem Substantia Nigra of Parkinsonian Brain," *Journal of Neural Transmission,* 74 (1988): 199–208.

75. James Penland, "Low Mineral Intakes May Affect The Psyche," *Proceedings of the North Dakota Academy of Science,* 1997, 50:57.

304    Notes

76. U. Merit and R. Rahamimoff, "Neuromuscular Transmission: Inhibition by Manganese Ions," *Science* (April 1972), 308–09.
77. Raymond Burk, "Selenium," in *Present Knowledge in Nutrition,* 5th ed. (1984): 323–24.
78. Beard, *op. cit.,* 616.
79. M. Welch Ross, U.S. Department of Agriculture Report on Selenium, Washington, D.C., 1986.
80. "Zinc Helps Regulate Chemical Communication Between Brain Cells," *Stanford University Medical Center News Report,* 30 April 1987.
81. T. G. Smart et al., "Modulation of Inhibitory and Excitatory Amino Acid Receptor Ion Channels by Zinc," *Neurobiology* (1994) 42: 393–441.
82. Alexander G. Schauss and Derck Bryce-Smith, "Evidence of Zinc Deficiency in Anorexia Nervosa and Bulimorexia," in *Nutrition and Brain Function* (Basel, Switzerland: S. Karger, 1987).
83. G. Danscher et al., "Increased Amount of Zinc in the Hippocampus and Amygdala of Alzheimer's Diseased Brains," *Journal of Neuroscientific Methods,* 1997 September 5; 76(1): 53–59.
84. M. P. Cuajungco and G. J. Lees, "Zinc Metabolism in the Brain; Relevance to Human Neurodegenerative Disorders," *Neurobiological Disease,* (1997); 4 (3–4): 137–69.
85. Ibid.
86. Baker, personal communication, *op. cit.*
87. R. M. Ortega et al., "Dietary Intake and Cognitive Function in a Group of Elderly People," *American Journal of Clinical Nutrition,* (1997 October); 66 (4): 803–90.
88. J. Warsama Jama et al., "Dietary Antioxidants and Cognitive Function in a Population-based Sample of Older Persons," *American Journal of Epidemiology,* (144, 3); 275–80.

## 9. Your Hungry Brain: Why You Eat and Why You Stop

1. Ruth Winter, "Appetite Control—The Secret Is at the Base of Your Brain," *Science Digest,* October 1980, 8–13.
2. J. Mayer, "The Glucostatic Theory of Regulation of Food Intake and the Problem of Obesity," *Bulletin of the New England Medical Center,* 14 (1952): 43–49.
3. A. W. Heatherington and S. W. Ranson, "Hypothalamic Lesions and Adiposity in the Rat," *Anatomical Record,* 78 (1940): 149–72.
4. M. L. Caldwell et al., "A Clinical Note on Food Preference of Individuals with Prader-Willis Syndrome," *Journal of Mental Deficiency Research,* 27(1): 45–49.
5. B. K. Arnand and J. R. Brobeck, "Localization of the Feeding Center in the Hypothalamus of the Rat," *Proceedings of the Society for Experimental Biology and Medicine* 77 (1951): 323–24.
6. E. Stellar, "The Physiology of Motivation," *Psychological Review,* 61 (1954): 5–22.

Notes    305

7. A. W. Logue, *The Psychology of Eating and Drinking* (New York: Freeman, 1986), 19.
8. G. Harvey Anderson, "Hunger, Appetite and Food Intake," *Present Knowledge in Nutrition,* 7th ed., eds. Ekhard E. Ziegler and L. J. Filer, Jr. (Washington, D.C.: ILSI Press, 1996), 13–18.
9. Ibid.
10. Ibid.
11. G. A. Bray, "Obesity, A Disorder of Nutrient Partitioning: The Mona Lisa Hypothesis," *Journal of Nutrition* 121 (1991): 1146–62.
12. Stephen Gislason, M.D., "Food Addition," *www.nutramet.com/zeno/addictive.htm,* 1/15/98.
13. Paula Geiselman, Donald Williamson, and Cheryl Smith, "Overeating Linked to Menstrual Periods" (paper presented at the Annual Meeting of the Society for Neuroscience, New Orleans, October 25–30, 1997).
14. Kelly Brownell, "Possible Genetic Answer as to Why Some People, Especially Women, Eat More and Gain Weight During Times of High Stress" (paper presented at a meeting of the Society of Behavioral Medicine in New Orleans, April 4, 1998).
15. Ellen Bratslavsky and Roy Baumeister, "The Cost of Not Eating Chocolate" (paper presented at the American Psychological Association Meeting, Toronto, August 19, 1996).
16. Mark Friedman, "New Perspectives on the Metabolic Basis of Hunger and Satiety," *Contemporary Nutrition,* 7 (May 1982).
17. Ibid.
18. Harry Kissileff, "Satiety," *Journal of Dentistry for Children,* S2(5) (1984): 386–89; H. R. Kissileff, "Chance and Necessity in Ingestive Behavior," *Appetite,* (1991 August); 17(1): 1–2.
19. Ibid.
20. Ibid.
21. Charles Pollak, interview with authors, Cornell Medical Center, Westchester, N.Y., November 1986.
22. B. Andersson and S. M. McCann, "Drinking, Antidiuresis and Milk Ejection from Electrical Stimulation Within the Hypothalamus of the Goat," *Acta Physiologica Scandinavica,* 35 (1955): 191–201.
23. Ibid.
24. Logue, *Psychology of Eating and Drinking, op. cit.,* 39.
25. Logue, *Psychology of Eating and Drinking, op. cit.,* 43.
26. Ibid.
27. Jan Oswald and K. Adam, "Rhythmic Raiding of Refrigerator Related to Rapid Eye Movement Sleep," *British Medical Journal* (1986): 292–99.
28. J. T. Metz et al., "Effect of Electrical Stimulation to the Human Brain (VMH) on Regional Cerebral Metabolism" (paper presented at the 16th Annual Meeting of the Society for Neuroscience, Washington, D.C., November 1986).
29. Dixie Farley, "Eating Disorders When Thinness Becomes an Obsession," *FDA Consumer,* (May 1986): 20–22.
30. Renfew Center (Philadelphia) Fact Sheet on Bulimia, 1986.
31. David B. Herzog and Paul Copeland, "Eating Disorders," *New England Journal of Medicine,* 313 (5); (1985): 295–303. David Herzog, "Eating Disorders: New Threats to Health," *Psychosomatics* 1992 Winter, 33 (1): 10–15.

32. Walter Kaye et al., "Elevated Cerebrospinal Fluid Levels of Immunoreactive Corticotropin-Releasing Hormone in Anorexia Nervosa," *Journal of Clinical Endocrinology and Metabolism,* (1996) 64 (2): 203–07.
33. Ibid.
34. Ibid.
35. Ibid.
36. National Institutes of Health, Consensus Development Conference, "Health Implications of Obesity," 5 (9).
37. "Just Looking at Food Can Make Fat People Fatter," *ADAMHA News,* 2 February 1980, 3.
38. Ibid.
39. "Dieting Can Slow Reaction Time," ARS USDA briefs, 1/15/98.
40. T. L. Burns P. P. Moll, and R. M. Lauer, "Genetic Models of Human Obesity— Family Studies," *Critical Review of Food Science and Nutrition* (1993) 33: 339–43.

# 10. Nutrients to Enhance Brain Performance

1. *Food Components to Enhance Performance,* Committee on Military Nutrition Research, Bernadette Marriott, ed. (Washington, D.C.: National Academy Press, 1994).
2. Food Components to Enhance Performance, 25.
3. Ibid., 28.
4. Gregory Belensky et al., "The Effects of Sleep Deprivation on Performance During Continuous Combat Operations," *Food Components to Enhance Performance,* Committee on Military Nutrition Research, Bernadette Marriott, ed., *op. cit.*
5. Bonnie Spring, "Carbohydrates, Protein and Performance," *Food Components to Enhance Performance,* Committee on Military Nutrition Research, Bernadette Marriott, ed., *op. cit.,* 321–23.
6. E. F. Coyle et al., "Muscle Glycogen Utilization During Prolonged Strenuous Exercise When Fed Carbohydrate," *Journal of Applied Physiology* (1986) 61: 165–72.
7. Paul Gold, Ph.D., "Glucose and Memory Enhancement" (paper presented at the Annual Meeting of the American Dietetic Association, November 2, 1996, Chicago, IL).
8. *The Concise Encyclopedia of Food and Nutrition,* Audrey Ensminger et al., eds. (Boca Raton, FL: CRC Press, 1995), 160.
9. Bonnie Spring, "Carbohydrate Craving: Clinical Implications" (paper presented at the 94th Annual Meeting of the American Psychological Association, Washington, D.C., 23 August 1986); Judith Wurtman, "Carbohydrate Craving," *op. cit.*
10. Peggy Borum, Ph.D., "The Role of Carnitine in Enhancing Physical Performance," *Food Components to Enhance Performance,* Committee on Military Nutrition Research, Bernadette Marriott, ed., *op. cit.,* 433–51.
11. Hollister Gruber, "Drug Treatment of Alzheimer's Disease," *Drugs Aging,* (1996 January); 8 (1): 47-55.

12. Carol Greenwood of the Department of Nutritional Sciences, University of Toronto Medical School, "Performance-Enhancing Effects of Protein and Amino Acids," 266.
13. E. Blomstrand et al., "Administration of Branched-Chain Amino Acids During Sustained Exercise—Effects on Performance and on Plasma Concentration of Some Amino Acids," *European Journal of Applied Physiology* (1991); 63: 83–88.
14. Greenwood, *op. cit.*
15. B. Sandage, Jr., L. Sabounjian, R. White, and R. J. Wurtman, "Choline Citrate May Enhance Athletic Performance" (paper presented at the American Physiological Society, 1992).
16. Chris Lecos, "Diet and the Elderly," *FDA Consumer,* September 1984, 23–25.
17. S. L. Ladd et al., "Effect of Phosphatidylcholine on Explicit Memory," *Clinical Neuropharmacology,* (1993 December); 16(6): 540–49.
18. Richard Wurtman, "Effects of Nutrients on Neurotransmitter Release," Food Components to Enhance Performance, *op. cit.,* 239–61.
19. A. J. Gelenberg; et al., "Choline and Lecithin in the Treatment of Tardive Dyskinesia: Preliminary Results from a Pilot Study," *American Journal of Psychiatry,* (1984); 136: 772–76.
20. D. C. Dorman et al., "Effects of an Extract of Gingko Biloba on Bromethalin-Induced Cerebral Blood Flow and Edema in Rats," *American Journal of Veterinary Research,* (1992 January); 53 (1): 138–42.
21. S. Hoyt, "Possibility and Limits of Therapy of Cognition Disorders in the Elderly," *Gerontology and Geriatrics,* (1995 November); 28 (6): 457–62.
22. Pierre LeBars, Martin Katz, et al., "A Placebo-Controlled, Double-Blind Randomized Trial of an Extract of Ginkgo Biloba for Dementia, *JAMA,* 1997 October 22: (278) 1327–32.
23. Chang Xu, Ph.D., Chinese Academy of Sciences, "Synthesis of Huperzine A Analogues and Their Inhibitory Activities of Acetylcholinesterase" (paper presented at the 206th American Chemical Society Meeting, Chicago, IL, August 25, 1993).
24. Alan Kozikowski, "An Improved Synthetic Route to Huperzine A; New Analogues and Their Inhibition of Acetylcholinesterase" (paper presented at the 206th American Chemical Society Meeting, Chicago, IL, August 25, 1993).
25. William Dicke, "Chinese Herb Remedy Curbs Alcohol Desire," *New York Times,* November 2, 1993, 14.
26. Georgetown University Report, June 20, 1997.
27. USDA Briefs, February 4, 1997.
28. Moriguchi N. Nishiyama, T. Moriguchi, and T. H. Saito, "Beneficial Effects of Aged Garlic Extract on Learning and Memory Impairment in the sensecence-acclerated mouse," *Experimental Gerontology,* 1997 January; 32(1-2): 149–60.
29. Tae H. Oh, Ph.D., professor of anatomy and neurobiology at Maryland, and Young C. Kim, Ph.D., from Seoul National University in Korea, "Effects of Ginsenosides Rb1 and Rg3 on Cortical Cells from Rats" (paper presented at the Society for Neuroscience Annual Meeting in New Orleans, October 29, 1997).

## 11. Diet for a Smart Brain

1. Edward Schneider et al., "Recommended Dietary Allowances and the Health of the Elderly," *New England Journal of Medicine,* 314, 16 January 1986; 157–60.
2. Elsworth Buskir, "Exercise," *Present Knowledge in Nutrition,* 7th ed., eds. Ekhard Ziegler and L. J. Filer, Jr. (Washington, D.C.: ILSI Press, 1996), 429.
3. Chris Lecos, "Diet and the Elderly: Research Points to Some Special Needs," *FDA Consumer,* October 1984, 27–29.
4. "Cholesterol-Lowering Drugs May Dull Your Edge," AP report, November 10, 1998.
5. S. Kalmijn et al., *American Journal of Epidemiology* (1997): 145, 1: 33–41.
6. Joseph Hibbeln et al., "Do Plasma Polyunsaturates Predict Hostility and Depression?" *World Review of Nutrition and Diet* (1997): 82: 175–86.
7. Tufts University "Diet & Nutrition Letter," Vol. 8, No. 9, November 1990, 1.
8. R. Wood et al., "Effect of Butter, Mono- and Polyunsaturated Fatty Acid–Enriched Butter, Trans-fatty Acid Margarine, and Zero Trans-fatty Acid Margarine on Serum Lipids and Lipoproteins in Healthy Men," *Journal of Lipid Research,* 1993 January; 34(1): 1–11; Marian Burros, "Now What U.S.? Study Says Margarine May Be Harmful," *New York Times,* October 7, 1992, 1.
9. "Health Doubts Cut Into Margarine Sales," *Wall Street Journal,* April 26, 1993, B1.
10. Ibid.
11. D. Kromhout et al., "The Inverse Relation Between Fish Consumption and 20-Year Mortality from Coronary Heart Disease," *New England Journal of Medicine* (1985): 312: 1205.
12. Jim Matthews, "Pharmaceutical Perspectives on Omega-3," (paper presented at Designer Foods II: Phytochemicals in Disease Prevention, sponsored by Rutgers University Department of Food Science, March 16–17, 1993, Piscataway, NJ).
13. D. Kromhout et al., "The Inverse Relation Between Fish Consumption and 20-Year Mortality from Coronary Heart Disease," *op. cit.*
14. C. Marwick, "International Conference Gives Boost to Omega Fatty Acids in Diet," *Journal of the American Medical Association* (1990 April 25): 263(16): 2153–54.
15. Ibid.
16. Buskir, *op. cit.*
17. Helen Whalley, "Salt and Hypertension: Consensus or Controversy?" *Lancet,* December 6, 1997, Vol. 350, 1686.
18. Melvyn Werbach, "Arthritis," *Nutritional Influences on Illness: A Sourcebook of Clinical Research* (Tarzana, CA: Third Line Press, 1993), 578–79.
19. "Keeping Americans Healthy Into the 21st Century" (A forum for media, presented by Healthy Choice and the Society for Nutrition Education, May 13, 1997).

# Appendix

## Labeling

A food label is a contract between us and the manufacturer. Like most contracts, it may be difficult to understand and what is not included may be as important as what is.

The provisions of the Nutrition Labeling and Education Act (NLEA) and the Dietary Supplement Act of 1992 are the first major change in food labeling regulations since 1974. As of May 8, 1994, food producers had to comply with most of FDA's new labeling requirements. (Advertising is not covered by NLEA; the Federal Trade Commission, however, has indicated it may apply the same criteria to advertising that FDA does to labels.)

Experts believe that these labels will lead to fewer diet-related diseases and lower incidence of cancer because shoppers will have the information they need to make informed food choices. The government estimates that over the next twenty years, the new labels will reduce national health care costs substantially by making it easier for the public to choose more healthful diets.

The new regulations have more realistic serving sizes. Instead of a food manufacturer presenting a low calorie or fat count for half a teaspoonful they will have to give the count for half a cup—the realistic serving size.

There will be many more products with labels to read because the regulations, for the first time, *make* nutrition labeling mandatory for almost all processed foods. Also, uniform point-of-purchase nutrition information will *accompany* many fresh foods, such as fruits and vegetables and raw fish, meat and poultry.

The FDA and USDA previously established a standard of identity for about 300 foods such as peanut butter, mayonnaise, and fruit cocktails, fixing the ingredients by law (*see* Glossary). Many of these foods were exempted from the need to list ingredients. The new labeling requires full ingredient listing for all foods, including those with standards of identity. It also allows manufacturers for the first time to produce healthier versions of some products and still use the recognized name. For instance a reduced-fat ice cream does not have to be called "imitation" or "ice milk" but can be called "low fat ice cream."

The FDA says under the new Nutrition Labeling and Education Act any term used to describe the nutrient content of a food will mean the same on every product on which it appears. Also, the list of acceptable claims now includes such descriptors as "free," "low," "light" (or "lite"), "reduced," "less," and "high." "Lean" and "extra lean" also have been defined and will apply specifically to the fat content of meat, including game meat, poultry, and fish (*see* Glossary).

The following are explanations set forth by the FDA of the new labeling changes: **Daily Values (DV)** comprise two sets of references for nutrients, *Daily Reference Values (Drives)* and *Reference Daily Intakes (RDIs)*.

## Daily Reference Values (Drives)

These are for nutrients for which no set of standards previously existed, such as fat, cholesterol, carbohydrates, proteins, and fibers. Drives for these energy-producing nutrients are based on the number of calories consumed per day. For labeling purposes, 2,000 calories has been established as the reference for calculating percent Daily Values. This level was chosen, in part, because many health experts say it approximates the maintenance calorie requirements of the group most often targeted for weight reduction: postmenopausal women.

Drives for the energy-producing nutrients are calculated as follows:

- Fat based on 30 percent of calories
- Saturated fat based on 10 percent of calories
- Carbohydrates based on 60 percent of calories
- Protein based on 10 percent of calories
- Fiber based on 11.5 grams of fiber per 1,000 calories

The DRVs for cholesterol, sodium and potassium, which do not contribute calories, remain the same no matter what the calorie level.

Because of the links between certain nutrients and specific diseases, DRVs for some nutrients represent the uppermost limit considered desirable. Eating too much fat or cholesterol, for example, has been linked to heart disease and too much sodium to the risk of high blood pressure. Therefore, the label shows DVs for fats and sodium as follows:

- Total fat: less than 65 grams
- Saturated fat: less than 20 grams
- Cholesterol: less than 300 milligrams
- Sodium: less than 2,400 milligrams

## Reference Daily Intakes (RDIs)

A set of dietary references based on and replacing the *Recommended Dietary Allowances (RDAs)* for essential vitamins and minerals and, in selected groups, protein. You will continue to see vitamins and minerals expressed as percentages on the label but these figures now refer to the Daily Values.

Here are the RDIs—once familiar to us as RDAs:

## REFERENCE DAILY INTAKES (RDIs)*

| Nutrient | Amount |
|---|---|
| Vitamin A | 5,000 International Units (IU) |
| Vitamin C | 60 milligrams (mg) |
| Thiamin | 1.5 mg |
| Riboflavin | 1.7 mg |
| Niacin | 20 mg |
| Calcium | 1.0 gram (g) |
| Iron | 18 mg |
| Vitamin D | 400 IU |
| Vitamin E | 30 IU |
| Vitamin $B_6$ | 2.0 mg |
| Folic acid | 0.4 mg |
| Vitamin $B_{12}$ | 6 micrograms (mcg) |
| Phosphorus | 1.0 g |
| Iodine | 150 mcg |
| Magnesium | 400 mg |
| Zinc | 15 mg |
| Copper | 2 mg |
| Biotin | 0.3 mg |
| Pantothenic acid | 10 mg |

*Based on National Academy of Sciences 1968 Recommended Dietary Allowances

The mandatory and voluntary dietary components on the new label and order in which they must appear are:

Total calories
    calories from fat
    calories from saturated fat
    total saturated fat
    stearic acid (on meat and poultry products only)
    polyunsaturated fat
    monounsaturated fat
    cholesterol
    sodium
    potassium
Total carbohydrate
Dietary fiber
    soluble fiber
    insoluble fiber
Sugars

Sugar alcohol (for example, the sugar substitutes xylitol, mannitol, and sorbitol)

Other carbohydrate (the difference between total carbohydrate and the sum of dietary fiber, sugars, and sugar alcohol, if declared)

Protein

Vitamin A

Percent of vitamin A present as beta-carotene

Vitamin C

Calcium

Iron

Other essential vitamins and minerals

If a food is fortified or enriched with any of the optional components, or a claim is made about any of them, pertinent additional nutrition information becomes mandatory. These mandatory and voluntary components are the only ones allowed on the nutrition panel.

## No Nutrition Information

Some foods are exempt from nutrition labeling. Due to space limitations, small packages such as a candy bar, do NOT have to provide nutrition information on the label. However the address or telephone number must be provided for shoppers who wish to obtain this material. Other foods that do not have to provide nutrition labeling include:

• Food produced by small businesses. (As mandated by NLEA, the FDA defines a small business as one with food sales of less than $50,000 a year or total sales of less than $500,000. The United States Department of Agriculture's Food Safety and Inspection Service (FSIS) defines a small business as one employing 500 or fewer employees and producing no more than a certain amount of product per year.)

• Food served for immediate consumption, such as that served in restaurants and hospital cafeterias, on airplanes, and by food service vendors (such as mall cookie counters, sidewalk vendors, and vending machines)

• Ready-to-eat foods that are not for immediate consumption, as long as the food is primarily prepared on site—for example, many bakery, deli, and candy store items.

• Food shipped in bulk, as long as it is not for sale in that form to consumers.

• Medical foods.

• Plain coffee and tea, flavor extracts, food colors, some spices, and other foods that contain no significant amounts of any nutrients.

• Donated foods.

- Products intended for export.
- Individually wrapped FSIS-regulated products weighing less than half an ounce and making no nutrient content claims.

Although these foods are exempt, they are free to carry nutrition information, when appropriate, as long as it complies with the new regulations.

# Index

# 318    Index